To my colleague, Dan

with gratitude for a job

done well and graciously.

Peg Nevin 5/24/73

THE MAKING OF A PSYCHIATRIST

THE MAKING OF A PSYCHIATRIST

DAVID S. VISCOTT, M.D.

ARBOR HOUSE

NEW YORK

FOR JOHN SPOONER

Give sorrow words; the grief that does not speak
Whispers the o'er-fraught heart, and bids it break.
—SHAKESPEARE, *Macbeth*

CONTENTS

AUTHOR'S NOTE

My INTENTION in writing this book was to give the reader a sense of what it took to become a psychiatrist. In order to do this there were several enormous problems to overcome. The reader had to be educated and taught a great deal of psychiatry. To do this in a straightforward way would, I felt, also be boring and unpalatable.

The solution, while obvious, was not easy. I decided to tell my own story about becoming a psychiatrist, not merely what happened outside of me but what changes occurred within me, so the reader could identify with what I was doing. This required a great deal of honesty and I was not sure that I wanted to reveal that much of myself. It became clear, though, that what I was doing and saying absolutely required me to be honest about many ideas and feelings I had either not really fully considered or had not been completely honest about before. The more honest I became about reporting my own feelings, the more honest I could be about discussing the profession.

THE MAKING OF A PSYCHIATRIST

INTRODUCTION—STIRRINGS

BEFORE I begin I have kind of a confession to make. I'm really not as much of a wise ass as I may sometimes seem. I only appear that way when a situation is very threatening to me. I suppose I always did. Like a lot of people, it's one of my defenses against being hurt. I've always been very sensitive not only to me being hurt but other people being hurt as well. Pain bothers me, anybody's pain. I've always wanted to help other people. I'm not sure even now that I understand why, but when I feel powerless to help, I feel terrible, and that's the time I'm likely to sound least serious.

My first clinical experience in medical school was the newborn ward in a pediatric hospital. I couldn't handle it. Most of the babies were dying or in pain and frequently nothing could be done about it. If I'd been a good little medical student I suppose I could have studied each detail about the diseases I saw and concerned myself with the diseases, not the kids. Some psychiatrists would call that "intellectualization." I would call it denial. I could barely stand coming to the ward. I also had a very difficult time in surgery and could not forget that underneath the green drapes the bleeding goop we were all merrily cutting away on was a human being. Dehumanizing people like that upsets me. I also got very upset when my patients died and not just because I might have missed something in their diagnosis or treatment as we all did from time to time. I always seemed to get too close. I had—and have—a very difficult time forgetting that patients are human, and I guess I became a bit overwhelmed when I remembered this fact—and so there followed this cover-up of mine, this tendency to a breezy, joking attitude. In time, as I felt more confident and, I suppose, less helpless, I was more able to do something about the confusion and despair I saw. I felt better about it all, more willing to let people see me as vulnerable, as warm and caring.

It seems as though I always opened up to people and was always interested in sharing something with them. Perhaps it was wanting to share a sense of closeness—or wanting to share a sense of loneliness. I'm still not sure.

I am telling you all this because I want to be honest about what I am going to say and I want it to be me who says it to you. I could change my style so that I would sound more respectable, more reverent, more of what you may think a psychiatrist should sound like; but it wouldn't be real and it wouldn't be me.

Actually, I am pretty concerned about putting you off, but that's a chance I'll have to take. I know people well enough by now to understand that in the end each person will see whatever he wants to in this; and no matter how decent a person I may be or how accurate my observations are, I realize there will be people who will think I'm a discredit to the profession, and fellow psychiatrists who'll race to throw the first stone.

You can't please everyone.

CHAPTER ONE

UP FROM MEDICINE: GREAT EXPECTATIONS

THE most beautiful sight in the world is the city of Saint Louis growing smaller in my car's rear-view mirror. For one horrible year of my life I was a medical intern at one of the most prestigious university hospitals in Saint Louis. There, among other things, I learned how long I could go without sleep before collapsing, how quickly my children could forget my name, and how easy it is for any marriage to slip to the brink of divorce when the husband is hardly ever home. I also discovered how little I knew about medicine, how little the other interns knew about medicine, and how little some of the staff doctors knew about medicine— and this was at one of the best hospitals in the country. God only knows what was going on at other places. . . .

At the moment I don't really give a damn about how much medicine I know because as the cornfields are beginning to blot out Saint Louis in the rear-view mirror, the memory of the revered, exalted portals of the hospital is fading. I am starting to feel better already.

I am heading east to the big city, to civilization where, I have been telling myself for these past twelve months, everything is going to be all right once again. I am going to begin my first year in residency in psychiatry at Union Hospital. You can take your one-hundred-hour, seven-day, four-night workweek . . .

Don't get me wrong, I don't hate medicine at this moment. It's just that I've never been well-enough rested to learn to enjoy it. I like psychiatry. At least I hope I am *going* to like psychiatry. I just can't see why I spent the past idiotic year killing myself. Up until right now

17

it seems I've spent most of my life in school fulfilling prerequisites and never being able to do what I really want and care most about.

I have a two-day drive ahead of me. One thing becomes clear as I pass by the alfalfa fields and the Burma Shave signs and that is that I don't really know one hell of a lot about psychiatry. I've read Frieda Fromm-Reichmann's *Principles of Intensive Psychotherapy* maybe six times and maybe a couple of dozen paperbacks over the year, ranging from R. D. Laing's *Politics of Experience* to something by Margaret Mead—I can't even remember the title of that one now. There really wasn't much time to read, my routine being largely consumed by work and a little sleep.

Most other interns tended to read such things as the results of what some research group in Copenhagen had discovered about clotting mechanisms in monkeys or what the Mount Sinai team had observed in kidney enzymes. This sort of thing was their daily diet and the hub of most of their conversations. They were very serious medical types, those fellows I interned with. I guess someday they will all become professors somewhere. They were all smart as hell, competitive, retentive, eager, thorough, and punctilious. Wonderful fellows, if you didn't mind their tendency to a bit of one-sidedness, their one-note quality.

I once announced, "Hey, Rudolph Nureyev is coming to town. Anyone want to make an evening of it?" After three or four of my associates asked "Who's he?" I ungenerously called them all lousy Philistines and made my own plans. But they really were nice guys, decent types. I know I must sound very cheeky and snobbish. I'm sorry for that, but remember I'd been very much out of my element for the past year and trying to feel superior to these other people was one of the ways I was able to keep my head together. The other way I kept my head together was by telling myself that the year would be over any day now.

Anyhow, by this time I know a lot of book knowledge about psychiatry from medical school. Hell, I can read as well as anyone else and I remember what I read so that's no great accomplishment. I enjoyed trying to do psychotherapy with the half dozen or so patients I worked with in medical school. I really did. Psychiatry was the only subject in medical school that felt like me. At least I could talk to people and relate to them as human beings instead of as "the gall-bladder in Room 1207." I felt for the first time that I could help a patient by being me, by being a person. It was a feeling I had always looked for.

I went to medical school because it seemed like a good idea at the time—too glib for you? It's not too far from the truth. When I was a kid I had all these corny ideas about becoming a kind family doctor who would sit with his patients saying reassuring things like "Now, now . . . there, there. He will get better soon. Don't you worry." Sweet ideas but not terribly realistic, as I learned in medical school. I also daydreamed about talking to parents and loved ones and comforting them. I had a full-blown omnipotent-benefactor fantasy. My sophisticated college and medical education made me feel embarrassed about it, but I don't think I ever really gave it up. Don't laugh. At least I admit to it freely. Some of the characters I went to medical school with were suffering from the same grandiose delusion to save the world and to be all things to all men, but they wouldn't and won't admit it. They get angry as hell when their patients don't accept their word as gospel or don't get better as quickly as they should. Patients like that can make a doctor and his fantasy look bad.

The picture I had in mind when I first decided to become a doctor wasn't at all the way it really is. The pressures of an overcrowded schedule are draining. The responsibility for another human life is frightening. The amount of material to comprehend and to be able to use is vast and often not much comprehended by many physicians. You begin to wonder where they ever dug up the guys in the bottom of your medical class. You feel sorry as hell for the people they'll treat and hope that they'll go into dermatology or medical publishing. Or, if you hate psychiatrists, which many doctors do, you hope that they'll go into psychiatry, where they can't *hurt* anyone. And you'll mean it.

Worst of all, you discover that the image of the kindly doctor, which may have seduced you into becoming a doctor, is gone. Your old family physician, the guy who trudged out into the cold at three o'clock in the morning and stuck his icy hands on your tummy, somehow disappeared. OK—maybe he didn't disappear, but he's become so scarce that when anyone finds him they write a story about him in the Sunday supplement, "Vermont Country Doctor Still Makes House Calls."

It's very sad, but if you're any good at all in medical school you're going to be pressured into becoming a specialist. The GP is a dying breed, they'll tell you, and they'll convince you to avoid becoming one by telling you there is too much knowledge for you to retain and still be competent. Anyhow, the competitiveness of medical school and the promise of becoming a big diagnostician somewhere gets to many of those lovely little dreams. To this day I am not certain exactly what a diagnostician does or if in fact such a subspecialty exists except in the eyes of some mother with a daughter of marriageable age. A lot of potentially great GPs are locked up in laboratories chasing fantasies of Nobel Prizes, studying enzymes which they incompletely understand and feeding their results to a computer that doesn't understand either. You don't have to make house calls for computers.

If you do become a GP, you spend your life trying to figure out when your first coronary is going to take place—so you become an internist instead. It's cleaner and usually there are fewer house calls. All the surgeons I ever met got up at five in the morning, operated for six hours, and then crammed dozens of patients into the afternoon and went around bragging about how hard they worked or how little sleep they were getting and how much money they were making. I wasn't enough of a masochist for that routine. I couldn't see being a pathologist. I had tried my hand at research for a while, but I hated the idea of not seeing patients.

There's a saying: "A psychiatrist knows nothing and does nothing. An internist knows everything and does nothing. A surgeon knows nothing and does everything. And a pathologist knows everything and does everything, but too late." Look, no one is perfect.

Actually I landed by chance on the idea of going into psychiatry. Being a psychiatrist seemed like a lot of fun. In medical school the psychiatric reading list was the only one I ever really enjoyed. A lot of the case histories were like short stories and some were pretty wild and sexy. I was an English major in college so it was right up my alley. To top it off, the hours on my medical school rotation in psychiatry were a breeze. Although I was officially finished with the day at two thirty, I usually stayed around longer. There were fascinating psychiatric emergencies. Each one seemed like a puzzle and no two were ever alike. I mean, I had seen about a dozen kidney stones when I was on urology and I couldn't tell one from the other. I really enjoyed talking to the patients about their lives; the old GP fantasy again, I suppose.

I applied for my psychiatric residency at Union Hospital a few months before leaving for my internship, which had to come first. One of the psychiatrists who interviewed me, an intense man with a face and mane like a lion, Dr. Gavin, listened very carefully without saying a word while I told him that I wanted to become a psychiatrist because it seemed like fun. He was silent for about five minutes while I crawled around in my chair waiting for him to tell me to get the hell out of there and stop wasting his time. Then he broke into a broad smile and said, "Very refreshing attitude," like he had just sampled a bowl of fruit. And he added, "We'd like to have you in the residency program."

I accepted on the spot. . . .

I really haven't learned very much about psychiatry in the year since that interview, but I know a little more about me. Still, knowing as little as I do, tomorrow I am going to walk onto the psychiatric ward in Union Hospital and be expected to act and talk like a psychiatrist.

What the hell do psychiatrists really do?

I never did like starting a new service or rotation. As soon as I had gotten used to a ward and worked out the problems with the patients and the nurses, it seemed it was time for me to leave for another ward in the hospital and learn to adjust again. This happened at least every other month during my internship and was always upsetting to me as well as to the patients and the nurses, who would often test you out with irritating and sometimes unnecessary calls, usually at three in the morning.

Just when you learned how to manage a difficult patient's problems it was time to move on. You would try to write comprehensive off-service notes, telling the intern who followed you what was going on and which problems he should look out for with which patient. But it would still take several weeks for him to get in control of the new situation, even though there was a resident assigned to each intern for supervision as well as continuity.

Actually it can get pretty hairy on a medical service at such a time, and it's not uncommon for the death rate to go up. This is especially true in the first weeks of July. That's the time when the new interns are just starting out fresh from medical school. If you have to go to the hospital for anything and have a choice, try to avoid going in the summer. Go when the odds are better.

My first rotation during my internship was to take charge of a TB ward at a local Veterans Hospital for one month. Each intern had to go there. Most of us hated it because we were so overworked. So what else is new? The very first day, I discovered that I was on night duty, the only medical doctor for some six hundred patients, and that I was also in charge of the emergency room. Only twenty-four hours earlier I was still in medical *school*. That first night I admitted six patients from the emergency room; two with heart attacks, one in diabetic coma, one with bilateral pneumonia, one with congestive heart failure, and a man with a bleeding ulcer. I ran my ass off examining these people, starting treatment, running tests in the laboratory. In the morning, as if by a miracle (color me a believer) the heart attack patients were comfortable, the diabetic was out of coma, the patient with congestive heart failure did me the dubious honor of urinating all over my brand new whites, but seemed out of danger. The patient with pneumonia no longer had a fever and both his lungs sounded much clearer (God bless penicillin), and the ulcer patient seemed to be stable. I was exhausted. I hadn't eaten or slept. I felt pushed to the limits of my skill and knowledge, such as they were, and worst of all I was terrified that the rest of the year was going to be like this.

At morning rounds I presented my new cases to the staff physician, Dr. Carlson, who looked like an intercollegiate wrestler. He just nodded a lot. I was very disappointed that no approving comments were made about what a great job I had done. For God's sake, I was a regular medical hero and no one even noticed. This is what they expect as a routine performance, I thought to myself. I am *never* going to make it.

To make matters still worse, during the day I would find requests on my desk to see patients on the surgical ward and to write consultation reports. Why me? Why didn't the other interns on the other services have this extra duty? On top of this each day I would be handed at least a dozen electrocardiograms to read. Again none of the other interns shared this privilege. I was becoming swamped and was struggling just to stay current with my work. Why was I being singled out as "slave of the year?"

The mystery of my extra work was revealed during my third week when another doctor reported to the hospital. He was the new chief resident and had just gotten out of military service. Dr. Carlson welcomed him warmly for a few moments and then his face took on an expression of sheer panic. "You mean," he said, pointing to me, "that *he's* the intern? My God! I thought *he* was the chief resident."

My God, indeed! The surgeons had been deciding whether or not to operate based on my consults. A rapid survey of my consults and electrocardiograms by Dr. Carlson and the new chief resident followed. To my breathless surprise and incredible pleasure, there were no additions or corrections made. Amazing! Just amazing! Oh well, Dr. Carlson made an honest mistake that anyone could have made. After all, the chief resident and I both had the same first names....

Once again, new beginnings frighten me. I am not at all sure what to expect the first day I report for my psychiatric residency.

Hell, I'm not even sure I remember how to get to Union Hospital.

CHAPTER TWO

INTRODUCTIONS:
WELCOMING COMMITTEE,
THE RESIDENTS, THE WARD

ACCORDING to the bronze plaque on the wall, the psychiatric ward of Union Hospital, Bamberg 5, was named for Harriet and Arthur Bamberg, who probably donated the funds for the building. It looked like every psychiatric ward I had ever seen, green walls, a day hall with a piano that was out of tune (the people who donate the damn things never give money to have them tuned), and patients lounging around. Everyone looked healthy enough but sort of sad.

I walked to the nurses' station, where the patients' records are kept, where medicines are dispensed, and where a doctor strange to a new service instinctively goes to look for something familiar. On the way, I saw some patients washing clothes in a small laundry room. Three or four people were milling around the corridor in front of the nurses' desk. I guessed that they were patients but they didn't look any different from anyone else.

"Can I help you?" asked a large lady who turned out to be Bella Grable, the ward secretary. She was sitting, pasting lab reports into the patients' charts.

"I'm Dr. Viscott. I'm looking for the other doctors."

"And you belong in there," she said pointing to a door across the hall, "so scoot."

You learned to take a lot on faith in this business. I walked toward the door.

"Excuse me, Dr. Viscott," said a very sad-looking lady in her forties using her urgent tone of voice. Everything she wore was brown.

23

A brown sweater, brown pants, brown blouse, and brown shoes. This is someone who likes to play it safe and not commit herself or take a stand, I said knowingly to myself, equating the color brown with blandness. I had read that in the *Reader's Digest* somewhere. I was playing psychiatrist and interpreting colors. What fun!

"Doctor, I couldn't help but overhear you talking to Bella. I know that you are going to be my doctor and take over for Dr. Jabers. I'm Mrs. Sacks and I want to speak with you as soon as possible. Right now would be best!" She looked angry and sounded very insistent.

"As soon as I have a better idea of my schedule," I began, "I will arrange a time, but right now I'm afraid I don't even know who my patients are."

"Oh!" She seemed disappointed. Her voice changed and she snapped at me, "You know, you don't seem to be very much of a doctor!" So much for all those theories about the color brown. She continued, but now shouting, "I don't think you're going to be able to do anything for me. Maybe I should have another doctor!"

Please, dear lady, give me half a break, I thought. I don't even know where to go to take a piss on this ward and you've already started to judge me. Look, give me a chance. You'll find out how little I know in time. Wait till you have all the facts before putting me down.

"Mrs. Sacks, we can talk as soon as I get a chance," I offered as pleasantly as I knew how.

"That's all you people say around here. I'll tell you one thing. You've got one hell of a lot of growing up to do to match Dr. Jabers. He's someone you should study. You don't look wet behind the ears yet."

I wasn't!

What do you have there, lady, ESP?, I thought. Get off my back and leave me alone. I moved closer to the door and reached for the handle. A good move, I thought. It would let me cut her off. I could make a final comment and slip right in. What an unreasonable bitch! "We can discuss it later on," I said, opening the door. I could see seven or eight people sitting around a large table. They turned and looked at me as the door opened. I started to walk in.

"I can tell you're not going to make it as a psychiatrist, Dr. Viscott," yelled Mrs. Sacks. "You're no goddamn good." Who needed this? All the eyes in the conference room were at me. Effie Sacks had waited until the door was wide open before yelling, "You're no goddamn good." What timing! What a beautiful way to begin!

A tall, smiling doctor, his belly hanging over his belt, got up and came into the hall. He was Marty DiAngelo, the third-year resident. "Effie, what's wrong with you?" he called after her as she beat a retreat back to the lounge. "That's lousy self-control," he added, and ushered me into the conference room. "Relax, kid," DiAngelo said to me, "you can't please everyone." So I was learning.

Larry Danielson, the chief resident, was sitting at the head of the table, patting his bald head with his left hand and shuffling through some papers with his right. "I see that you have just met one of your patients, Dr. Viscott. I'm pleased that you two have hit it off so well."

Everyone started to laugh. "Everyone" included two nurses and one student nurse and the three other first-year residents I would be working with.

Bertram Feinstein had hair down to his shoulders and a long beard. He didn't look like a typical M.D. He had a Harvard College and Harvard Medical School degree as well as a Peter Bent Brigham Hospital background (another hallowed portal).

"Hello," said Bert. He was the only other resident to say hello, the others just waved or nodded. Apparently they were sizing me up. All residents sized each other up and worried about how much more everyone else knew than they did. They acted very cool because they didn't want to appear like the idiots they felt like. Usually the residents who didn't feel like idiots at the beginning were the ones who got into trouble—they were the authentic card-carrying idiots.

Bert Feinstein seemed to be a warm and pleasant person who had a great deal of common sense. He wasn't afraid to ask questions when he didn't understand. He was honest and fun to be with. Bert always had something in his mouth—either food, candy, gum, a cigarette, a cigar, a pencil, or rolled-up paper. He introduced himself as an "oral character type," which seemed fairly self-evident. This first morning he had a stack of doughnuts in front of him and was offering them around, but he acted so pleased when anyone refused that no one had the heart to take one. Bert really needed his doughnuts.

Danielson put his papers down and looked at Bert. "What are you operating here, a coffee shop?" he asked playfully in the tone a teacher uses to patronize students. He was trying to be funny and also trying to be one of the guys. This was very hard for him to do because he was in direct competition with Marty DiAngelo who was much funnier. DiAngelo had been in residency for three years and thus should know just about as much as Danielson. Actually he knew a lot more, but had no vested interest in proving it to anyone. Danielson continued, "We are going to go right around the table so that everyone can introduce himself. And say something about yourself that gives us an idea about who you are and what you are like." I'm sure that you know this routine. It's usually impossible to remember what the others said; at best you remember yourself trying to be as clever as possible.

"You go first," said DiAngelo to Danielson. "I've known you for years and I couldn't make a distinctive statement about you. Why don't you tell us a little about yourself." DiAngelo then laughed and said, "I'm Marty DiAngelo and I just made *my* introduction."

Danielson began again, trying to maintain some sense of dignity and assert his superiority over DiAngelo who was, after all, under his authority. "I'm Lawrence Danielson."

"Is that what your name is?" interrupted DiAngelo. "It was only yesterday you told the nurse on Surgical 3 that you were Clint Eastwood's brother." Nurses' laughter. It was pretty obvious that everyone liked DiAngelo.

"I am also the chief resident," Larry Danielson continued. "I run the ward and make sure that everyone is doing what he is supposed to and I—"

"Am very sensitive about being called 'baldy,' " interrupted Marty DiAngelo.

"Dr. DiAngelo," said Larry, trying to be good-natured and funny, "is not actually a resident here. He's just an example of what you are supposed to keep patients from turning into." Audience groans. It looked like Danielson would be making bad jokes all year long.

"I'm Terry O'Conner," said an extraordinarily attractive, shapely strawberry blonde. "I'm one of the nurses who has to put up with this nonsense. No, really, Larry, you know I love you." Terry O'Conner was always getting into difficulty with young male patients who would develop a crush on her and grab at her in the laundry room or in the nurses' office, where she sometimes talked with patients. Terry contributed to these assaults by her bouncy walk and her generally seductive manner, but she honestly seemed unaware of it all. Each new pass a patient made came as a surprise, but only to her. Everyone grabbed at Terry, everyone.

It was my turn to say something and you already know how new situations upset me. I'm usually pretty bold about introductions but, having been upset by Mrs. Sacks' attack and the confusing display of personalities before me, I said only, "I'm David Viscott and I just met Mrs. Sacks. Hooray for me!" DiAngelo clasped his hands and held them over his head.

"I'm Bert Feinstein," said Bert Feinstein, I think. I'm not sure. His mouth was full.

"D. J. Marley," said a thin, fine-featured woman somewhere in her mid-twenties. Hell, we were all in our mid- to late twenties, except maybe Larry. D. J. Marley did not even say, "I am D. J. Marley." She just said, "D. J. Marley." That's all she said.

D. J. Marley was the first woman resident in five years to grace the dingy halls of Bamberg 5. Grace isn't exactly the right word. Nothing is exactly the right word for anything D. J. Marley did.

I imagined D.J. to be one of these superbright female medic types I had run into from time to time. How did I know she wasn't a nurse? Well, nurses are generally softer and almost always give themselves the benefit of a first name or a Miss. And this gal was just too tight, too fitted together for that. Also none of the nurses seemed to know her. The nurses kept passing little notes to each other. That was how people communicated in psychiatric conferences.

I imagined that D. J. Marley was one of these gals who was vale-dictorian at Sarah Lawrence, probably had a degree in philosophy, spoke three or four languages fluently, published several papers in a field in which she was already famous, and had a following of dozens of former professors who constantly wrote her begging her to return when she'd done with training. I knew the type. I could spot them a mile away. They intimidated me. Actually they scared the shit out of me.

Larry smiled uneasily, "Welcome to Bamberg 5, Dr. Marley." Terry turned and gave a look to the other nurse, Amanda Little, which indicated that she recognized Larry's special welcome as flirting. Amanda was a huge, powerful black woman who nodded a lot and looked very serious about everything. I guessed that you didn't try to joke around with Amanda Little. At least I wasn't about to.

Stanley Lovett, M.D., the other first-year resident asked, "Dr. Marley, are you in any way related to the famous neurosurgeon at Johns Hopkins?" Lovett was trying to score points. Lovett was always trying to score points. You could catch it early from his tone of voice.

D. J. Marley did not bother to turn around to look at Lovett, who was sitting away from the table in a corner of the room. She smiled icily and said, "No. Are you?" Lovett looked very confused. Marty DiAngelo just looked up at the ceiling to make sure it was still there.

Stanley Lovett, M.D., had wanted to become a psychoanalyst from the day he first could pronounce the word correctly twice in succession. It sounded good. It must have sounded real good. Stanley Lovett, M.D., was everybody's favorite psychoanalytic candidate.

Let me explain what that means. The process Stanley, Bert, D. J. Marley, and I were beginning was a psychiatric residency. It would take three years to complete, in which time we would work with patients in a general hospital ward for a year, this first year, and then work in a state hospital the next year, and finally spend a year in the Union Hospital outpatient clinics. After these three years of training we would be free to go our several ways and practice psychiatry. We could take an additional year of training, which was not required, or do research. In any case, after three years we would be full-fledged psychiatrists, trained to diagnose and treat patients. Although all psychiatric therapies were taught, the Union Hospital program stressed the use of psychotherapy, treating patients by listening to their problems, asking questions, and helping them understand how their feelings, actions, and wishes were related.

If we wanted to, we could apply at any time to a local psychoanalytic institute to train to be a psychoanalyst. If one of us was accepted he would begin his own psychoanalysis with a teaching analyst; this would entail lying on his back one hour a day, five days a week, and telling all his innermost secrets. If after a year the analyst felt that he was not too crazy in the head, he would allow the analytic candidate to attend seminars while continuing his analysis. After four to seven more years, depending on how complicated the analysis was and how well the trial analyses of the candidate's two to four patients were going, he would be free to practice psychoanalysis and probably be old enough to collect social security at the same time.

In classical psychoanalysis the patient lies on his back saying whatever comes into his mind while the analyst sits behind him and listens, saying very little. Eventually the patient develops feelings about the analyst, which are interpreted as the basis for understanding what the patient feels about other people. This takes many years and is not particularly more effective than psychotherapy. It is limited to certain kinds of patients who should not be psychotic and are able to afford paying six or seven thousand dollars a year. Also, in order to be an analyst one must be able to sit quietly and to remain unknown to the patient.

By now I think you realize that's not very much in keeping with my personality. I like to talk to patients, to share ideas and feelings with them. Analysts like to remain anonymous or as they put it, mainly silent. They love to hide in shadows.

Stanley Lovett, M.D., was practicing being an analyst by sitting in the corner and listening. He was a first-year resident just like me except that he had applied to and had been accepted into the psychoanalytic institute and had begun his teaching analysis with Dr. Fletcher. He already felt superior to the rest of us. He would never miss an opportunity to talk about his own personal analysis. When he needed an excuse for being rude he would tell us he was going through "something difficult in the analysis." He never referred to it as *my* analysis. He always said *the* analysis as if it were some sacred vessel. Although he talked a lot and used a lot of jargon, he really said very little about himself.

For instance, Stanley would describe Mrs. Sacks' outburst at me as "a failure of the anxiety-binding defenses to operate effectively with a resultant displacement of the unresolved hostility from Dr. Jagers to Dr. Viscott as part of the process of decathecting" (translation: releasing emotional or mental energy, previously attached to an object or person). Anyone else, wishing to be helpful, would say that Mrs. Sacks was hurt and upset that her old therapist had left and was angry at her new doctor for trying to take his place.

The two statements mean exactly the same thing, but if you always think about patients in the language of jargon rather than feelings, you make it more difficult to think of them as human and to identify with them. The use of jargon turns me right off. It's good to know jargon if you want to write a lot of papers or if you have to show everyone how bright you are or if you need something to hide behind when you don't know what's going on. A lot of psychologists use jargon, especially those with little experience treating patients. Whenever someone uses a lot of psychological jargon around you it is a sign of two possible dangers: first, they may be afraid of getting close to you and dealing with you as a human being with real feelings or, second, they may be trying to impress you. You don't need a mental health professional like that, although that's the kind that impresses committees and school boards and often gets hired because they sound good.

The conference room door opened and Jackie Rose, the head nurse, walked in. Amanda cleared her throat, Terry sat up straight, Larry looked serious. Jackie sat down. She stared at us. She looked like a head nurse. She weighed a ton and a half and you could always tell when she was coming by her heavy footsteps. When you found out

Jackie's age you said, "She's only thirty-three! I thought she was much older." The Jackie Roses of this world are all born old. There just isn't time in one lifetime to grow into what they become.

If a patient were threatening to harm himself and suddenly made a dash toward an open window, he'd land smack into Jackie Rose, somehow there as if from out of nowhere. She would belt him to the floor with those big hamlike arms of hers. The patient would just sit there dazed while she yelled, "You must be some kind of dumb sonofabitch to think I would let you jump through one of *my* windows. Nobody has ever made it through a window on *my* floor. And if they did, I would be right there on the sidewalk and beat the living daylights out of them." Then Jackie would make her standard (and most dreaded) threat, which involved sitting on the patient, which she actually carried off on one or two occasions with magnificent results. She had more power to make a person believe in himself than anyone I had ever met.

Legend has it that Jackie Rose could really paste you one. I never saw her hit anyone, but rumor had it that during the winter of '59 when she was accosted by three young toughs on Washington Street, only she walked away. She was also the warmest, most sensitive, most gentle person on the nursing staff, if not the entire psychiatric service. She knew intuitively and effectively how to act with patients. She never said a great deal about the theory behind her actions, but she was usually right. She taught a course in the nursing school and supervised student nurses on the ward. She had written a manual on psychiatric nursing. Every resident secretly read Jackie's book and learned more from it than from some of the texts we were required to read.

Once she grabbed one of Lovett's patients, Mrs. Beyers, who had been acting very crazy. Jackie yelled at her to start acting sane, meaning to eat meals on time, keep herself tidy, and stop screaming on the ward. Jackie acted after waiting two weeks for Stanley Lovett, M.D., boy psychoanalyst, to find out everything that had happened to the lady in early childhood in order to get a complete psychological developmental history so that he could be sure that he would do and say the right thing at the right time. Of course Lovett hadn't yet actually done anything for Mrs. Beyers. He still didn't think he knew enough and Mrs. Beyers refused to talk to him. Meanwhile, Mrs. Beyers continued to be a terror. So, Jackie followed her around making her clean up after herself. In three days Mrs. Beyers began to talk sense. Lovett was furious and reported Jackie to his supervisor,

Dr. Jerome Gelb, who smiled at him tolerantly. And Dr. Gelb was an analyst, which is some kind of poetic justice.

Jackie Rose either hated or loved you. You were never in doubt. It really didn't make that much difference, because you always knew what to expect from her and could make allowances. She was consistent. She might hate you but she would never do anything that would undermine you or your work with a patient. She was very much a professional. When her feelings got in the way, she admitted it openly. She was a very real person. She would even tell patients that she did not like them and why, doing it in a straightforward way. They sometimes got more out of her real anger at them than they would ever get from the feigned sympathy and phony empathy that some of us therapists offered.

"Larry," Jackie began, "Have you made your opening pitch so we can get down to business?"

Danielson looked down at his papers and began rubbing his head. "I haven't gotten around to much, except introductions," he said. You could see in a minute who was really running this ward, just from Jackie's tone of voice and from the speed of Larry's hand over his head. This looked like it was going to be an interesting clinical year. "I have some papers to give to the residents," Larry added, and hurriedly began to pass out some schedules.

The first four single-spaced pages contained the details we were required to cover and comment upon in our standard psychiatric evaluation of each patient on that ward. It looked like an invoice for the fittings of the *Queen Mary*. Besides name, age, and the other usual vital statistics, the list included such items as appearance, gestures and mannerisms, perceptual functions by the dozen as well as a myriad of intellectual functions, feelings, defenses; and the presence and absence of some hundred details which characterize people, such as associations, speed of conversation, logical vs. illogical progression of thoughts, and the inventing of new words (neologisms). Just to indicate the presence or absence of these details would take a week, providing the patient was completely cooperative. And if you did take the time to comment on each one you would have no time left to find out what was bothering the patient. I suddenly felt pressured.

I could just imagine sitting down with some lady who'd just lost her uterus on the subway coming over to the hospital and asking her, "Do you ever invent new words? Would you mind counting backward from 100 by 7s for me? Are you afraid of heights? Who was the last president? Do you ever feel you are floating away from reality?

What kind of dressing would you like on your word salad? And oh yes, lady, I almost forgot, how did you manage to lose your uterus on the subway?"

You have no idea how terribly confusing it all can be at the beginning of a new rotation, in a discipline you are unfamiliar with, trying to learn the ropes, talking about ideas that are strange to you, and then to be handed a sheet containing hundreds of points which you are expected to cover in your reports. It's overwhelming. You think that everyone else knows exactly what to do and you feel that you don't know anything. You can bet your Phi Beta Kappa pin, junior year yet, that D. J. Marley knows exactly what to put down and where and will probably find some mistakes on the form. My point is I felt I didn't know anything.

"Also," continued Larry, thumbing through his papers, "I have a list of the on-call schedules. Each of you will be on one night in five and every fifth weekend."

That seemed like a dream come true. I'd have time to find out what the name of my youngest child was. I think it was Patty or Penny or something like that. It began with a P, I'm sure of that. I have a picture of her somewhere in my wallet taken during the daylight hours so I could remember what she looked like when the sun was out. I can remember one six-day period last year when I did not see her at all.

"And," Larry continued, "I have the ward schedule so you will know what times you have open to see patients." Marvelous! I could find time to talk to Effie Sacks.

The ward schedule was very crowded. Every day at nine there was Larry's conference for discussing general problems on the ward. Then there was a case presentation and discussion daily from ten thirty to twelve. We would meet with the two ward supervisors, Dr. Gelb and Dr. Alex Karlsson, and discuss patients. In the second half of the conference a new patient would be presented by the resident who had evaluated him. Patients were formally presented about one week after admission. Each resident was required to write a study of the life of the patient he evaluated. They could be extensive, sometimes as long as eight or ten typewritten pages. Each month there would be a different staff physician who would listen to the case presentations and comment about what he thought was going on. Then he would interview the patient and make you look like an idiot. Not because that was his intent, but because he was really so much better. It can be very discouraging to see an experienced interviewer in

twenty minutes get exactly the right information from a patient which
you missed in eight hours of interviewing. So much for the mornings.

Four afternoons each week there were teaching seminars of various kinds. Mondays there was a group dynamics seminar—whatever
the hell that was.

"What is a group dynamics seminar?" asked Bert.

"*You'll* find out," said DiAngelo menacingly.

"You learn about group therapy," said Terry O'Conner, sweetly.
"I'll be in it this year with you guys." That sounded nice.

"You learn about group therapy by being in group therapy," said
Jackie Rose, "and judging from some of the people in this room," she
continued looking straight at Lovett, "it might do them a world of
good."

"I don't understand," said Lovett, looking threatened by the prospect of discussing his feelings in front of other people. Lovett used
the phrase "I don't understand" a great deal.

"You will," taunted DiAngelo. "You'll be cured."

"Get on with it, Larry," Jackie said.

We continued to go over the schedule. On Tuesday there was a
seminar dealing with the theory of psychodynamics, in which the patterns of behavior were dissected. There would be much discussion of
the meaning of fantasies and dreams. Lovett would expound and would
tell us about what he had read and what he thought it meant as if he
were the only one who could really understand the material, him
being a psychoanalytic candidate and all. Lovett had an autographed
copy of one of Freud's early papers and also had an autographed copy
of a paper by Harry Stack Sullivan, the great American psychoanalyst.
He was also reported to have an autographed copy of the Gospel
according to Saint Matthew with margin comments and corrections
by Jesus Christ himself.

Wednesdays, Grand Rounds were scheduled from four to five
thirty. These consisted of an elaborate case presentation or a guest
lecturer, some noted authority in the profession, usually followed by
a question-and-answer session. All the bigwigs in the medical school
participated, and the residents competed with each other to ask the
most brilliant question, designed more to reveal the questioner's IQ
in a favorable light than to illuminate the subject. "Attendance is
mandatory," said Larry. "You have to sign the attendance sheet. Dr.
Noyes checks the attendance sheet each week." Dr. Noyes was chairman of the Department of Psychiatry at the medical school. He acted
as if his finest hour came during World War II and he never quite got

over it. He tried to run the department like an army division. He would introduce the guest speakers as if he were turning us all over to the command of a great general. The attendance sheet to him was like a report from the battlefield. I really rebelled against this kind of stupidity and used to sign the attendance sheet with a different phony name each week. I reformed, after a while, and signed the same phony name each week. I signed *George F. Handel.*

Thursday afternoons were filled with seminars which covered a wide range of topics from research to the physical methods of treating emotional disease. Following the weekly ward meeting just after lunch on Friday the afternoon was free. If you had no patients scheduled you were free to go. Apparently whoever planned this schedule loved long weekends. That was great! Who knows, I might even get to know all my kids by name.

"Don't forget to leave some spare time open," warned Larry. "You'll spend from three to four hours a day treating patients and you have to leave two hours a week for supervision. You'll also be spending a few hours a week following up patients after they've been discharged. And you have to be sure to leave time to write notes, keep your records in shape, and spend time with the nurses."

It was beginning to look like a lot of work all over again. In addition to having his own doctor, each patient on the ward was assigned to a nurse who also acted as a therapist. Naturally you were expected to spend some time each day with your patients' nurse-therapist. Some of the nurses were excellent therapists and could make you feel like a rank amateur; but almost anyone at this stage could.

One of the customs on the ward was that the residents ate lunch together and took a whole hour doing so. Lunch was almost a social event. It was more than that. It was one of the ways residents would symbolically fill up after being drained by patients. It was a reassurance session.

"Look. Enough of all this crap for a minute." Jackie was getting very impatient. "I have a patient out here who is about to tear my place apart."

"Well, why the hell didn't you say so?" asked Larry.

"I knew it was your big first day with the new residents and I know how much you like to impress them."

Larry looked irritated, patted his bald head, and said, "Well, we might as well discuss it. If you gentlemen . . . and lady," he added conspicuously, remembering D.J. Marley, "are ever going to learn about what really happens on a psychiatric ward, you might as well start now. Tell us what's going on, Jackie," he said, putting on the doctor-in-charge voice that he saved for occasions like this and for impressing his mother-in-law.

"Roberta Goldman is throwing books around the day hall and screaming that she's going to punch out some windows. She's terrifying the other patients."

"Well, that is a problem," said Larry, checking through his papers, looking for something. "How would you handle this situation, Dr. Lovett?" he asked after a moment.

"I don't understand what you mean," said Lovett, putting down his pipe.

"How would you handle Roberta Goldman?" repeated Larry.

"Well, I'd want to know more about her; why she was in the hospital; why she is upset now, what her past history was like, what kind of difficulties she's had. It would take some time."

"She's a twenty-five-year-old lady who is in the hospital because her husband can't stand her anymore and is trying to divorce her. They've had trouble for years. She's very dependent and very immature," offered Larry, who impressed me for the first time by having all that pertinent information at his fingertips. I supposed he really knew all of the patients. Which was pretty reassuring. "Well?" said Larry, staring at Lovett.

"I guess she sounds like a borderline psychotic" (translation: showing psychotic traits but not yet out of touch with reality), said Lovett.

"Maybe, maybe not," said DiAngelo, "and so what if she is?"

"I don't think she is," said Amanda Little, who was Roberta's nurse-therapist.

"Why don't we ask Andre, the aide, for his opinion?" said Jackie sarcastically. "Meanwhile she'll tear my beautiful ward apart. If you want me to go out there and handle it for you, Dr. Lovett, I will. Maybe we *should* call the aide." There were three aides on the ward, all from Oberlin College, very bright kids, who really didn't know a hell of a lot. But neither did I, I felt. Anyhow they were nice kids and the patients enjoyed talking to them.

"Well, Dr. Lovett, what are you going to do about this lady?" said Larry.

I looked at Bert, who seemed as pleased as I that we weren't being put on the spot like that the very first day. But I couldn't understand why Lovett was getting it so rough and so suddenly. What had he done?

"Well," Stanley Lovett continued, "I still think I would want some more information. She should sit down and talk about how she feels."

"If she could sit down and talk about her feelings," said Amanda, "I don't think she would need to act so violently." Lovett winced.

"Meanwhile, my ward . . . my gorgeous ward," said Jackie, pleading for action. Although Jackie sounded urgent, I noticed that she seemed very much relaxed in all the confusion and almost seemed to enjoy creating the pressure.

"You won't have any time to sit down with this woman," said Larry. "Amanda is right, she expresses herself by acting violently."

"Oh, I see," said Stanley Lovett, M.D., who really didn't see at all. "She's acting out her feelings and displacing them onto the objects in her environment. Such weak ego controls!"

"That's it. That's it exactly," said DiAngelo, rolling his eyes back. "Wow!" I began to stare at the ceiling with DiAngelo.

"I feel that the best one can do with people like this is to demonstrate to them how inappropriate their actions are and to draw firm lines of what may and may not be tolerated," said Bert, trying to get Lovett off the hook.

"Tell her to shape up," I said. For this I went to medical school?

"Bravo," said Larry. "Now, Dr. Lovett, go out there and firmly draw the limits of appropriateness for this crazy lady."

"Hey, why me?" pleaded Lovett, looking like the hapless pirate in the movies who drew the short straw and would be killed by the others and buried with the treasure.

"Because, Dr. Lovett," said Larry, checking his papers again, "Mrs. Goldman is one of the patients assigned to you. I admitted her two nights ago."

Jackie Rose got up and opened the door and beckoned to Lovett. Amanda Little also moved. "Uh, uh," said Larry, shaking his head. "Amanda has to stay here. It's your baby, Dr. Lovett. Good luck." Lovett left, following behind Jackie, pale as a ghost.

Bert grabbed the last doughnut out of his paper bag and pushed it all into his mouth, maybe so he wouldn't have to answer any questions if asked. I just looked at the ceiling, wondering when my turn would come. I felt someone staring at me.

D. J. Marley was looking right at me and started to smile, a big, very pretty, very sexy (did I have an imagination), very warm, very nice smile. D. J. Marley started to giggle. D. J. Marley started to laugh without even an attempt to cover it up.

Even DiAngelo, cool and matter-of-fact and experienced, seemed surprised, concerned. Danielson, not knowing what to do, started rubbing his bald head. Amanda Little, who said nothing unless asked directly, and when asked said next to nothing, kept looking from Larry to Terry and back, trying to find some clue how to act. Terry O'Conner seemed to think it was funny but wiped the smile off her face every time her eye caught Larry's.

D.J. Marley was howling. She was cracking up!

"OK," said DiAngelo, who was the only one willing to talk. "What gives?"

The question was answered by a renewed burst of D. J. Marley laughter. "Oh, my God," she tried to begin, but couldn't. Larry looked very worried. D. J. Marley noticed that Larry was getting panicked and stopped laughing—just like that. She shook her head and with what seemed a near superhuman effort said, "And I thought I'd seen the last of doctors playing childish games when I finished my internship."

Everyone was relieved that D. J. Marley was not about to break apart in some acute manic psychosis, and there were even one or two soft laughs.

"If you only knew," said DiAngelo, "this is where the real game playing begins."

"Yes," said D. J. Marley, "here you can't even tell the doctors from the patients. That's the game, telling them apart."

CHAPTER THREE

FIRST PATIENTS, FIRST ENCOUNTERS

THE moment I stepped out into the hall I bumped into Effie Sacks. She was standing right next to the conference room door, waiting for me to come out. "You can see me now, Dr. Viscott," she informed me.

"I think so," I said, "but first I have to find out where my office is."

Effie Sacks did not look at all pleased. I walked to the nurses' station. It was crowded because the other residents were reading the assignment list posted on the bulletin board to find out who their patients were. I should read my patients' charts and get familiar with their histories before interviewing them. The right way to do things. Nice and leisurely. Without this pressure Effie Sacks was giving me.

"You want to go for coffee?" asked Bert Feinstein.

"You must be kidding," I said. "Do you see the look on the lady behind me?" I pulled Effie's chart from the rack.

Bert turned and looked at Effie. "What did you do, scratch her new car in the parking lot?"

"That's one of my patients. She expects me to see her immediately."

Bert tapped me on the shoulder and whispered, "Spend a few minutes with her and tell her you plan to study her case very thoroughly and that you'll be speaking with her in greater detail later. I used to work as an aide at the Hartford Institute for Living when I was in college. I know all the right lines. Just ask me."

Everyone seemed to know what to do but me. D. J. Marley had just finished copying down the names of her patients and was removing their charts from the rack. She caught my eye and gave me a pleasant look. Then she smiled again. What the hell was it with her? It was an interesting smile, almost breaking into a laugh again. What was going on?

"Did you see your list of patients?" D.J. asked. She assumed that I hadn't. "You've got some surprises."

"What do you mean?" I asked, my stomach turning and dropping.

"You'll see." She smiled a sweet, nonmalicious smile which I took as malicious and not terribly sweet.

I walked over to look at the list. Why was it everyone here knew something that I didn't know?

"Dr. Viscott!" shouted Effie Sacks, startling me. "Are you going to see me or not? I want to be seen right now or I'm going to walk out of this hospital."

"Dr. Viscott knows you want to see him," said Bella Grable, the secretary, quietly. "He'll be with you as soon as he can. I haven't even given him his office keys yet." Bella was very soothing. She fumbled around in her desk drawer and pulled out some keys. Each had a tag.

"Thanks," I said, taking the keys, secretly wishing that Bella had never found them. I didn't have a chance to look at the list. I felt squeamish. Bert had learned a tactic I didn't think of. D. J. Marley knew something I didn't about my patients. It was all unnerving. One of the tags read '"on-call room" and, I assumed, opened the door to the room where I was to sleep the nights I was on call. Another had a tag, "office 4." The third key had no tag. "What's this one for?" I asked.

"The little boys' room" said Bella. Effie Sacks smiled. The idea of my getting a key to "the little boys' room" must have fit perfectly into her view of me. "It's around the corner." Bella pointed in the other direction toward the day hall. I put Mrs. Sacks' chart under my arm.

"Mrs. Sacks," I said, like a salesman in a fine fur salon asking a patron to "Come this way, please." Mrs. Sacks and I walked down the corridor. I wanted to say something to her like "Have you been here long?" or "Do you like it here?" or "Do you have many visitors?" These are the pleasant social remarks that come easily with friends or even with strangers. They are difficult remarks to make to someone who is supposed to be your patient when you are supposed to be her psychiatrist. I mean, I knew psychiatrists were supposed to act in a certain way with their patients, but I didn't know precisely what that was. So I kept quiet and we walked in silence down the hall. Obviously I studied every door we passed to see if it had the number 4 on it.

There was a sound of great confusion coming from the day hall, the sound of people shouting, of furniture bumping against the wall and the sound of a foot dragging across the floor. Office 4 was just before the day hall. I opened the door, turned on the light, and Effie Sacks stormed in ahead of me. I took a peek around the corner into the day hall to see what the confusion was all about.

"What are you going to do to me?" screamed a disheveled blonde woman to Dr. Stanley Lovett, M.D., who was in the middle of his baptism by fire. She was Roberta Goldman and was knocking books from the bookcases and making a mess. Lovett winced as each book fell to the floor. D. J. Marley was sitting in a chair at one end of the day hall. When she caught my eye she smiled that funny smile of hers. She was taking everything in. Amanda Little was shaking her head. Jackie was talking to two other patients, acting as if nothing was happening but really watching Lovett out of the corner of her eye.

I felt better. Someone was under more pressure than I.

I entered my office for the first time. It was small, about the size of a jail cell. It had no windows. The ceiling was ten feet high with pipes running across, all painted green to match the walls. The walls were bare. The office was furnished with a wooden desk that looked as if it had been used as a wartime barricade. In front of the desk was a swivel chair, which I would soon discover squeaked whenever it moved and would give me away any time I felt uneasy or restless talking to a patient, acting as a built-in lie detector. A molded plastic chair stood next to the desk. It was furnished with Effie Sacks.

Well, what do I do now?

"Dr. Viscott, I demand to know why you think you are qualified to help me."

What the hell do you say to an opener like that? Should I give her a list of my credentials? I could tell her about all the books I'd read and how my extensive clinical experience had led me to the conclusion that many of the popular notions of psychiatry are not valid, such as those sometimes mentioned in the *Reader's Digest*. I had credentials all right, credentials that qualified me to become a resident in psychiatry, but not much else.

I could intone "I am a doctor," using the voice I used in my junior high school production of *Our Miss Brooks* when I played the principal. That might go over big. It was the tactic that I had seen some of the attending physicians in my internship use. They got respect from their patients who thought they must know so much merely because they were doctors. I hate *playing* doctor.

Effie Sacks was just glaring at me. "Well, aren't you going to answer my question? Or are you one of these sit silent and stupid types?"

Jesus, lady, I can't understand why you are so pissed off at me! I know, I know, I'm not Dr. Jabers. You are so goddamn angry I can't think.

"Mrs. Sacks," I began pleasantly. Could I be pleasant when I was frightened! "You seem very angry at me. And I really don't understand why." The hell with telling her whether I am qualified to help her. That's my business.

"What do you mean I seem angry?" she shouted. It was at this point that I discovered that my office was also furnished with an incredible echo. The place rang like a giant Chinese gong.

"You seem very angry at me," I repeated, "and you really don't know anything about me."

"I know enough. I can tell that you don't know your way around."

"I just got here," I said, interrupting apologetically. What the hell is the matter with me, apologizing to this lady? I hadn't done anything. This goddamn chair squeaks like hell! And it's uncomfortable!

"I meant what I said when I said you weren't wet behind the ears yet," she snapped. "I know that you're just starting your residency. I know that you don't know anything. Dr. Jabers really knew my case."

Ah, those glorious two words, "my case." How often was I to hear them spoken by patients. When Effie Sacks said "my case" she wanted to attribute her action and feelings to a disease over which she had no control and for which she should not be held responsible. So if Effie Sacks was nasty to you, you were supposed to think of it as "her case's" fault and not hold it against her. From Effie Sacks' point of view anyone who expected her to be reasonable, to wait her turn, or to be considerate was not only stupid because he did not understand "her case," but was cruel as well because he was picking on her when she couldn't help it.

How do you deal with this? What the hell did Dr. Jabers tell her? I wanted to open the chart and read his off-service note, but she would probably start screaming at me because I had to look something up.

I recalled that during my internship I had once taken a medical history from an old Jewish lady who had been taking a drug that was totally unfamiliar to me. I opened up my pocket manual to look it up and she started screaming, "Oy, oy. Here I am, a sick person, dying, and they give me somebody for a doctor who has to look up things in a book. Go away and get me a doctor who already knows. . . ."

"Well, what did Dr. Jabers tell you about . . . your case?"

Effie Sacks stopped glaring at me. Her look softened and for a moment she almost didn't look angry. She sat back in the chair and took a deep breath, pursed her lips, and turned to me.

I had gotten through to her! I could tell, by the relaxation of all her muscles, the abrupt change in mood, the change in her posture and facial expression. It was distinctly warm, sad; perhaps she was even thankful I had reached her.

Effie Sacks smiled at me and said, "It's none of your goddamn business what Dr. Jabers told me or what I told Dr. Jabers."

I hated Dr. Jabers' guts. Stanley Lovett, MD, would call that a displacement of my angry feelings toward Mrs. Sacks onto Dr. Jabers.

I also hated this squeaky chair.

"Excuse me," I said, opening up Mrs. Sacks' chart, looking for Dr. Jabers' off-service note. Good man, Dr. Jabers, you have big round handwriting. Looks like a woman's handwriting. Maybe Jabers was a passive, feminine guy and she digs his type. Ah, here's the note:

"June 30—Off-service note: Mrs. Sacks is a 32-year-old." Thirty-two. Look at that woman. She can't be thirty-two. As my mother would say, I'd hate to be hanging since she was thirty-two. "A 32-year-old woman with a passive aggressive personality, passive dependent type; who is addicted to alcohol. The present problem began with her discovering that her husband was unfaithful. She has attempted to control him by acting helpless, and her anxiety by drinking. Therapy is aimed at helping her control her feelings and understand her role in driving him away." I put the chart down.

A tough one. OK, so now what do I do?

"Well, this is my hour, you're supposed to spend time with me, not with my chart. You have very bad manners, Dr. Viscott."

This lady is feeling hurt and angry and I don't know what to do about it. Maybe I should just sympathize with her and tell her that I understand how tough it's been for her lately. Funny, I don't feel so angry at her. Why?

"I'm sorry, but I felt I should read Dr. Jabers' off-service note, his summary note to—"

"You mean you just read it? In less than a minute?" she interrupted.

"It's customary for the doctor to write a one-paragraph summary when he leaves a service."

"Dr. Jabers *must* have written more than one paragraph about me." What did I open my big mouth for? "I was Dr. Jabers' favorite patient. He told me so himself."

Right away I knew that had to be pure bullshit. I may not have known much, but I knew that a psychiatrist doesn't generally tell a patient that she is his favorite patient. Obviously, this lady thinks she was Dr. Jabers' favorite patient because she *needs* to be someone's favorite. After all, her husband is screwing around and she feels abandoned. No wonder she's angry. She feels Dr. Jabers has abandoned her too. Because he couldn't help it, since he was just following orders, so to speak, she can keep thinking of Jabers as the nice guy. So what does that make me? I'm not too crazy about my role already. What is supposed to happen?

"Dr. Viscott, you have a lot to learn. Dr. Jabers had a great deal to say about me and he said it well and he said it clearly. He understood my case. Obviously you don't."

She's right. I don't really. What if I told her?

"Mrs. Sacks, there's no use pretending that I understand everything about you. I don't. I just arrived. I haven't had the time to sit down and give your case the serious attention it deserves or to read Dr. Jabers' notes quietly and think them over. I'd like a chance to help you, but you have to give me a little time to get to know you better."

Effie Sacks was looking at me as if I had just slapped her. I could tell I had said something wrong, but I wasn't sure what. She looked so hateful.

"Dr. Viscott, that's the first reasonable thing you've said. I'd like you to study Dr. Jabers' comments. It'll be very helpful to you in your training. You can learn a great deal from him. Someday he'll be a very important psychiatrist."

So much for my ability to read Mrs. Sacks' facial expressions.

"Dr. Viscott," she began, "will you give me a weekend pass? I want to go home." It was Thursday. I didn't know the regulations about weekend or overnight passes or even if Mrs. Sacks was allowed to go home.

"I'll have to look into it," I said. Mrs. Sacks put on an angry smile. "I just don't know enough about you right now. I'll check right away though," I said almost servilely. I felt Mrs. Sacks' magic working on me. She had done me the great favor of behaving decently for a moment, and out of gratitude for that passing pleasantness I could feel myself acting extra nice. It was a little unreal. I hate feeling like a phony. I felt as if the conversation were taking place in a foreign language that I understood incompletely and was pleased just to be able to communicate at any level.

What was wrong? If I were a fourth-year medical student on my psychiatry rotation I could have been much firmer and could have said, "You'll have to wait until I decide." The power of my own convictions had abandoned me. I just wasn't sure about anything today.

"Have you been home for a weekend before?" I asked, thinking this was the best way to get my bearings, and stalling for time.

"Of course," she snapped.

"I see!" I'm going to buy a can of household oil and fix this damn chair before I go out of my mind. "You could make my work easier by telling me something about yourself. How you got here, for instance."

"I came by automobile. . . . Oh, can't you get all this from the chart? God, I hate you psychiatrists and having to tell my story over and over again. I'm not getting anywhere!"

"You psychiatrists" is correct. That is what the lady said. I'm a psychiatrist. I may have been here only one hour, but I'm a psychiatrist. That's great! That and a dime will get me a cup of coffee, but nothing will ever get this lady to talk.

"It would be helpful—" I began again.

There was a loud knock on the door.

"Come in." It was Jackie Rose.

"I have to see you right away," Jackie said.

"Mrs. Jabers—I mean—Mrs. . . ."

"Mrs. Sacks," corrected Mrs. Sacks. "I understand. You really don't want to talk with me. Jackie is always butting in. You could tell her to wait. Dr. Jabers would have."

"Dr. Viscott, please." Jackie was pushing. Effie got up slowly and lounged toward the door. Jackie stepped in. "Effie, it's very important. You can see your doctor later." Jackie shooed Effie out and closed the door behind her.

"Dr. Viscott, I need you in the day hall to take care of Roberta Goldman."

What had happened? My God, something must have happened to Dr. Lovett. I know he seemed frightened when I looked in the day hall. Maybe he flipped out. God! Losing a resident the first day.

"What about Dr. Lovett?"

"It was a mistake."

What was a mistake? To accept him as a resident? To throw him in with the lions like that? "What was a mistake?" I asked.

"Roberta Goldman is *your* patient, not his. Bella read the list wrong."

That was just what I needed, just what the doctor ordered to cheer me up after my abortive meeting with Effie Sacks.

"What am I supposed to do?"

"Well, like you told Dr. Lovett in conference, get her to shape up." Jackie smiled.

I'll never give anyone advice again as long as I live.

The day hall was a mess. Roberta Goldman had thrown books all over the place. Maybe a hundred or so. When I walked in she was standing in the corner, still taking books out of the bookcase one by one and watching them drop.

"Okay, Dr. Lovett, you can go. Your replacement has arrived," Jackie announced. Stanley Lovett, MD, was still white as he walked over to me.

"She's severely negativistic (translation: resistant to advice) and probably a schizophrenic who is symbolically tearing the world apart," he said. "Nihilistic (translation: under delusion that nothing exists)," he added as an afterthought on the way out.

Good for you, Stanley.

"I'll leave. It's not good to confuse authority objects," he said, pronouncing a concept almost one hundred percent nonsense.

Chicken!

D. J. Marley was still in the same seat as before, reading her patients' charts. Apparently her office was not vacant yet. She smiled at me. I walked over toward her, looking for support. D. J. whispered, "I told you you'd have a surprise. Lovett didn't know the first thing to do. God, he's horrible. Like a stick. Don't worry, you'll be better. I can tell."

"How can you tell?" I asked D. J. Marley.

"I can tell. People with blue eyes aren't usually sticks."

One thing I have always admired and am helpless before is a truly scientific mind. Jackie beckoned to me. Roberta was standing with her back to us, still removing books from the bookcase and dropping them one by one. Are you ready, folks? Here I go.

I walked toward this woman and stepped over some books. I

raised myself up onto the bookcase to get a comfortable seat to watch. I was suddenly reminded of when I was a kid watching the girls jump rope, calling out each skip.

"One hundred and forty-three," I said, making a game out of it. If someone acts like a child, deal with them like a child.

Another book fell.

"One hundred and forty-four," I said.

Another book fell.

"One hundred and forty-five."

Roberta Goldman kept dropping books.

"One hundred and forty-six."

She pulled the books out one by one with her middle finger, held each between her index finger and thumb, bent the wrist and released —perfect form!

"One hundred and fifty. Congratulations," I said in a bright announcer-like voice, as if I was about to reveal the prize Roberta had just won. "That's one hundred and fifty books in the world-record time of less than twenty-three minutes."

Roberta Goldman stopped. Her hands were at her side. She became completely still. After a moment she turned around to see where the voice was coming from. Roberta Goldman was staring me right in the face.

Roberta Goldman looked wild. She could have played Ophelia in *Hamlet*. Her long blonde hair was everywhere, over her eyes and face. She had no color in her face and her skin looked a little waxy, perhaps a bit masklike. She had enormous eyes, but they seemed lifeless, like two big holes that went straight to the back of her head. She looked more in my direction rather than at me. I felt as if a statue had suddenly come to life and turned toward me. I was waiting for it to attack.

I decided to make as light of the situation as possible. Roberta Goldman had just thrown a temper tantrum; now what would I do if my daughter Penny had thrown a temper tantrum, I thought. If you emphasize the negative points with a kid you're lost. You can't win. The kid will just get more obstinate and negative. You've got to accentuate the positive, eliminate the negative, and don't mess with Mr. In-between. You have to use everything you know to help people. And there's nothing wrong with common sense, even if you can't find a scientific theory to back you up.

"I'm Dr. Viscott," I began. Roberta Goldman continued to look right through me. "I guess you're pretty upset." All of a sudden I didn't know what to say. I had forgotten what I planned to do. Was I going to treat her like a child? Was I going to play games with her? What was I doing? I could see D. J. Marley out of the corner of my eye staring at me. Jackie Rose was playing cards with two patients at a table to the side. She was also keeping her eye on me.

I bent over and picked up one of the books from the floor, Richard Halliburton's *Royal Road to Romance*. Halliburton was a great world traveler who would try anything and was last seen sailing into the sunset in a Chinese junk. "Hey," I asked, "do you know this book?" Roberta Goldman's stone face actually reacted. Nothing spectacular, she responded by wrinkling her brow. "It's a great book," I continued. "I read it in junior high school. It's about the adventures of a great world traveler. I used to read it over and over again. It was a good escape."

Roberta Goldman was looking at the book in my hand, not in the direction of the book in my hand, but actually at it. At least that's what I thought. "Sometimes," I continued, trying to tie this all in with her temper tantrum, "people need to escape from unpleasant situations for a while to get their bearings." I started leafing through the book, half remembering an incident Halliburton described on a train in the Himalayas that I thought was great when I was a kid. "There's a part here about the wildest train ride," I said. I hadn't read this book in years and here I was getting into it again. Talk about escaping! Roberta Goldman seemed interested in what I was saying. "This guy Halliburton fascinated me," I continued, "he was always looking for something that no one else had done, for something new. Something that was especially his and no one else's. He knew how important it was to be free."

What the hell did Larry Danielson say was wrong with this woman? I can't remember. Here I am in the middle of the day hall talking about a book I barely remember to a crazy woman who will probably hit me with something in a minute. I don't know anything about her. What did Larry say? Marriage troubles is all I can remember. Amazing how well-informed we doctors are, isn't it?

"You know, I think you'd like this," I said. "It's a good book."

I handed Roberta Goldman the book. That is, I extended my hand and touched her hand with the book.

Roberta Goldman, card-carrying wild woman, took the book. She looked at it for a moment and then looked at me, a little puzzled. I had a brilliant inspiration. I picked up two or three books from the floor and said, "Why don't you put the Halliburton book aside and I'll help you put the other books back." I made a statement assuming she was going to put the books back and I said it as nicely as I knew how, without any punishing quality to my voice. The lady was out of control and I was trying to help her get back in control without humiliating her. Just the same way I would with my kid.

Roberta Goldman held the three books I handed her, but did not put them away. So I picked up one or two more and put them on the shelf myself. She watched me for a moment. I really get involved in anything I do and must have looked very industrious.

Roberta Goldman watched me put books away for several minutes. "Thirty-three," I said, pretending I had been counting.

"Twenty-one," said Roberta Goldman. "You've only put away twenty-one."

My God, she was actually counting! At least she was interested. A good sign.

"Just checking to see if you were paying attention," I said, looking at her and smiling. "By the way, what's your score?" I added.

"Three," she said finally, putting the Halliburton book aside and sticking two others on the shelf.

"It must be a hell of a lot of fun dropping books like that," I remarked, chuckling. "You really seemed to get into it." I don't know why I brought up the subject again. I guess I was still afraid that she would start throwing books again and I wanted to show her I was able to talk about it with her. So I made light of it. She did seem to be having fun dropping them, as a matter of fact, thinking back on it. I mean, the way she pulled them out and dropped them with two fingers did seem a bit put on for effect.

Roberta Goldman smiled and then pretended that she hadn't and then she smiled again and laughed through her nose, pretending that she hadn't. And then she just laughed out loud. "I guess it looked pretty stupid," she said.

"I've seen worse," I said.

"I," she began to choke up, "I don't think I'm in very good control of myself these days. . . ."

"You looked like you were in perfectly good control dropping those books," I said, handing her another book.

"No! I wasn't. I mean, I shouldn't have to drop books." She squeezed the book, as if debating whether to throw it.

"You were upset," I said, watching her put the book back on the shelf.

"People who are upset don't drop books like that if they're normal." She ran her hands over the books on the shelf, as if testing her self-control.

"When people are upset they do silly, stupid things. It doesn't mean they're abnormal. It just means they're upset."

"I've been so out of control though." She was kneeling on the floor, staring at all the books around her, feeling ashamed.

"Take a look at what good control you're showing now putting the books back. You get more in control with each book." What a great statement. Who knows, maybe I do have a feel for this business.

Roberta put several books away one at a time and filled a shelf. She smiled a pleasant smile, relieved that she had regained control.

"Now *that's* thirty-three," she said, trying to be cute, "not what *you* call thirty-three." Roberta stood and began to pick up other books and carry them a dozen at a time to the shelves. "By the way, you really didn't count one hundred and fifty books before, did you?"

"No. I just guessed." I started piling books in a stack.

"Are you going to be my doctor?" She looked at me very calmly. Somehow she had managed to grow eyes where the black holes in her head had been. Roberta Goldman's complexion actually didn't seem pasty and she had pretty good color. She also had freckles. Roberta Goldman was very pretty. Funny how you don't notice something like that when a person is in a rage. All that adrenaline pumping and all.

"Yes, I am going to be your doctor," I said.

"That's nice."

I thought it was nice too.

"I think that's nice, too," I said.

Just one minute! I don't understand something. Is this the same woman that a moment ago Jackie reported was threatening to punch out windows? What did I just do? All of a sudden I felt very confused and unsure of myself. Maybe I should have been proud of myself but I didn't know what I had just done. Was I merely being glib with her?

"I have to go to a meeting," I said, noticing the time. "We'll talk later."

"OK," said Roberta.

D. J. Marley got up as I walked past and followed me into the corridor. "Super," said D. J. Marley. I shrugged.

Jackie's heavy footsteps caught up with us. "Dr. Viscott, you did a nice job with her," said Jackie, "but you didn't do it the way you advised Dr. Lovett."

"What do you mean?" I asked, slowing down for her.

"You didn't tell her to shape up," said Jackie.

"What do you call that technique?" asked D. J. Marley.

"I don't know," I said.

I didn't.

"I must see you right away," demanded Effie Sacks, who was still waiting for me in the corridor.

"I'm going to a meeting," I explained. Effie's face darkened. She turned and walked rapidly to her room and slammed the door.

"What do you call *that* technique?" asked D. J. Marley.

"I don't know that either."

I didn't.

Dr. Alexander Karlsson and Dr. Jerome Gelb were in charge of the meeting and sat at the head of the table. Danielson took a seat next to Karlsson. The cast was the same as before.

Jerome Gelb was my supervisor. Although he asked people to call him "Jerry" he was probably the last person in the world you would ever think of as having a nickname. He was a Jerome. A Jerry is someone you went to college with years ago and occasionally run into in a cocktail lounge, laughing about all the good times you shared. Jeromes are not Jerrys. Jeromes are doctoral candidates, commissioners of departments of public utilities, and senior partners in law firms, or in the case of Jerome Gelb they are practicing psychoanalysts who supervise residents in psychiatry.

Alex Karlsson, on the other hand, was never thought of as Alexander. He was a genial, friendly, outgoing type who was not at all concerned about how he was supposed to appear. The two supervisors balanced each other very nicely, although I had little contact with Alex. Gelb was interested in hearing residents discuss details about patients which seemed to prove the validity of Freud's theories, such as slips of the tongue which revealed unconscious ideas. Gelb was especially fond of dreams and would spend hours interpreting them. Alex was more concerned with how to manage patients and how to help them make use of what you understood about them. You learned a lot from Gelb, but you sometimes didn't know what to do with what you had learned. It was rather abstract. You would understand the patient's dreams better and the meaning of some of his actions, but often it would be hard to translate that knowledge into something that would help him grow.

"I think it would be a good idea to tell them who we are, Jerry, and a little bit about what we expect," Alex began.

"Sure," said Gelb, reaming his pipe and nodding.

"I'm Alex Karlsson and I'm the co-director of the ward with Dr. Gelb. I will be supervising Dr. Marley and Dr. Feinstein, and Dr. Gelb will supervise Dr. Viscott and Dr. Lovett. These conferences are really supposed to be for discussion of ward problems and specific cases, but for this month we'll be using them to help you folks get acquainted."

"That's right," said Gelb. "I'd like to mention that it's nice to have a woman in training for a change."

"Indeed it is," said Alex Karlsson.

D. J. Marley smiled.

"Well, what shall we talk about?" asked Karlsson.

"Why don't you tell them about Mrs. Goldman, Jackie?" said Larry.

"Mrs. Goldman was admitted two days ago. She hasn't been evaluated yet," began Jackie. "She is in a difficult marriage situation. Her husband is threatening to divorce her. She was a law student when she got married, but gave it up so she could work and send her husband through school. Now he wants to drop her and she feels defeated."

"What's the problem?" asked Alex.

"She's been crying," said Jackie, "and feeling very helpless and trapped and out of control. Everything she's counted on in her life seems to be falling through for her. She started to feel desperate and began throwing things around and wrecking the day hall, threatening to punch out windows." Jackie sat back.

"Did she actually break any windows?" asked Alex Karlsson.

"No," Jackie answered. "She just threw some books around."

"What did you do about it?" Karlsson asked.

"I was asked to manage the problem," said Stanley Lovett, lighting his pipe. "I found her in the day hall very confused, striking out, tearful and destructive. I tried to appeal to her to control herself, but it seemed the more I tried, the more resistive she became. She started taking books off the shelves one by one and dropping them deliberately. I couldn't do anything with her."

"Well, what did you do?" asked Alex.

"Well," Lovett said hesitantly, "nothing. The ward secretary came in and told me that she had made a mistake and that Mrs. Goldman was Dr. Viscott's patient. I couldn't do a thing with her. She's the most negative person I've ever met."

"She seemed attracted to Dr. Viscott," said Jackie.

"Are you *positive*, Dr. Viscott?" asked Marty DiAngelo, turning to me.

"That's very funny, Marty," said Gelb, referring to Marty's pun on positive and negative. "And you know punning is supposed to be a sign of a very high IQ, Marty."

"I heard that, Jerry," said Marty.

A resident on a first-name basis with his supervisor. I was envious.

"And what did you do, Dr. Viscott?" asked Gelb.

I told him.

"Very nice," said Karlsson. "You gave her permission to be angry and accepted it as part of the way people are."

"You know, the book dropping is very interesting," said Gelb. "In some way it must represent to her the dropping of her academic career for her husband and her husband dropping her."

Now that's something I wouldn't have thought of. It sounded at once a bit pat and farfetched.

"How would you use an understanding like that?" I asked.

"When she's more in control," Gelb said, "and mentions that she is upset with her husband for wanting to drop her or with herself for dropping school, you could point out how upset she was when she was dropping books. It's helpful to show patients how their actions in the present sometimes symbolize their feelings about events in the past. It's as if they're trying to resolve their past feelings by acting in the present. Like Mrs. Goldman, it is almost as if she wished she were the one dropping someone—perhaps her husband—instead of it being the other way around."

"Of course, we don't know that much about her yet," said Dr. Karlsson. "Tell me, Dr. Viscott, why you decided to act the way you did with her."

"I don't know. She just seemed to be playing games and I decided to borrow her style of dealing with me. I mean, I just played a game back."

"Well," said Dr. Gelb, "I feel you intuitively made use of her style of behavior rather effectively."

This was very strange. I really didn't know what I was doing and people were telling me I had done something right and rather complicated. Everything seemed so vague in this business.

CHAPTER FOUR

WILL FAILURE
SPOIL HAROLD PARKER?

HAROLD Parker was my third patient. He was a businessman from a prominent New Hampshire family who was under great pressures. Within the same month his wife left him, his business, which had been on the skids for years, was being threatened with bankruptcy proceedings, and he turned fifty-five, the age at which his mother had committed suicide. There was so much going on that I didn't know where to begin. His chart was packed full of notes, formulations, and suggestions. He seemed very transparent and very vulnerable. He was also very anti-Semitic, which is why he was assigned to me. Dr. Gelb felt that working with D.J. Marley would be too difficult for him because of the difficulties with his wife. Since Viscott sounded the least Jewish of all the residents' names, I was elected. Surprise! Dr. Gelb, guess what?

Problem: How does a young Jewish psychiatrist deal with an anti-Semitic patient? I asked Dr. Gelb.

"That's quite a sticky problem. We felt *sure* you weren't Jewish. You don't *look* Jewish. Play it by ear, I guess."

That's reassuring, I thought. "What does that mean?" I asked.

"It means you point it out to him when he mentions it and talk about it and ask him if he thinks it will get in the way."

In other words, play it by ear.

Mr. Parker had been a sportsman all his life. He hunted, played tennis, squash, and golf, and had a yacht. He also ran scared, very scared. He went to Hebron and then to Rice, majoring in the art of being sociable. He graduated and went into the family business just as the bottom fell out of the stock market at the beginning of the Depression. His father had carried on the family name "in commerce," as they spoke of business in his social circles. Because Mr. Parker had no brothers he was expected to follow the tradition. His grandfather had been the brains of the family business. In the year after he joined the company his grandfather and his father both died of natural causes, but Mr. Parker felt both deaths were probably related to the Depression. He was left with several million dollars and a company he neither knew how to run nor cared much about. He felt he could not sell the company because it would be giving in to weakness, something he had learned to resist both on the playing fields of Hebron and Rice and on the squash courts of his club. However, he yielded easily to the temptation to drink himself into oblivion when pressures beseiged him, which was frequently.

"Mr. Parker, I'm going to be taking over from Dr. Meredith and will try to be as helpful to you as I can."

"Good, good," he said, reaching over and touching me on the knee with his hand, tapping me twice.

"Is there anything that you would like to bring me up to date on?"

"No, no. Everything's about the same. Everything's fine!"

Everything's just great, according to Dr. Meredith's off-service note in the chart: "the bank and his lawyers are getting together this week to consider arrangements for auctioning off his factory; his wife is demanding more money than he can possibly pay; the nurses have seen him drawing doodles of guns and knives, which Dr. Meredith suspected may be either in remembrance of his mother's suicide or in anticipation of his own; and his latest series of liver function tests suggests that he may have cirrhosis." Other than that, Mr. Parker was just fine.

"How do you expect your business affairs to turn out?" I asked, trying to find out how he really felt.

"Oh fine. They'll work out well," he said, and tapped my desk twice. I noticed he also tapped his left foot twice. "Why shouldn't they turn out well? I've got some good boys taking care of the shop for me." By "boys" he meant Edgar, the manager who had tried to run the company for the past thirty years while putting up with his interferences. Harold Parker knew in his heart that he was incompetent but did not know that everyone else also knew it, and so spent much of his life trying to save face unnecessarily. Unfortunately he felt a compulsion to put his own personal stamp on each and every business deal, contract, and arrangement that his manager tried to put together.

Almost without exception his contribution ruined the plans. He was forced to deplete his capital just to keep the business going and was finally running out. When the situation recently became worse he had to decide whether to sell the business or invest his remaining capital in it. The "good guys" were about to leave a sinking ship.

It was fairly easy to find out how most people would feel under similar circumstances. You just asked them and they would tell you that they felt depressed, hopeless, helpless, panicked, or worthless. Those are the general feelings most people have when they have suffered serious losses and believe they are about to suffer still greater ones. To find out how Harold Parker felt about his present situation was much more difficult.

Harold Parker was an obsessive-compulsive neurotic. He was a man who did not feel in control of his feelings most of the time and struggled to keep them in check. He was a man who was also out of touch with his feelings. He could barely express anger when he felt it. He was terrified of appearing weak. He believed that a man always had to appear strong, sure of himself, and be able to lead and carry that ball into the end zone. Noble characteristics! Maybe, but not when they were that inflexible and not when they prevented a person from showing human feelings.

Harold was not really unfeeling. He had a lot of feeling, but it was all bottled up inside him. His constant dread that he was out of control made him spend so much of his energy in keeping up appearances that he had eroded away much of what was good and had only appearances left.

In order to control his inner world Harold Parker had developed an intricate system of rituals which he repeated to ward off bad luck, bad thoughts, or bad feelings. He had a compulsion to repeat his actions or to touch objects a certain number of times to prevent his plans from going bad or to keep his angry thoughts from hurting someone. He lived by the kind of magic in the old rhyme that kids repeat when walking down a sidewalk. "Step on a crack, break your mother's back." Although he couldn't admit his bad feelings toward anyone, he would often find himself performing a ritual to prevent harm from coming to someone he didn't like. Harold would not be able to understand that it was he who wished harm to come to that person in the first place.

When his plant manager, Edgar, first told him that his company was going down the drain years ago, Harold Parker started chanting to himself, "Edgar will have his health, Harold will have his wealth," and he would touch something solid twice. Sometimes once with his right foot and once with his left. Or twice each. Over the years he acquired a considerable number of these magic rituals. They in turn began to take up more and more of his time, to the point where he spent most of his day thinking about his rituals and little if any time thinking about ways of solving his problems. He dealt in magic signs and rituals and expected a magic answer which would set everything right again. It was as if he believed in salvation, deliverance, divine intervention. It was extremely difficult for his lawyers and business manager to deal with him, since he rejected most of their plans out of hand because they did not magically make everything right.

Here I was, a first-year resident with a little experience in life, less in psychiatry, and I was a member of the ethnic group my patient liked least. How was I supposed to help him? What could I possibly do or say that would make life easier for him?

I needed to know if Mr. Parker was suicidal. What did his doodles of knives and guns mean? Maybe he was just angry. Maybe he was thinking of doing himself in. His mother *did* kill herself.

There was nothing so frightening to me as a patient who could kill himself. I felt very pressured to find out as much as possible to make sure that I was doing the right thing. I knew I didn't have very much power over a patient's actions. Some patients will kill themselves no matter what you do, but I still wanted to do what I could.

When you suspect that a patient is suicidal you begin to see suicidal meanings in everything he does. If a depressed patient took four aspirins for a headache it would not be unusual to hear supervisors or other residents refer to this as evidence of a suicidal wish.

Psychiatrists see many suicidal gestures, incomplete or symbolic suicidal attempts such as a patient driving a car a hundred miles an hour in bad weather. The suicidal gesture is also familiar to laymen, who respond to it by saying, "What are you trying to do, kill yourself?" The point is that when a depressed patient whom you suspect might be suicidal takes long solitary walks to the seashore in winter, or drives into the mountains until his car runs out of gas, you tend to view it with concern. Concern, hell, you're terrified because the patient may be about to kill himself and because you don't want to be at fault for missing important clues.

I was looking for the important clues with Mr. Parker, although I wasn't certain I knew what those clues were. The ten sure ways to tell if a patient is going to kill himself weren't listed in any book. Mr. Parker was unable to talk about his feelings of depression and helplessness, and so it was even more difficult for him to talk about actual feelings of self-destruction.

When you are a resident in psychiatry you learn very quickly that most people occasionally have some self-destructive feelings, even suicidal feelings. People tend to deny that they have suicidal thoughts but at one time or other most people feel that the world would be better off without them, that they are causing more harm than good, or that they are more trouble than they are worth; such feelings are just part of being human and reflect feeling badly about oneself. If you've never felt this way about yourself, the chances are that you aren't really being honest or, like Mr. Parker, you believe you can't admit to such feelings because that would be an admission of weakness.

"What do you think is going to happen with your company, Mr. Parker?" I asked.

"I think things will turn out well, as they always do. It's a sound company." He tapped my desk twice again and smiled an artificial smile, the kind of smile I was sure he had given to his teammates at Rice when Clemson was beating them by four touchdowns with only three minutes to play. I could hear him saying, "Don't worry, we'll make it somehow."

"Who's running the company while you're here?" I asked. Obsessive-compulsives usually want to be in control.

"I'm running it," said Harold Parker, tapping his right foot once. Once? Where's the second tap? I was pretty sure there would be another tap coming. There's *supposed* to be another tap coming. The first tap supposedly symbolizes a bad wish and the second supposedly erases it. Where was it? Maybe he didn't tap his foot magically at all. Maybe he just liked to tap his foot. Maybe I was reading a lot into all of this. Maybe this was all bullshit. Paying attention to so many details of a patient's behavior was tiring.

"You're running the company from here?"

"I'm on the phone a couple of times a day to Edgar. He's my manager. That's how I'm running it." Mr. Parker tapped my desk twice.

"How do you run your company usually?"

"I call Edgar a couple of times a day. I don't usually go into the office every day. Maybe two or three times a week and have lunch with Edgar or his son, Eliot. Eliot's a great squash player. He's an 'A' player. I'm only a 'C' player. I used to be a 'B' player, but you know, getting older. Can't keep running around with the younger guys." Mr. Parker smiled.

That was a complete surprise. Mr. Parker looked bright and animated when he talked about squash. I wouldn't have expected him to be able to admit he was getting older and wasn't as good as he once was, but he apparently felt good enough about himself to do so.

Bright idea! This guy feels good about sports and little else in the world. Judging from Dr. Meredith's history, there was nothing else he liked. Dr. Meredith had written a twelve-page summary of Harold Parker's life and had covered almost everything in detail except Mr. Parker's sports activities. Hell, what's wrong with talking with the guy about the things he does well?

"Mr. Parker, you seem to be quite a sportsman."

"Oh, well, I wouldn't go that far," Mr. Parker said, still smiling. How about that, he can even afford to be modest. His self-image was higher as an athlete than as a businessman. You didn't need to be too bright to figure that out.

"You seem to have accomplished a great deal in sports," I said.

"Well, I was one hell of a halfback at Rice. I was injured my senior year so I didn't get to play the entire season. But I scored an average of eight points a game in the five games I played. I once scored two touchdowns in one quarter against Clemson. But you know, they never had much of a football team." He could talk about his accomplishments and even put them down a bit.

"Two touchdowns in one quarter," I said enthusiastically. I'm not what you would call a big football fan. I enjoyed the pageantry of the football games when I was a student at Dartmouth. I liked the fall foliage, the pretty girls, and the parties, but frankly I couldn't give a damn whether Dartmouth won or lost. I liked to see a long pass play or a long running play but I didn't care which side made it. Still, I could appreciate a man scoring twice in one quarter. It was probably the high point of Mr. Parker's life. He'd been slipping down ever since.

"That must have been a big moment for you," I added.

"Not really." He smiled. "Actually I just took the ball from Muggsy Harris and went for short yardage over the middle each time. The boys on the line made some pretty big holes to go through. Really, doc, even *you* could have walked through them without padding. The big moment for me was winning the club member-guest three years ago. I had three birdies in a row and two pars on the last five holes to pull ahead of the leaders. A finish like Arnold Palmer."

"Wow!" I said. I restrict my golf to a bucket of balls twice a year at a driving range. "That's great!"

"Yes, it was fantastic. I never felt so strong." He looked pleased, recalling the past.

Harold Parker went on to tell about the hole in one he made five years ago, the time he broke par playing with a borrowed set of clubs, his yacht, his interest in sponsoring Little League teams, and his regret that he hadn't learned to ski when he was a kid. I mentioned that skiing was my favorite sport. Harold couldn't get over it.

"I went up to the top of Cannon Mountain with a group of friends. I took one look down those slopes and said, 'Baby, that's not for me.' I don't know how you do it, doc."

"You don't go straight down all the time. You go from side to side. You can take it easy. You learn to control yourself."

"And you still fall down and bust your ass," said Harold, laughing.

"But you do that in any sport."

"You fall farther and bust more skiing, doc. I can tell, and you're out of control a lot." Aha!

We talked about tennis and the advantage of steel over wood tennis rackets. Harold preferred wood. I was amazed. I had begun the sessions expecting to be bored and here he was being lively, even entertaining, and talking about interesting events in his life. This was so different from the picture that Dr. Meredith painted in his report. Meredith focused on all the events that were undermining Mr. Parker.

Whoops! Meredith is probably right. There is a great deal undermining Mr. Parker. He is in a situation over his head and he may be suicidal. Harold Parker is a man who never should have gone into "commerce." He is just not cut out for it. He is a sportsman and that's what he should have remained. Why didn't he join something like the International Olympic Committee years ago and live on the interest from his money? Why did he follow a career that wasn't his?

Was Harold Parker suicidal? I couldn't tell yet. He was indeed upset about the possibility of losing his business and couldn't face his feelings.

I let him tell me about his positive accomplishments in order to let him feel good about himself. Actually this made the sessions with him much easier for me to take, too, since we both had a lot

in common. That is, we liked some of the same sports. Bit by bit
his feelings about his failures came to the surface.

The anti-Semitism turned out to be no problem at all. It was a
cover for Mr. Parker's envy of Edgar, his plant manager, who had
been running his business for the past thirty years. Mr. Parker
found it simpler to be angry at Edgar for being Jewish than at himself for not being more adept in business. He never seemed particularly interested in knowing whether I was Jewish. For that
matter, he didn't seem to care if anyone else was either—just Edgar.
(For example, it never stopped Mr. Parker from inviting Edgar's son
to play at his club.) I guess that was understandable. Mr. Parker
would have hated anything Edgar was.

Well, next stop, Dr. Gelb, to find out what all this *really* meant.

CHAPTER FIVE

WHAT'S IT ALL ABOUT, DAVID . . . ?

During my first supervisory session with Dr. Gelb I felt *I* was being evaluated. I sensed that Dr. Gelb was trying to determine what sort of person I was, what my hangups were, how much I knew, and what he would have to keep in mind when dealing with me.

"What do you think of your experience so far?" he began in a friendly voice.

"I think it's going to be a great year. I really like what I've seen." For some reason I felt inhibited. I was silent.

"About Mr. Parker, David. You've seen him now."

"Four times," I said, a little anxious, staring straight ahead, acting like a difficult patient.

"Four times...What do you think?"

"He seems like someone who has been out of his element all his life. He should have been a professional sportsman. He played varsity football at Rice. He's an excellent golfer and it sounds like he's a good tennis and squash player. I don't think it's possible for him to change now, but it sure seems like he missed the boat." I couldn't believe how anxious I felt.

"Why do you suppose he didn't become a sportsman years ago?" asked Dr. Gelb.

As I sat back in the wing chair next to Gelb's desk to think, I relaxed a little and noticed the office for the first time.

Dr. Jerome Gelb was in his early forties. He had a short well-groomed beard which had considerably more gray in it than the hairs on his head. He smoked a pipe. More accurately, he smoked many pipes and had a pipe collection on his desk. He usually sat in a large Danish modern swivel chair. I was sure that it did not squeak. It wouldn't *dare* squeak when he was sitting in it. Near his chair was *the* couch. Jerome Gelb was a psychoanalyst and had an analyst's couch in his office, a threatening little thing. It was a brown leatherette couch that was coming apart a bit at the seams. A threadbare and dingy Oriental rug lay on the floor. The office was filled with pieces of pre-Columbian and African art. Little statues everywhere, just like Freud's office. I once saw a picture of it. There were several color photographs on the wall. One, I think, was of Mount Kilimanjaro. The others were jungle scenes. A large tapestry, probably African, covered the wall next to the couch. There was a large ceremonial mask on the wall opposite the couch. Patients lying on the couch would look at this grotesque mask five days a week. I imagined that it would probably influence their train of thought or give them nightmares or maybe even cure them. Who knows, if it works, keep it.

Dr. Gelb was an African art nut. He was an African nut for good reason. His wife, Mara, was a black woman fifteen years his junior. It was his second marriage and her third. He apparently felt that getting involved in the art of her culture helped him get closer to her feelings. Mara was involved in community organizing and worked in a multiservice community center. I wondered if she had pictures of rabbis on the walls of her office. Mara and Jerome lived on the outskirts of the ghetto in a modest townhouse that they spent over $50,000 remodeling.

I had forgotten the question.

"I'm not sure I know what you're asking," I said, pretending I hadn't forgotten. I was really caught up looking at all the ornaments in his office.

"What made Mr. Parker go into the family business when he had other talents?" Gelb asked.

"I guess he didn't want to disappoint his father by appearing weak," I said. "The grandfather was the brains in the family. Mr. Parker's father didn't seem too well-suited for business."

"You could point out to Mr. Parker," Dr. Gelb suggested, "that his father was afraid of facing the business alone. You could tell him that he has done a better job than his father by sticking with it so long.

"You know, David," continued Gelb, having difficulty getting his pipe going, "I suspect that Mr. Parker was so overwhelmed with his father's death and so resented the responsibility thrown on him years ago that when his father died Mr. Parker was unable to ventilate his angry feelings. As a result, he has spent his life since then trying to find acceptable ways to let the anger out but can't seem to do it. His angry thoughts frighten him and he invents rituals to bind them down."

Dr. Gelb was puffing away merrily and very happy with his newfound insight about Mr. Parker. Psychoanalysts love their insights. They are like gifts that they give to themselves. Dr. Gelb went on, "I wonder if discussing the deaths of his father and grandfather again would open up anything new. I suspect those deaths are far removed from him by now. It might be a good tack to take for one session. Who knows?"

I was very excited about this. I imagined helping Mr. Parker reach his lost feelings about his father and grandfather and give up his business and do something with sports.

"Wouldn't it be great if I could help him break away from the old rut and do something in sports for himself?" I asked.

"Well . . . I'm not sure who that would benefit most. You or Mr. Parker," said Dr. Gelb, deflating me pretty good.

"I don't understand," I said.

"Mr. Parker has been living his life just the way it is now for a very long time. You can try, as I said before, but don't be too disappointed if you fail. Remember, you have to keep your goals and his goals separate in your mind. You don't want the patient trying to live his life just to please you. Remember, he couldn't please his own father."

I felt really put down, but it was clearly good counsel. I didn't intend to push Mr. Parker into competitive sports.

"What's going on with you and Mrs. Sacks these days?" Dr. Gelb asked, switching rather abruptly.

"Well, I suppose you've already heard about her weekend visit home."

"Yes, I understand it didn't go too well. Tell me how you decided to let her go home." Gelb's pipe was out again.

I felt on the spot. "I gave Mrs. Sacks a weekend pass because I felt she could manage it. She'd been pressuring me the entire first day. Dr. Jabers had been thinking about letting her go home, so I figured that it had a good chance to work out. Anyhow, I felt it was worth a try." I was embarrassed over my rather feeble reasoning.

When a decision works well, people often don't question your reasoning. When a decision doesn't work out, no reasoning seems adequate.

"I take it you went through her chart carefully?" asked Gelb. He seemed very stern suddenly. I felt it was somehow my fault that Mrs. Sacks got into a fight with her husband and then started drinking heavily. She returned to the ward drunk and noisy. Marty DiAngelo was on duty the first weekend and told me that she was even more obnoxious than usual. He hadn't believed such a thing was possible.

"I went over it very carefully," I said, almost apologetically.

"Perhaps Dr. Jabers should have been more explicit about his concerns. He felt Mrs. Sacks would start to fight with her husband to confuse the situation. He wanted to make sure that they got together only on this ward, with a doctor present to referee and point out what each was doing. That's what I wish you had done. How did it go when you saw her today?" Gelb sat back and listened.

"Well, I had spoken to Terry O'Conner, who is her nurse-therapist, before I saw her. Terry had a pretty good idea of what went on at home. Apparently Mrs. Sacks only talks when she's drunk."

"And remembers very little afterward, you'll discover. What did you say?"

"I said, 'Good morning, Mrs. Sacks, I understand you really had quite a time for yourself this weekend.'"

"What?" Gelb suddenly sat upright in his chair. He took his feet off the ottoman and stared at me. "That was exactly the wrong thing to say."

My mouth went dry and my heart started pounding. What did I say that was so wrong?

"You said 'quite a time'?" Gelb asked disbelievingly. I nodded.

"That has the worst sort of ring to it. It sounds as if you're making fun of her. She didn't go out and get drunk because she wanted to. She went out and got drunk because she felt helpless and unable to manage her life in any other way. The fact that she became drunk and obnoxious only means that she failed again at trying to deal with her husband. Your comment makes it sound like you see her as someone who is being delinquent or just out having a good time."

I felt terrible. "I had no intention of giving that impression," I began. "When I said, 'I understand you had quite a time,' I really meant, 'Let's talk about what was going on.' I guess Mrs. Sacks pressures me and makes me feel on the spot, always demanding something from me. Maybe I was glad that her weekend didn't work out. But I really didn't mean any harm." I was getting a bit overwhelmed. I had no idea that I had said anything so bad. I just wanted to get Mrs. Sacks to talk.

"I would have said something very different," said Gelb, leaning back in his chair and fumbling in his pockets for a match. "I would have said, 'I understand you had a difficult time this weekend.' It would convey the idea that her drinking failed to meet the problems of a difficult time at home. And it would give an opportunity to discuss her troubles. Do you understand the difference?"

"Yes." There was a huge difference. Suddenly I began to realize what a psychiatrist was supposed to do and say, to align with strength and try to understand weaknesses. I was not at all certain that I would ever be that much on top of the situation to respond that way all the time, especially under pressure.

How could I be sure what I was doing or saying was correct? Dr. Gelb's approach not only showed a desire to help but also a useful attitude. I knew a helpful statement pointed out the problem and sympathized with the patient in an accepting way. But how the hell could I make statements like that all the time?

"Well," Gelb went on, "what did she say after you said that?"

"She told me about her husband's behavior and how much he had upset her. She also mentioned she saw his date book and noticed he'd circled his girl friend's birthday, when he had forgotten her last birthday."

"What did you say?"

"I asked her how she felt about that and she said, 'How do you expect?' "

"And?"

"I said, 'Hurt.' She nodded and started to cry."

"Well, apparently Mrs. Sacks doesn't pay as much attention to your opening comments as I do. Or more likely, you probably didn't sound so critical to her. She wouldn't have been so open with you if she felt you were unsympathetic."

Although Gelb reassured me a little with that last statement, I still felt miserable. I could hardly remember feeling lower. I'm usually not that sensitive to criticism, but Gelb's comments really cut into me, and not because that was his intention. I felt miles and years away from being a decent psychiatrist.

Also, my flip attitude was bothering me. I know I've already told you how it reflected my being unsure. But I didn't like to think that it got in my way to this extent. Even though my comment didn't seem to affect greatly my relationship with Mrs. Sacks, it bothered me a great deal because it represented a part of me that didn't seem to be under *my* control. What if Mrs. Sacks had taken my comment at face value and decided that no one could understand her? I would have done her a serious disservice.

I felt that to be a good psychotherapist I would have to analyze carefully every statement I made to a patient to be sure that I wasn't giving the wrong impression. This seemed almost impossible to do. At that stage of my training I just didn't know enough and I couldn't see how I could ever know enough to be sure I was always right. And if I finally did learn how to act and what to say, I doubted that there would be anything left of my spontaneity.

The road to becoming a psychotherapist seemed as technical as becoming a specialist in any other branch of medicine, and yet more vague. Jerome Gelb had a great deal of technique at his disposal and he displayed it during supervision, leaving me feeling limp. He must be so damn perfect in therapy, I thought. All of a sudden I wanted to be a patient in analysis with him.

Dr. Gelb got up from his chair and moved to his desk. I imagined he was going to fill out some special forms that he kept in his center drawer for getting rid of bad residents. I could picture him reaching for a pen and reporting me in red ink, just like my third-grade teacher did once when I cut up in school. One of the girls had written "Brush your teeth every day" on the blackboard and when the teacher left the room I talked my friend Saul Ottenstein into erasing "teeth" and writing "bra" in its place. (Come on, I was only eight.) The girl told on us. The principal reprimanded both of us and said she couldn't believe that the sons of two professional men could act this way. She questioned whether we would ever amount to anything. Saul's now a surgeon in Baltimore and, according to my mother, doing very well. I guess I didn't amount to anything because here I was, still expecting to be reported in red ink.

Dr. Gelb pulled out his right-hand desk drawer and then the left, looking for something. My God, he *is* going to get something, I thought. He finally found a piece of brown paper and pulled it out. It was a bag with his lunch. Boy, can guilt make you paranoid. . . .

What does a psychoanalyst, the husband of a young black activist, bring for lunch every day, I wondered. Soul food? Dr. Gelb brought the same lunch every day, a Swiss cheese sandwich on dark bread with lettuce and mayonnaise. Why is this so important? Well, I'm a little embarrassed to tell you this, but because deep in my heart of hearts I must secretly believe that you are what you eat, I began to eat a Swiss cheese sandwich on dark bread with lettuce and mayonnaise every day for lunch, and I usually skip lunch. I also promised never to call Bert Feinstein an oral character again.

I had been pardoned. I was not reported to Dr. Noyes, the head of the department, and was spared the dreadful ceremony, which, given Dr. Noyes' military demeanor, I imagined would be as upsetting as being drummed out of the corps like Jose Ferrer in *The Dreyfus Affair*. I could see myself having all my degrees pulled away from my name, and being expelled to roam the world as a layman. . . .

As a matter of fact, Dr. Gelb didn't seem particularly interested in pursuing the matter after he made his point. He opened a thermos and poured a cup of onion soup.

"How did your earlier sessions with Mrs. Sacks go?"

"Well, she once began by asking why I felt qualified to help her."

"Good old Effie Sacks. She's tough. What did you say?" asked Gelb, sipping his soup.

"I pointed out that she seemed angry and that I would like to know why."

"Good. Avoid answering a question like that. Always look at the style in which the comment is made. The question often doesn't matter. The sentence only serves to carry the patient's feelings. Examine the feelings, point them out, and try to find where they really come from."

"I also pointed out I was interested in Dr. Jabers' comments, that I needed more time to consider what he wrote. She seemed pleased with that. I thought it would be a good idea to talk with her about some of Dr. Jabers' comments as a way of helping her deal with Dr. Jabers leaving her."

"I think she could use that opportunity to discuss her feelings of being left alone," said Gelb. "After all, her husband left her too."

How do you like that? I had the same idea as Dr. Gelb when I saw her. Not so bad for a beginner.

"I thought so too," I said in my professional tone of voice, trying to make Gelb believe that I would never again say "I understand you had quite a time this weekend."

"I'd continue to discuss her feelings of loss with her," continued

Dr. Gelb. "I wouldn't be surprised if you discovered she had a lot of childhood losses, but I don't think she'll ever let you close enough to her to tell you.

"And what about Roberta Goldman?" Gelb asked, his mouth full. Somehow watching Gelb eat made me feel relaxed.

"I've been trying to gather a history on her. I'm supposed to present her to Dr. Gavin this week."

"What have you found out about her? I guess you're off to a good start with her. Terry O'Conner said Mrs. Goldman mentioned that she likes you and that you seemed like a nice person. That's important in any therapeutic relationship."

"From what she's told me I can only piece a little together. I've been sympathetic and a good listener. I'm mostly interested in getting our relationship off to a good start, so I haven't been digging too deeply."

"Well, you'll know more when you present her to Dr. Gavin next week. You'll like him. He's very good at digging out details." Gelb had finished his sandwich and was wiping his lips with a napkin. "Is it one o'clock already?" he asked. "Well, I'll see you later in the week."

On the way out I bumped into Bert Feinstein and Marty DiAngelo.

"You want to join us in a spot of lunch?" asked Bert.

"I think watching you eat would be an experience," I said.

"It is," Marty remarked. "This is my second lunch today. I'm going again just to see Bert eat."

We got on the elevator. A patient from the ward, Mary Larrabee, a fat schizophrenic former nun, was standing in the back of the elevator, hallucinating and saying the "Our Father" to ward off demons. She was Marty's patient.

"Hi, Mary," Marty said. "Do you know Dr. Viscott and Dr. Feinstein?"

"Pleased to meet you, Father," said Mary.

"Same here," said Bert Feinstein.

"Hello," I said.

"You going to the coffee shop?" asked Marty.

Mary was hallucinating.

"Mary!" Marty almost shouted to get her attention. "Are you going to the coffee shop?"

"Oh, yes, yes. I . . ." and she drifted off.

I really admired DiAngelo. He was very natural with patients. He just acted like himself and tried to be helpful to them. Actually, it was a great deal more complicated than that. Marty had two years' experience compared to my one week and had resolved many of the self-doubts and crises I was now struggling with. He felt comfortable about himself and he understood enough about psychological symptoms to relax and take things as they happened. He felt he could handle almost any psychological problem that came his way and he didn't feel he had to prove himself. He was content to let patients have their symptoms and not feel he'd failed. Sometimes Jerome Gelb could learn from him.

The doors of the elevator closed. The elevator jerked downward. A typical hospital elevator. I imagined how a patient would feel riding on it right after a barium enema.

"Very smooth," said Bert.

"Hail Mary," said Mary.

The elevator stopped. The doors did not open.

"Damn," said Marty, "we're stuck between floors. This elevator is always going on the fritz. Don't worry, Mary, I'll press the alarm bell."

"Oh, no," said Mary. She went on hallucinating. Marty pressed the bell. "*Hoc est corpus meum,*" said Mary.

"How long will we be stuck here?" I asked.

"Not long," said Marty.

The elevator phone rang. Marty answered it. "It's for you," he said, handing the phone to me with a smile.

"Very funny," I said.

Marty explained the situation to the operator.

"*Kyrie eleison, Christe eleison,*" Mary intoned.

"The elevator repairman will be right here, Mary," said Marty.

"Holy Mary, Mother of God, pray for us sinners now and at the hour of our death," Mary continued. "You have to pray. We all have to get on our knees and pray to God. Let's say the Act of Contrition together. Let's pray together. Please, it was like this in the convent. When one of the sisters didn't pray, she ruined the prayers for all of us. If we do not pray together, we will all be damned."

"Mary," said DiAngelo, trying to calm her down, "It's only the elevator."

"What if I pray in Hebrew?" said Bert.

"I'll beat you up," whispered Marty. "And where I come from, you learn how to do that by instinct."

You can see for yourself how little an Ivy League education and a medical school degree add to a chap's polish, not to mention his sense of contradiction. I mean, how do you learn an instinct?

"*Benedictus in Domine,*" said Mary.

I could hear the strains of the Benedictus from the Mozart *Requiem* running through my head. Bert and Marty were staring at Mary.

"Mary," asked Marty, "do you feel OK? You know nothing is going to happen to you. This is only an elevator and we are all going to the coffee shop. I'll buy you a coffee when we get there. How do you like your coffee, Mary?"

"We are all going to hell. There is no absolution," said Mary.

"Mary, stop that crap!" said DiAngelo. "You're acting like a crazy religious nut." Mary became quiet. DiAngelo whispered, "Try saying that to a nun in my neighborhood some time, especially if you're a Jewish shrink. Zap, your friends have a five-thousand-dollar funeral to go to."

Mary had stopped; in fact, she looked calm. Marty's yelling was therapeutic. The Mozart *Requiem* kept repeating in my head. This is great, Mary's not hallucinating but if the music doesn't stop, I will be.

The door opened and we were assisted out by an embarrassed worker.

"You got here fast this time," said Marty, looking at his watch. "You beat your old record by eight minutes."

"We were working on it and I forgot to put up the out-of-order sign."

"Come on up to Bamberg 5 afterward," said Marty. "I'll give you a free psychiatric examination so you can find out where all your secret hostilities come from." He gave the workman an obscene gesture, with a smile, and it was returned with a laugh. "He never fixes it right," said Marty. "I got caught in it for an hour last fall. Real bad. . . . I was with Dr. Noyes!"

We walked into the coffee shop. Marty ordered coffee and a piece of pound cake for Mary, her reward for not acting any crazier on the elevator.

"How do you like Gelb as a supervisor?" asked Bert, sitting down.

"He seems pretty sharp," I said, and told them about my blunder with Mrs. Sacks and Gelb's critique.

"That sounds like a fairly big point. I would have missed it completely," Bert said.

"So would I," said Marty, "and so would Gelb if he were seeing the patient."

"What do you mean?" I asked.

"Look," said Marty, "when you're seeing patients it's hard to be on top of everything they say. Especially in your situation. You guys are brand new at this. You're wondering if you're doing the right thing and you feel pressured. It's hard to make the perfect comment at a time like that. And you don't know that much about the patients and little about psychiatry."

"More accurately," said Bert, "we know nothing."

"Right!" I said, enjoying the support I was getting from Marty.

"And," Marty continued, "you're right there in the middle of it all as it's happening. If you were my supervisor, David, and I came to you with a statement like the one you made you'd find a way to say it differently too. It's like Monday-morning quarterbacking."

"I still would have missed it," said Bert, eating a pickle.

"Yes," said Marty, "but you went to Harvard."

"What's that got to do with it?" Bert protested.

"You Harvard guys are so theoretical you can't even take a shit in the morning without considering which part of the colon is involved."

"Nice dinner talk," said Bert, resuming his attack on the other half of his sandwich.

"Don't worry," Marty laughed, "when you guys start supervising medical students you'll be picking up their mistakes right and left, the poor bastards. Lovett isn't going to wait too long before he tells you what you're doing wrong." Marty pointed to the side.

Stanley Lovett, M.D., and Terry O'Conner, R.N., had just walked into the coffee shop. They found a table near us. Terry waved hello.

"Lovett's making a play for Terry," said Bert.

"The line forms at the left," said Marty. "Everyone makes a play for Terry at least once during the year. Terry never knows what's going on until you're sitting on the couch in her apartment taking your shoes off and sipping a drink."

"And then—and then?" said Bert, pretending to pant.

"And then," said Marty, "she asks you what you're doing with your shoes off. She's a classic hysterical type. They're all alike. They come on the sexiest, most-ready-to-pop-into-bed women in the world. They all kiss with their eyes open and their mouths closed. It would serve Lovett right."

"Ha!" said Bert, who was eavesdropping on Terry's and Lovett's conversation, "he's really coming on. I think he's making a pass."

"What'd he say?" asked Marty.

"Lovett just asked Terry if she thought Mr. Gentry was a pseudo-neurotic schizophrenic or a true schizophrenic."

"I would have slapped him," I said.

"You guys won't believe this," said Marty, "but he's the kind of guy who'll finally make it with her."

"And he won't even be trying," I said.

"Neither of them will," said Marty. "It'll be an accident. When it's over they'll need someone to tell them what happened."

"Like Dr. Gelb," I offered.

"Yes," said Marty, "and he'll tell them how he would have done it differently."

CHAPTER SIX

CASE PRESENTATION

ROBERTA Goldman and I got along well. More accurately, she enjoyed talking with me but did not enjoy discussing her problems. Each time I asked a specific quesiton she would go silent and a distant look would come over her and I would worry she was about to turn into a book-dropping fiend again. I was new at this and a bit timid and often found myself backing down. As a result I wasn't getting enough information to write a complete report, and I had to make a detailed presentation to Dr. Gavin in about a week. I had to push her.

"Mrs. Goldman, I know you don't like talking about your past and would rather discuss other things, but I really need to know some facts," I began.

"Do we have to? It's so boring." Anything Roberta Goldman didn't like was boring to her.

"When did you first notice that something was wrong in your marriage?"

"When Gary told me he wanted to divorce me."

"Not until then?"

"I just told you, when he said he was going to divorce me." She lit a cigarette and stared across the desk at me. "Gary is a very nice guy. I just don't know why he would want to act this way."

"Did you ever have any problems with him before?"

"What are you, a broken record? No! We always got along just fine. Perfectly fine. It came as a complete shock to me—" Roberta stared at the wall.

I leaned back in my squeaky chair and said, "I know you think I'm being repetitive but it sounds very strange to me that you wouldn't know he had begun to feel differently about you before he told you so."

"I didn't know." Roberta looked very irritated.

"Did you ask him why he wanted to get a divorce?"

"No."

"How come?"

"Because I was yelling and crying at the same time. I was just so upset."

"What about when you felt more in control of yourself?"

"I never felt enough in control of myself to ask him."

"Would you like to know why he wanted a divorce?"

"No, I would just like him back and to stay with me."

Roberta did tell me that she had a brilliant college record. She married her husband during her first year of law school, against the wishes of her mother. Her husband, Gary, was studying architecture. He said he wanted to have a family and was strongly opposed to Roberta continuing in law school. He believed a woman's place was in the home and Roberta gave up law school to stay at home.

"There's something I just don't understand, Mrs. Goldman. Why did you give up law school to stay home?"

"I didn't stay home. Where'd you get an idea like that? I went out and I worked. I put Gary through school," she said, changing her story.

"But what about law school?"

"You sound just like my stepfather."

Stepfather! I didn't even know she had a stepfather!

"I don't understand."

"Look, Dr. Viscott. I had it right up to here with law school. I had to play the competitive female and I just didn't like it. I went to law school because my parents wanted me to. Do you understand that? Well, I was looking for a way out but I just couldn't disappoint them. Anyway, I have a very difficult time speaking up to my mother. My mother still tells me what to do. I don't like to give in, but unless someone helps me out I go along with her just to avoid the fuss. Gary stood up to my mother for me, and when he asked me to marry him I felt it was a good opportunity to get out of the house *and* law school. Now is that so terribly complicated to understand?"

"No, it isn't, but why couldn't you just tell your mother you didn't want to go?"

"Have you ever met my mother? You go and tell her something she doesn't want to hear and see how she makes you feel."

"How would that be?"

"Like two cents, like you had just taken out her heart and cut it into ribbons." Which sounded like a secret wish of Roberta's. "She has a way of making you feel so guilty you do exactly what she wants."

"Then how do you feel?"

"Worse—trapped. Like I felt in law school."

"Did you ever feel trapped in your marriage?" I asked, figuring if she felt trapped in going along with mother she just might feel trapped in avoiding what mother wanted. Often people who react to others rather than acting on their own find themselves forced to decide among several choices, all of which are unsuitable for them.

"No, why should I have felt trapped in my marriage? What are you leading up to?" Roberta Goldman looked very annoyed. Here come the books, I thought. So what if the books do start falling? Why should I let her intimidate me? After all, I'm only trying to help her understand how she contributes to her own troubles.

"Before you said you felt you got married just to avoid your mother, not because you really wanted to get married."

"You mean you think I married Gary just to get out of my house, that I didn't really love him."

"I didn't say that."

"I heard what you said." Roberta paused a moment. "OK, it's partly true, but I still love Gary. He wanted to take care of me and didn't want me to do anything but be a woman to him. It was very appealing."

"I don't understand," I said. "You just told me you worked to put him through school after you got married. That doesn't sound like not doing anything."

"I was helping him. That's all. I was being a helpful wife. I wasn't really doing anything for my career. I was putting my career second to his, and I liked it that way."

"But you said he was taking care of you. It sounds more like you were taking care of him. Or have I heard this all wrong?" I already knew Gary wasn't taking care of her emotionally, beyond speaking up to her mother. Talk about confusion!

"Look, you're confusing everything." Roberta was sitting on the edge of her chair. "I was just helping him out at the beginning."

"When did you stop working?"

"This spring. I wanted to have a baby and stay home from work."

"How did Gary feel about that?"

"What do you think he felt about that?" she snapped.

Would I have asked if I already knew? Her nastiness was just her way of avoiding questions. I suppose I could put up with it, but it was getting on my nerves.

"Did he want you to have a baby?"

"We discussed it. We discussed it many times."

"And?" I asked.

I was just going to be silent for a bit.

So was she.

"Well, are we just going to stare at each other?" she asked.

"What did you and Gary discuss about having a baby?"

"Just that."

"Did Gary seem interested?" Boy, was that a stupid question. Of course he was interested. "I mean, what did he think of the idea?"

"He said he liked it. . . ." she began, but didn't elaborate. I felt she'd implied the opposite.

"Did you feel he had some reservations?" I said, playing my hunch.

"Maybe. I don't know, you're putting words in my mouth."

This was one confusing story. Why did she get herself in a situation like this? She couldn't stand her domineering mother so to get away she married some guy to dominate her. Except he turns out to be the weak one and she the strong one!

By the time the day of the presentation to Dr. Gavin rolled around I didn't know very much more about Roberta Goldman. Dr. Gavin still looked as lionlike as he had when he interviewed me for my residency a year and a half ago.

All psychiatric case presentations were pretty much the same. They begin with the chief complaint, a formal statement identifying the patient, stating the problem as much as possible in her own words.

"Roberta Goldman is a twenty-five-year-old married woman with no children who complains she has been losing control of herself for the past two months," I read aloud to Dr. Gavin and the other residents. I noticed that Stanley Lovett was taking notes and smiling to himself, obviously looking for ammunition to shoot me down. The little sonofabitch. It was bad enough to have to be the first resident to represent a case, and that the first visiting physician in rotation was Dr. Gavin, with a reputation for being a stickler for detail. Marty DiAngelo tried to peek over Lovett's shoulder to see what he was writing, but Lovett covered his notes with his hand. DiAngelo just shrugged to me.

In the next part of the presentation, the Present Illness, I told how Roberta quit her job and wanted to have a baby and how ambivalent her husband was about the idea. I reported the skimpy past history Roberta gave me to Dr. Gavin ("Why do I have to go into that now?" or "What has that got to do with my problem?") and said that I had backed down, spent most of the time with her trying to find out what was going on in the present. I gave a brief summary of her medical history and continued with a report of her mental status, a description of how she appeared and reacted.

"This is a very bright woman who seems willing to talk with her doctor but not about her problems. She is eager to find simple solutions but is unwilling to endure the frustration of looking at the role she plays in her difficulties. Her associations are logical and she stays on one train of thought until she comes to something painful for her. Her memory for recent and distant events seems unimpaired. She shows no evidence of any form of psychosis. Abstraction, judgment, and reasoning are good. Her reality sense is intact. She seemed depressed in the first sessions, but less so recently. Her major defenses appear to be rationalization, denial, avoidance, and intellectualization," and dropping books, I thought, but didn't say.

"What about her hospital course?" asked Gavin, who hadn't said a word for the past twenty minutes.

"She seems to have more control over herself," said Terry O'Conner, her nurse-therapist, "and except for being upset the first few days she's been no particular problem. She seems pleased to be in the hospital and happy to have decisions made for her."

"Well, Dr. Viscott, what do you think?" asked Dr. Gavin, waiting to hear my formulation. A psychiatric formulation should try to show how the patient's symptoms and problems relate to her life history and how the events of the present are symbolic of events in the past and finally it should suggest a diagnosis.

Well, what did I think?

"Mrs. Goldman is a passive-dependent, passive-aggressive woman who married a man on the promise that he would take care of her and assume responsibility for all her decisions. She also hoped to escape from her controlling mother. Unfortunately the role she now finds herself in is opposite from the one she bargained for and she is expected to care for her husband in the way that she originally wanted her husband to care for her. When she decided that she wanted to stay home to have a baby and stop supporting her husband, he rebelled and decided to abandon her. Now she finds herself in a worse situation than the one she avoided by getting married in the first place." What a boring, uninteresting presentation this was. I was even putting *myself* to sleep.

"Are you satisfied that you understand why she is the way she is?" asked Dr. Gavin.

"No. I find her very difficult to interview."

"Well, perhaps, but what do you think I should specifically look for when I interview her?"

"I'm not sure. That's a hard question."

"Of course it's a hard question," said Gavin tolerantly, "but unless you've formulated some goals before you sit down to interview a patient, you won't get any of the right answers because you won't be asking the right questions."

Stanley Lovett sneered, as if to say he already knew that.

"What questions do we want to know?" Gavin asked. "First, why is her reaction to her husband's wish to leave so overwhelming? She is certainly a bright woman who is capable of a great deal more. I just wonder. She must have known her husband was unable to take care of himself when she married him. The story you gave, Dr. Viscott, is very interesting. How stupid do you think a woman would have to be to marry a man with the hope of being cared for and then get a full-time job, act as wife and cook and all the other things she was to him and still not know she wasn't getting what she bargained for? Don't answer that. It's not a matter of being stupid. It's a matter of being psychologically blind. She has such a powerful need to feel taken care of that she fools herself into believing that she is being taken care of when, in fact, she is the one who is doing the caretaking. This woman thinks she must pose as a passive person in order to get by. She's afraid to be active even though when she is, she does well.

"The moment she suggests she wants to have a baby he threatens to leave. She must have known he was like this when she married him. Why did this woman pick someone who would abandon her? You pointed out how she avoids painful thoughts and refuses to talk about her past. Well, she probably wants to avoid thinking about a time when she was abandoned."

"But then why would she pick a man who would abandon her at the slightest stress?" asked Bert.

"Because," said Gavin, "she couldn't deal with a feeling in the past, she is forced to recreate situations in which the feeling recurs in the present."

"Like a repetition compulsion," said Stanley Lovett, scoring a point.

"I think," Gavin continued, "that her husband threatening to abandon her is a symbol of a previous abandonment. Her reaction to it in the present, which you described as so helpless and childlike, sounds like a replay of the feelings she had when she was much younger."

That was a very complicated theory. How could anyone prove it? "How can you demonstrate that?" I asked.

"By asking the right questions," said Gavin. "I'd want to know if she has ever been abandoned. Has she?"

"Not to my knowledge," I said. "Her mother and father have always been together. She did once mention, though, that her father was her stepfather." I'd forgotten to follow that up.

Gavin was immediately interested. Lovett, taking his cue from this, put down his pad of paper for a moment and nodded as if he had predicted it all. "What happened to her real father?" good old kick-them-when-they're-down Stanley asked.

Talk about feeling like an idiot. "She dropped that offhandedly while I was trying to get my bearings on another point. I guess I neglected to follow up. I was trying so hard to make sure I had all the right information according to the standard evaluation form that I guess I missed it."

"Maybe," Marty said, "she's one of those masochistic women who tries to punish herself as a way of feeling a loss she can't face." He added, "A neurotic substitute."

"She didn't seem that way to me," said Larry Danielson. "I thought of her more as a passive yet angry woman who was simply afraid to assert herself without the cover of another person's responsibility."

Everyone was flexing their interpretive muscles, showing off, playing "Psychiatry on Parade."

"What do you think?" Gavin turned to Lovett.

Lovett put down his paper and looked at Gavin. "I think I would agree with you," said Lovett.

"I'm just hypothesizing. I have no proof of anything yet," Gavin commented. "What about you, Dr. Marley?"

"I think," said D.J., "that there must be a pathological relationship between this woman and her mother. She seems caught in a love-hate bind and finds herself paralyzed. She relied on a marriage to an inadequate man to free her from mother. I would like to know more about the relationship between her mother and real father. I suspect that mother was castrating toward him and forced him out. I suspect that Mrs. Goldman probably identified with her real father and was afraid her mother would turn against her too. All she knows is that she's afraid of being anything that mother can attack."

D.J. was smart. No getting away from it. Jackie Rose nodded. She approved of D. J. Marley.

"Well, let's bring her in and interview her," said Gavin.

I walked out of the conference room to find Mrs. Goldman.

"Mrs. Goldman," I began, "Dr. Gavin is ready to see you."

"Do I have to go through with this? I'm sick of seeing a new doctor every ten minutes."

We walked down the corridor to the conference room.

"I don't want to go." Roberta Goldman stopped.

"What?" I knew what she said. I just wanted her to have a chance to retract it, without making a scene.

"I don't want to go in—all those people staring at me."

"The reason that a patient is interviewed in conference," I explained, "is to get as many new ideas as possible. I know how difficult some of your problems are and several heads are better than one." What I wanted to say was, you've got to go, Mrs. Goldman. You'll make me look like an idiot if you don't. You are my first presentation and everyone will think that I don't know how to manage patients. Come on, be a sport. Help a guy out. OK, so it is a little uncomfortable talking in front of people. I'm not sure I would like to do it myself, but it's a chance to get another opinion and to— let's face it, it's a teaching experience for me and the other residents and it's a chance to see a very excellent psychiatrist and get his opinion.

Actually, it *was* an excellent way of reviewing a case and determining the goals of therapy.

"Mrs. Goldman," I tried again, "I know you'll be a little nervous. You wouldn't be human if you weren't, but it's such a good opportunity to find out more about your problem. I told you I would present your case in detail, so it's not as if you are a stranger to these people. They're all professionals and they all understand."

"Well . . . if you think it will help."

"I do." I felt as if I were talking a relative into authorizing an autopsy.

Mrs. Goldman finally walked into the conference room.

"Mrs. Goldman, this is Dr. Gavin," I said and sat down.

"For a minute I thought you weren't going to come in," said Gavin.

"I thought about it," said Roberta.

"What were you afraid of?"

"Talking in front of all you people."

"That's understandable. How do you feel sitting here right now?" Gavin reached across the table for an ash tray and lit up a cigar.

"I feel alone."

"How do you mean, alone?"

"Alone, I just feel alone. You know what this is like!" Roberta was getting sore. Who could blame her?

"Yes, but I want to know what it's like when *you* feel alone. I know what I feel when I'm alone. No two people feel alone the same way."

"I feel up against everyone else, all by myself."

"Who should be here with you so you wouldn't feel alone?"

"I . . ." said Mrs. Goldman, and she became silent.

"What was that thought you just had?"

"I didn't think anything."

"Come off it, Mrs. Goldman. You just had a very sad thought. Who should be here with you? Who were you thinking of?"

"Look, I don't have to take this. Why can't I just get up and go out of the conference room?"

"You can get up if you want and leave, and I suppose you can take that feeling of loneliness with you. You know what, Mrs. Goldman, I'll bet you carry that feeling of loneliness with you all the time."

Mrs. Goldman was very fidgety. She lit up a cigarette.

"Share my ash tray," said Gavin, puffing on his cigar.

"Thanks."

"Who were you missing a moment ago?"

"Is it that important?"

"Yes! It's that important!"

"I was missing a Raggedy Ann doll I had when I was a kid."

"Do you miss the doll a lot?" said Gavin softly.

"Well, not really, but I sometimes see pictures of the doll in my mind."

"Who got you the doll?"

"My mother."

"When?"

"Oh, I guess I was seven. We lived in Providence."

"Why did you get the doll?"

"We were moving to a new apartment and my mother thought

I would be lonely. It was a new neighborhood. None of my old friends were there. It wasn't as nice a neighborhood as the one we left. I had to double up with my younger sister."

"How come?"

"We couldn't afford the old place anymore."

"Why?"

"Why do you ask so many questions? I can't see what this has to do with my being upset or having to go in the hospital. I can't see why a grown man is wasting his time asking me about a Raggedy Ann doll or about why I had to move. I think it's stupid. I don't want to sit here."

"You certainly are getting very upset over questions that you feel are trivial."

"It's not the questions, it's just that I'm upset about wasting my time talking to you and talking to Viscott and talking to Terry. I'm not getting anything out of all this."

"Mrs. Goldman, why did your family have to move?"

"Because my father left and we didn't have enough money," she said, trembling now.

"And when your father left how did you feel?"

"Alone." Roberta was bent over.

"The way you feel now?"

"Yes." She started to cry.

"Where did your father go?"

"I don't know. My mother never told me."

"What did she tell you?"

"She just said that he went away."

"Why did you think he went away?"

"I don't know."

"Did you ever see him again?"

"No." She started crying uncontrollably.

"You must miss him a great deal," said Gavin, unleashing her feelings.

"Oh, I do. If he were here, everything would be different. He would know how to handle my mother." Gavin handed her a Kleenex. She blew her nose. He did not comfort her, he just sat there smoking his cigar and waited.

"Mrs. Goldman, how often do you think about your father?"

"I think about my stepfather. He's a mess. My mother runs all over him, but I never think about my real father."

"I take it your mother couldn't run all over him."

"No, but she could push him out. I wanted him to stay so much."

"Why?"

"Why? That's a stupid question. Why does anyone want a father?"

"Why did you, is the question."

"To take me for what I am and not try and change me the way my mother does. I always thought that if he were around he would have kept me from making so many horrible mistakes. I get so afraid of being myself. I've been hiding the real me for so many years that I don't even know who I am anymore. I just want everyone to get off my back."

"What about your husband?"

"He's abandoning me, too."

"He's abandoning you, too?" said Gavin. What beautiful technique and so damn natural! "You feel your husband and your father *are* abandoning you? That's an odd way to talk about something that took place in the past. You mention it as if it's still taking place. Perhaps you feel it is."

"I do," said Roberta. "God, I feel the same now that I did when my mother told me he was leaving and I had to double up with my sister."

"How's that?"

"Why is he doing this to me?"

"I'm not sure I know who you mean, your husband or your father?"

"Everybody," Roberta said, and she broke down in tears again.

Gavin sat quietly, waiting for her to stop. "Mrs. Goldman, I think many of your problems now have to do with the past feelings about missing your father. You seem very lost without him and have many unanswered questions about him. They need to be answered before you can solve any of the problems in the present. I think your father is still as vivid in your mind and as influential as he ever was. This is something that you will have to spend some time working out."

"Is that all?" Roberta asked.

Gavin nodded. I got up and opened the door and walked out into the hall with Roberta.

"Oh, I feel just horrible," she said, but she added, "Will I be seeing you today?"

"In the early afternoon." I walked back into the conference room.

"That's a very interesting lady, Dr. Viscott," said Dr. Gavin.

I looked around the conference room to see if everyone thought I was some kind of moron for giving such a crummy presentation compared to Gavin's interview. What an amazing interviewer! He had full control of everything. He pushed her as far as he liked. When she cried he let her cry, and yet he was sympathetic when he needed to be. I felt sick to my stomach. I would never be able to interview anyone like that. Maybe you have to be an analyst to be that good, I thought.

Bert Feinstein whispered in my ear, "You wanna apply for an Ob-Gyn residency with me? I understand they have a lot of openings."

"What do you think now?" Gavin asked me.

"I think she'd like to be herself," I said. "She's not like her mother and she's not like her stepfather. I guess she hopes that if she ever found her real father she'd discover she was like him and that it would be all right to be herself. The feeling of loneliness she has is a feeling of not being like anyone else."

"Also," added Gavin, "of not even being like herself."

"I think," said Bert, "that she's torn between wanting to be something that pleases her mother and hating her mother for pushing her father out. She wants to be like her father but is afraid that if she is, mother will push her out too."

"Well," Gavin said, "what are you going to do with this lady? She is an excellent candidate for long-term therapy, bright, young, not psychotic and I'm sure she'll become more and more verbal in time."

"I guess," I began, "she should talk about her feelings about her father, what he means to her, how she managed without him all these years, what she thinks has become of him, and why she thinks he left her without saying a word. Then, I think we have to discuss what's going on in her marriage, how it relates to the past."

"It may be a good idea," said Gavin, "to see her and her husband together to get some idea of what's going on. You might also want to interview her mother. You can learn a great deal from even a short session with someone's mother. Don't be one of these psychiatrists who says he never sees the family. You can see whomever you want in a patient's family, just don't discuss anything the patient has told you, ever. That's the only rule. . . . Yes, Dr. Danielson."

"It seems to me," Larry offered, "that one could focus on her strengths and do quite well. Remember, she has virtually been supporting herself since she got married so she really is very independent. You should point that out to her."

"Let her know she is strong," added Gavin, "but not all alone. If anyone is doing the abandoning, she is. She could have predicted her husband would leave if she ever made strong demands on him. She knew he couldn't take that. Let her know you feel she has more control over her life than she recognizes and that you believe she can do a great deal more for herself."

"I don't know about the future of this marriage," said Terry. "Her husband has been on the ward only once since she's been here. He's very angry at her. He even screamed at her in the day hall a couple of times. He just can't stand her being sick. It scares and angers him."

Terry sent me a note, "I think Mr. Goldman is a creep." Terry really knew where it was at.

"Well," said Gavin, "I would agree with these comments." Gavin left and smiled as he did, obviously pleased with himself.

D.J., Bert, Marty, and I sat down at lunch. We were getting to be a foursome. Sometimes Lovett joined us, but then the conversation always seemed to switch to Lovett's ideas and Lovett's point of view.

"He's fantastic," said D.J. about Dr. Gavin. "He's so intuitive. He's so bright. God, could you imagine what it would be like to be able to interview like that anytime you wanted."

"Or to have his kind of insight at a cocktail party," said Bert.

"Or to know how hard to push or where to push," I said, and added, "I think I'm going to puke."

"Do you mind turning your head?" said D.J.

"How do you learn to be like that?" said Bert.

"God, I really admire that man," said D.J.

"We know, we know," said Bert.

"How come you're smiling, Marty?" I asked.

"I've heard this conversation before, two years ago, the first time I heard Gavin interview a patient. I felt crummy and stupid too. Gavin's really great, but he also puts on a show for your benefit. He likes snowing the young residents. OK, he *is* good at it and you do learn, but he's not like that all the time. He gets up for these conferences and he puts a great deal of effort into it. Look, kids, he's only been doing his thing for the past twenty years and he's been doing it in an academic setting. Don't be so down, David. As far as early psychiatric evaluations go you did pretty good. He usually tears them apart."

"Really?"

"Really!" reassured Marty. "Feel better?"

"Yes."

"Then get your goddamn spoon out of my soup. By the way, I'd listen to his suggestions. If he said a patient was a good candidate for long-term therapy, I'd consider it very seriously."

CHAPTER SEVEN

EVENING DUTY

Evening duty was shared equally by all the residents. The nights we were on call we were expected to stay on the hospital grounds or leave a telephone number where we could be reached in an emergency. After finishing with my work on the ward I would usually go to the on-call room in the hospital dormitory. It was a fancy name for a room with a telephone, a bed, and a dresser. Why it had a dresser I didn't understand, because the most any of us would use the room for would be a weekend. But I certainly needed the bed and the hospital certainly needed the telephone.

The room was very uncomfortable and cramped. We were promised a larger room as soon as a resident from one of the other services who had a permanent room in the dorm left for a rotation at another hospital. Meanwhile, we were stuck with the place. I liked to stretch out and nap before dinner. Being on night duty entitled you to a free meal at the hospital cafeteria. It absolutely had to be free because no one in his right mind would spend good money on that food.

I always ate dinner with residents from the other services. I found that no matter how friendly I got with the other residents, they tended to look on being a psychiatrist as a little like being a charlatan or magician. Psychiatric residents referred to each other as "shrinks." Some residents from other services referred to us as "spooks" and some used less complimentary terms, all supposedly in good fun but hostile as hell at the same time. Other residents also liked to get psychiatrists to defend what they were doing.

"Tell me," said Frank Howland, a surgical resident, one night at supper, "do you guys ever do anything for a patient?"

"What do you mean?" I said. "Why, we do miracles."

"I dunno," said Frank, "I couldn't stand just talking to a person knowing that would be all I could do for him. Don't you ever get the urge to do something like cut?"

"Yes," I said, "but it's not usually therapeutic."

"I think you guys are full of crap," said Frank.

"Not all the time," said Les Ahearn. Les was the medical resident on call that night. He was not only well informed about medicine, he also knew a great deal about psychiatry. Les was excellent at making psychiatric diagnoses and sympathetic to the problems psychiatrists had to face. Les was also one of the few residents who knew how to use and profit from a psychiatric consultation. He would ask the psychiatric consult specific questions and was interested in learning how to manage the patient better. Some residents called in psychiatrists to see their patients by way of a threat. "If you don't start cooperating we'll have to call the psychiatrist to see what's wrong with you," these jolly fellows would say. That's a hell of a way to begin an interview, with the patient expecting you to try to prove he's crazy. No wonder we were often resented.

Actually, a lot of psychiatrists caused these problems with other doctors. When they got called as a consult to see a patient they frequently wrote a very long, often obscure report in the chart which was chock-full of jargon. They frequently didn't summarize their recommendations in simple, easy-to-understand language. They forgot that once a doctor was outside of your specialty he had to be treated like a layman. You couldn't expect a third-year surgical resident like Frank Howland, who was all caught up in discovering new surgical approaches for reaching posterior thoracic structures, to remember the few hours of psychiatry he had in medical school or to want to take the time to read an extended literary note in the chart. Howland needed a few sentences in the chart that might go like this: "Patient is very dependent and hostile, needs (1) TLC (tender loving care) from nurses who should visit frequently to reassure him, (2) a brief two- or three-minute summary from his doctor each morning telling him how his case is improving. *Please* stress the positive points and play down negative ones. Remember he *is* improving and should always be reassured of that. Tell him setbacks are expected in the normal course of the disease. . . ."

Howland would not even bother to read a note beyond these few

lines. If you didn't write something helpful you were just wasting
your time, aggravating the patient, alienating the other doctor, and
undermining the usefulness of your future consultations.

When Larry Danielson described night duty to us he told us to
expect to find some of the other house officers hostile and uncooperative. That was the way many people reacted to psychiatrists. "You see,"
said Larry, "many of these guys have enormous authority problems of
their own. They refuse to think about a question, their way of acting
or practicing medicine. They want to be left to their rigid ways. When
you walk onto the ward they are afraid you'll find something wrong
with them. Let's face it, everyone secretly feels he is crazy." I was
prepared for Frank Howland.

"Look, shrinko," said Howland, "I have never had a psychiatric
consultation in the past two years that was worth a damn. I just got a
lot of bullshit from you nuts about the patient's defenses this or the
patient's defenses that or you tell me that the patient is Oedipal or
that he's acting out. What the hell am I supposed to do with that? All
you bastards care about is showing off how much you know to each
other, but as far as I can see none of you can apply what you know
and help the patient. But what can you expect, the people who write
psychiatric reports are psychiatrists. Almost all of the psychiatrists I've
met were out of their heads. They certainly were often crazier than
their patients. I think its a prerequisite for going into psychiatry that
you have to be proved committable. You guys are really a poor excuse
for the profession. They should take psychiatry out of medical school
and put it in the department of archeology or anthropology with the
other witchcraft."

"I feel the same way," said George Maslow, the obstetrical resident,
a very handsome guy who called all his patients "dear." George Maslow
had the nickname "Back Passage" Maslow because when he did a rectal
examination on a patient in labor to determine the position of the
baby's head, he would say, "Now, dear, I'm going to put my finger in
your back passage so I can tell how the baby's doing." He was too
embarrassed to say "rectum" or "vagina." He called the vagina the
"front passage," but "Back Passage" stuck as a nickname because it
was so much more evocative. Maslow hated the nickname. Howland
once asked him if he would prefer to be called "gotcha." Maslow hated
the joke.

"The young women that I see," Maslow continued, "sometimes have
emotional problems during pregnancy and afterward, but it usually
is short-lived. The only time I have trouble with these patients is when

I call in a shrink. He talks to them about what it means to be a mother and how do they feel about having a baby and all that shit. Before you know it they get the patient so upset she's ready for the funny farm. I think that there are a lot of so-called psychiatric problems that are really nothing more than people's ordinary reactions to life. I don't see any need to call in a psychiatrist every time someone gets upset. Everyone gets upset. What are the people in the ghetto supposed to do when they get upset, call in one of you clowns for fifty bucks an hour? You guys don't do a hell of a lot more than a good friend who sits and listens anyway."

"You could argue the same way about obstetricians and midwives," needled Les Ahearn, who was digging into his second helping of meat loaf. As far as anyone could tell, Ahearn was the only person in the history of the hospital who routinely ate seconds of meat in the hospital cafeteria.

"Chew with your mouth closed, Les," said Frank Howland, "you're making me sick." This from a man who spent eight hours a day looking at bloody entrails.

"I like the food here," said Les. He really did.

"Come on, Viscott, do you really believe in a postpartum depression?" asked Maslow. "I've seen maybe two in the last three years. I think it's a lot of shit you guys imagined to drum up business."

"Like fibroids," Les said, needling back.

"I never bother to ask help from shrinks," continued "Back Passage" Maslow. "You think a woman has the time or inclination with a new baby in the house to go and spend time in a psychiatrist's office? Bull. The problem will go away in time. All psychiatric problems do."

I really didn't feel up to defending psychiatry at that point, and anyway, I certainly wasn't going to waste my energy trying to convert Maslow. Andre Lumen, the Oberlin college student who was working as an aide, sat down at another table with Lynn Baker, the student nurse from Bamberg 5. When the other residents left to get back to their services, I joined Andre and Lynn for coffee.

Lynn was adorable, bright-eyed, and interested in everything. She had been working with Mr. Parker and, according to my suggestion, talking with him about his positive accomplishments, giving him that special ego boost only a young woman can give a man. If you could find a way to bottle that and sell it . . .

"Hi," said Lynn. She had a way of making "Hi" a six-syllable word. It would take almost three seconds for her to pronounce it. I love enthusiastic people. Andre Lumen looked confused. He always looked confused. Andre wanted to be a clinical psychologist and took his college sabbatical leave as a psychiatric aide to find out what it would involve. He still hadn't found out much.

"Gee," said Lynn, "Mr. Parker really is a nice man!"

"What do you mean by that exactly?" asked Stanley Lovett, sitting down with us.

"I just mean he's nice to talk to. I go for walks with him in the neighborhood."

"Can you be more specific," Stanley said in his best inquisitor-examiner tone.

"This question is worth twenty-five points," I said, "so think before you answer it, Lynn." Stanley looked sore. "By the way, Stanley, what are you doing here at night?" I asked.

"I had to spend some time with a new admission. Mr. Green. He's a very depressed man."

"You expect any problem with him tonight?"

"No, I doubt it, but he does seem to be wavering between giving up his defenses and just barely holding on," said Stanley, patting a stack of notes he carried with him.

"You mean he looks like he's about to crack up, a nervous break-down?" asked Andre.

"I guess," said Stanley.

Laymen use the term "nervous breakdown" to describe almost any emotional illness and they think it's usually caused by overwork. Most nervous breakdowns really describe a person who is unable to cope with stress and as a result gets anxious or depressed. Stanley didn't like very many people, and Andre and Lynn were among those he didn't like most—Andre because he used lay terms and Lynn because she was enthusiastic and eager, traits which secretly frightened him. Like I said, I really loved Lynn, and enjoyed working with her.

Matter of fact, working with student nurses could be great fun. If you treated them like human beings, which many prima donna resident types didn't, they could be among the most helpful people on the staff. They had considerable time to spend with individual patients. If you took pains to give them practical suggestions, student nurses could be invaluable, but if you ignored them they could and often did screw things up terribly.

"I thought your remark to Mr. Parker was great," I told Lynn.

"What did you say to him?" Andre asked.

"That anyone who went through what he went through would have felt worse than he did," Lynn said, "that he showed real guts in sticking it out and that he must have a very, very strong character to do that." Lynn was proud of herself; so was I.

"But poor judgment," said Stanley. "Look how he ignored reality. I don't see his effort as indicating any great particular strength."

"What would you tell him?" Lynn said.

"It's not what I would have told him," said Stanley, avoiding the question. "It's just that I feel much more pessimistic about this man. He seems to be set on undermining everything he does in life."

"He's great at sports," Lynn said. "A natural winner. That's not undermining."

"How do you explain that?" I asked Stanley.

"Overcompensation," said Stanley dogmatically. "A classic example of a reaction in excess of the necessary amount to make up for a known deficit."

"That kind of talk is what makes us all so popular. It ought to be censored. Look, Stanley, Parker thinks he has to be strong and powerful, a real big man all the time," I said. "I've been having Lynn tell him it's OK and even important for a real man also to be tender and understanding and warm, and to get him to admit that he doesn't know everything and to understand that doesn't mean he's worthless. Now if he could admit that his business manager knows more than he does and follow his advice he would be a helluva lot better off. I also told him that he'd have more time to himself, more money, less worries about his business and be able to do more in sports, or work with a boys' club."

"I don't think a psychiatrist should poke into a man's life and make value judgments," said Stanley. "I think you are imposing your will on this man."

"What am I supposed to do? Not comment about the things I see that are so obvious to me and that he through no fault of his own can't see at all? He's been making the same mistakes all his life. Why is it wrong for me to tell him that he seems to like something better than what he's doing? And why shouldn't he try it? I think he can learn to come to terms with being a less than adequate businessman and accept the idea a person can't be good at everything and believe that because the business was right for his grandfather doesn't mean it's right for him."

"I think you are dangerously overstepping your grounds as a psychiatrist," repeated Lovett. "Your role is to sit there and to listen and to put together the pieces in this man's life so that you will have a valid working formulation of how his mind and defenses work. Now,

you and I know that that takes time. You've seen this guy for a couple
of sessions and you apparently think you know all about him."

"No, not all about him, but enough to know that he's barking up
the wrong tree and that he would be much happier doing something
else. What's wrong with telling him that and helping him discover
how he feels about the new possibilities and, if he decides he wants to
change, helping him to do it?"

"Sounds like you have a counter-transference (translation: therapist's feelings about the patient) problem here, Dr. Viscott, but you
are so defended against it you can't be honest with yourself. You
know, you really ought to consider going into psychoanalysis to find
out what makes you so headstrong with patients and so anxious to make
them get so much better. It's the patient's job to get better, not yours.
I explain that to my patients. I tell them that I want to help them, but
my help will come mainly through my silence and my listening to
them, trying to clarify what they say to me."

"You treat all patients like that?" asked Lynn.

"Pretty much. I feel the psychoanalytic model for treating patients
is the most helpful and objective."

"And the one that doesn't make you reveal anything about yourself," said Andre Lumen, out of nowhere.

"Don't confuse technique with defense," said Stanley obscurely,
trying to put Andre down.

"But what if your attraction to the silent psychoanalytic technique
where you reveal little of yourself is nothing more than your defense
against getting involved with the patient," I said, trying to nail Stanley.

"Now who's being defensive, doctor?" said Lovett. "I'd really
think about undergoing psychoanalysis yourself to resolve your own
hostilities. It might do you a world of good."

"Stanley, can I ask you a question?"

"Go ahead!"

"Why the hell don't you call me by my first name like everyone
else? I won't bite you. I might even buy you dinner."

Stanley didn't comment. Lynn started laughing.

Lynn, Andre, and I walked back to the ward. The cafeteria was
on the fourteenth floor so I decided to walk down the nine flights of
stairs. This was another form of identification with Jerome Gelb.
Besides eating Swiss cheese sandwiches, Gelb also walked up nine
floors to the cafeteria for exercise at least once a day—well, a sort of
reverse identification anyway. Lynn decided to race me down and
Andre followed. We all reached Bamberg 5 out of breath. Several

patients led by Effie Sacks tried to find out from the nurses what had happened to get us in such a peculiar human state.

It was really incredible. If psychiatric patients saw their doctors or nurses acting in a way not readily understandable to them, they panicked. They expected you to act like a doctor all of the time. Part of educating patients involved teaching them you were only human and like them had feelings, depending on how comfortable you were with yourself, that you might or might not share with them.

The rest of a patient's education included understanding such fine points as, everyone gets mad, at least irritated when they're hurt; or suffer a loss; and that you should tell whoever hurt you that he did so, as soon as possible, so that your anger doesn't have a chance to build up and to make you feel guilty because guilty feelings build on themselves and can depress the hell out of you. You also taught patients that anxiety comes from anticipating a loss or hurt and that their job was to help you discover what that loss or hurt might be. Your job was to teach them to cope with it.

It sounded terribly simple, but therapy really was complicated. Patients were often guarded and didn't want to admit they had problems or were weak and needed help. They sometimes so distorted what they told you it was really difficult to know if they were reacting to something real or imagined. Doing therapy was like learning to see a new view of the world. In some sense I felt like a theater director putting scenes from a patient's life in a new order that made a clearer sense, taking feelings in the present that seemed out of place and relating them to the events in the patient's past that originally caused them.

To sit silently as Lovett inevitably preferred seemed terribly wrong. I guessed he was imitating his own analyst. Some of Lovett's patients were psychotic. I mean, they had a very poor sense of who they were and what was real. Talking with a passive silent physician afraid to react like a human being almost always makes psychotics worse.

There were two nurses on the evening shift, Candy Bourke and Helen Doran. Candy was bright, self-assured, and sexually aggressive with the house officers. She was always good for a laugh, especially one at other people's expense. She would often cuddle up to me when I was about to sign out to the dormitory and in a raspy voice say, "Keep your door open for me, big boy, I know the way." Her partner,

Helen Doran, had been engaged for three years and was beginning to show signs of desperation that girls feel when they sense that their plans are not going to turn out the way they want. Helen was moody and tearful and often found it difficult to talk to patients or to be helpful to them. She spent most of her time checking and dispensing medicines. Helen was a mousy, polite, self-effacing but sincere person. She had the personality of a toad that had fallen under a steamroller and preferred to be left alone.

Nurses' rounds at night were an opportunity to find out how everybody else's patients were getting along. Helen always listened while Candy read the nurses' ward notes. I also reviewed the patients' charts because (1) I was very nosey; (2) I liked to see what other doctors were giving their patients; and (3) I wanted to have some idea of what problems to expect.

"Let's see," said Candy, "We are fourteen patients tonight. OK, Roberta Goldman's husband will be up to see her tonight. He's putting in a command performance."

"I want to see him when he gets to the ward," I said.

Helen wrote that down.

"She had a quiet day," Candy said. "She's been sort of crying since her presentation to Dr. Gavin. Terry says she was talking about her father letting her down a lot. She took it very hard."

"I can understand that," said Helen, apparently sharing similar feelings.

"Mary Larrabee," said Candy. "Now that woman is driving me bonkers. She's DiAngelo's patient. If she doesn't stop going around here all the time with her Hail Marys and all that crap she's going to get me committed."

"She blessed me twice," said Andre Lumen.

"My theory," said Candy, "is that she gets especially religious when she has a juicy sexual thought. I think she's probably both hetero and homosexual and gets upset whenever she gets close to a man *or* a woman."

"But she's a former nun," protested Lynn, showing a bit of her naiveté.

"Nuns have a sex life too," I said, "even if it's unconscious."

"Gee," said Andre, "I never had a nun interested in me before."

"There's always a first time," said Candy. "She's on 100 milligrams of Mellaril four times a day and she doesn't seem to be any quieter."

"How long has she been on it?" I asked.

"Two weeks," Helen said.

"Well, it sometimes takes a little longer for it to act," I said. If a patient's medication was not enough there was an unwritten policy that the doctor on night duty would not alter the medication or dose without speaking to the patient's doctor, unless it was an emergency or the patient developed a severe allergic reaction to the drug. I watched Mary Larrabee buzz by the desk, which we could see through the half-closed office door. She seemed agitated, irritable, and was offering prayers. "Maybe she could stand a higher dose . . ." I said, and wrote a brief note in the chart. "Pt. shows irritability, restlessness. ? if dose should be increased or perhaps decreased." I told the assembled that sometimes on this drug patients get restless and more difficult to manage. That's what *I'd* been told.

"So you're not going to do anything for her tonight, are you, hero?" said Candy disdainfully.

"If she can't sleep we might increase her sleeping medication," said Helen.

"Bobby Jacklin—" Candy began.

"That's *my* patient," said Lynn, showing pride of ownership. "He's a very disorganized schizophrenic boy, Dr. Lovett's patient. He's regressed and stays in his room all day. I try to get him to go out and talk about school and his plans, but he refuses."

"Try talking about him brushing his teeth, keeping his clothes and room clean, and helping him with that," I suggested. "When people are that disorganized, they often can't care for themselves, need help organizing their lives. I wouldn't talk about anything serious yet, it's too soon. Right now he needs someone to tell him when to blow his nose."

"You should hear what Dr. Lovett is discussing with him," said Lynn angrily. "He puts him through a third degree every day as if he were trying to discover the causes of schizophrenia, and as if Bobby were the only available patient. I think he's making him worse."

"What medication is he on?" I asked.

"He's on 30 cc. of Milk of Magnesia at bedtime if he wants, and 100 mg. of Seconal for sleep. Nothing, in other words."

These two medications were part of the standard orders all residents wrote when patients were admitted to the hospital. The minimum standard. No doctor wrote orders in another doctor's order book. Even supervisors didn't write in the order book. It was acceptable, however, to write notes in the patient's chart describing any findings you thought would be important for the patient's doctor to know.

Bobby Jacklin needed a great deal of help and probably could have used some phenothiazines, potent tranquilizers which had an antipsychotic effect. If I wrote a note in Lovett's chart, it would just be inviting a battle. He really thought he knew it all. He was going to take on schizophrenia all by himself without drugs. That's not an impossible task, but even when doctors with many more years' training than Stanley Lovett treat such patients without drugs, the results aren't usually anything to brag about. Certain tranquilizers are very helpful. In my humble opinion, a Bobby Jacklin should be given something stronger than a room in Union Hospital and daily sessions with a doctor whose tactic was to be silent lest he miss a golden word. Especially since Jacklin hardly talked himself.

"And now, here's your beauty, David," said Candy, "Effie Sacks."

"I went for a walk with her today," said Andre Lumen. "We went to a bakery and picked up some cookies for the other patients on the ward. I guess she felt sad about the way she acted last weekend."

"I guess she's expecting to go home next weekend and wants to make up with her husband," I said. "I had two long talks with her this week. She seems to get the idea she's making her husband desperate with her drinking. I think she deserves another chance to go home. The worst she could do would be to fail, and if she does, well, she's gained something too."

"That sounds good," said Lynn very enthusiastically. Candy stared at Lynn for a moment and then at me to see if there were anything going on between us. Candy turned back to her notes, winking at me.

"Arthur Green," Candy began. "He was just admitted this evening by Dr. Lovett. I don't know what's wrong with him. . . . Let's see . . . it just says he's depressed. . . . Oh, he's on suicidal precautions. Did you know that, Helen?"

"No!" said Helen, getting anxious.

"Christ! Who's minding the store?" I said.

"Andre," Candy said, "why don't you go out and see that Mr. Green is settled into his room. Help him unpack and give him a tour of the ward. Just stay around him. He's depressed. That's all I can tell you right now." Andre left.

There were several kinds of suicidal precautions on Bamberg 5. Most were written when a depressed patient was newly admitted and the resident wasn't sure if he was suicidal. When a patient became dangerously suicidal, someone was assigned to be with him all the time. Generally, patients felt more comfortable when doctors intervened like that. They were afraid they lacked self-control and, aware of it or not, wanted to be protected from their self-destructive thoughts. Andre would spend a few hours with Mr. Green, and if he suspected anything he would ask me to see him.

"Joseph Murphy," said Candy, "is still anxious and pacing the floor. He's having some kind of side reaction to his phenothiazines. I think he could use some more Cogentin." One of the annoying side effects of the phenothiazine tranquilizers was Parkinsonian symptoms: stiffness, drooling, and tremors. Cogentin often relieved these side effects. Mr. Murphy's history was that he got anxious each year on the anniversary of his wife's death and needed to be hospitalized to regulate his medication. He was Bert Feinstein's patient and was driving Bert crazy demanding a magic cure for his anxiety. He'd never accepted his wife's death, so each year it was like facing it all over again.

"Betsy Lewis," continued Candy, "is also Dr. Feinstein's. She's still a pain in the neck. She develops all of these conversion symptoms whenever she thinks she isn't getting enough attention. Today she collapsed in the day hall three times and pretended she was paralyzed. She made a big commotion and everyone ran over to pick her up."

"That's probably the wrong way to handle her," I said. "What does Dr. Feinstein suggest?"

"He's asked us to let her lay there." Candy smiled.

"OK," I said, "if that's what he wants."

"You should try to pick her up sometime," said Helen. "She weighs a ton—all dead weight."

"Well," I said, "if she falls down when I'm on duty, follow Dr. Feinstein's orders; ignore her and leave her lying on the floor, wherever she is. Don't let the other patients help her. If she wants to move she'll have to do it herself." Just like the way you treat a negativistic child, I thought to myself. You don't reward obstinacy with attention.

"Ernie Stone is next," said Candy.

"I love that kid," said Lynn, "he's such a neat kid."

Ernie was sixteen and the youngest patient on the ward. He was admitted to the hospital for intense feelings of depersonalization, feelings that he was not really himself, that he was an observer outside himself watching everything he did. This feeling is not terribly uncommon in adolescents but was more severe in Ernie.

"All quiet with him for the moment," said Helen.

"Rosa Bottone is one of Dr. Marley's patients," said Candy about the next patient. "She is a lady from the South Shore from Kingswell. She has a severe depressive reaction. She also has another serious problem—she's a patient of Dr. Ciriello."

"What does that mean?"

"Dr. Ciriello," said Helen coming to life, "is one of the biggest nothings that ever happened. He has one of these electric shock practices where he sees a hundred patients a week, evaluating them for shock therapy, and then gives them all shock therapy on the premises as outpatients. He practically advertises. He's like Dr. Delwin. Did you ever hear of him?"

"No," I said. "I never heard of him."

"Well," said Helen, getting very angry and red in the face, probably unusual for her, "he's a butcher. He calls himself a psychiatrist but he really does nothing more than shock everyone who comes into his office. The only reason Mrs. Bottone is here is because after over a hundred shocks during the last two years she seemed to get worse and he didn't know what to do with her. She was admitted one week before you new residents came."

"What did Dr. Marley order for her?" I asked.

"She's taken her off all medicine for the time being and had her scheduled for a neurologic examination. Dr. Ciriello still comes to the ward and gives his opinions and writes orders in the chart. Dr. Marley just tells us to ignore them, even though Mrs. Bottone is still his private patient."

Whenever a patient was admitted to a teaching hospital by a private doctor, the patient was considered to be under the care of the resident or intern assigned to him. The attending physician could make suggestions and discuss the patient with the house staff, but he was not allowed to write orders or prescribe treatments for the patient. He was entitled to write notes freely in the chart giving his opinion. If he didn't find things to his liking he could complain to the head of the department. I'll say one thing for Dr. Noyes, he might have been a stuffed shirt, but when it came to protecting the rights of a Union Hospital resident with his patient, he was just fine.

"I don't expect any trouble with her tonight," said Candy. "Jud Cain is another of Dr. Marley's patients. He's really handsome. He's supposed to be a psychopath, some kind of con man."

"What's he doing here?" I asked.

"His mother died recently. After the funeral he left suddenly for Zermatt and pretended he was an expert skier and gave lessons to rich tourists who thought he spoke English well. When he came back to the States he was broke. He got a job in a used-car lot selling cars not always the property of the lot's owner. Dr. Marley thinks it was a way to invite punishment for his guilt feelings about his mother's death. At the moment he's quiet, doesn't seem any trouble." Psychopaths were notorious for causing dissension in the ranks.

"Then there's your patient, Mr. Parker, who'll be going back to work tomorrow," said Candy.

"Make sure he takes his sleeping medication a half hour early so he gets a good night's sleep. It's his first full day back on the job."

"Mr. Paul Gentry is Dr. DiAngelo's patient," Candy continued, going down her list. "He's a chronic schizophrenic who's been sick since he was a kid. When his therapist, Dr. Linquist, went on vacation he decompensated. He does this every year. He works as a movie usher. He sees his doctor twice a week and watches TV. That's all he's ever done."

"It *should* be a simple life," said Helen. "After all, he's a simple schizophrenic."

"Simple schizophrenics," I said, "are reclusive, asocial, often nonverbal people who function at the lowest levels of society with little feeling or warmth. They are frequently hoboes. They sometimes live in hippie communes where they can be anonymous." Lynn nodded. She obviously knew a few.

"The last patient is also Dr. DiAngelo's," Candy continued. "Sarah Meyers is a nice little lady. She has an involutional psychotic depression. That's fancy talk for her persistent delusion that she has a penis in her mouth. According to Marty she can describe it exactly in every detail, how long it is, how round, how hard. It's always the same. Supposedly when she was sixteen she used to work in a delicatessen. One evening after work her boss forced her to take his penis in her mouth. She claims she was too frightened to resist, although her boss never used any real force. This happened maybe twenty times. She never thought about it again until the past month or so. She's in the middle of her menopause. Her kids have left home and she feels very depressed."

This one was right out of the books. In menopausal depressions, patients' old unresolved sexual guilts often returned like a reawakened corpse. Mrs. Meyers felt guilty because she was not really a helpless victim. She may have been the first time, but she could have avoided the other times simply by quitting work. Marty had told me a little about her.

"Can you believe it," Marty had said, "she says that in all her married years she never once performed fellatio on her husband. She says she wouldn't have dreamed of such a thing, and to wake up one morning believing that she had a penis in her mouth was too much."

"It must upset everything this woman believes in about herself," I had told Marty. "She sees herself as a sweet grandmother type."

"But it's not just that delusion about herself. It's also the outrageous (to her) idea that she, Sarah Meyers, used to suck off her boss behind the counter near the pastrami, and maybe liked it. It's the 'liked it' part that bugs her. She's going crazy thinking what kind of a woman am I to have thoughts like this and to be so angry at my daughter."

"She seems better," said Helen. "I'll say one thing, I'll be glad when she stops talking about that penis of hers. You know, it embarrasses me a little." Helen shrugged, not ashamed to admit she was embarrassed.

"Well, that's it," said Candy. "I don't think there'll be too many problems on the ward tonight. I don't know enough about Mr. Green, the new patient yet. But I'll drop in and talk to him. We should find out whether we need to put him in a room opposite the nurses' station to keep a closer watch on him."

We all walked out of the office to the nurses' station. It was only seven fifteen. Andre Lumen had been with Mr. Green for a half hour. I walked into Mr. Green's room. His roommate was Mr. Parker.

"Oh, hi there, doc," said Mr. Parker cheerfully, wearing the smile he put on when he was starting to get anxious. "Tomorrow's my big day back at the old grind." He got up off the bed and walked toward me. "I'm a little scared," he said, and tapped me twice on the shoulder.

"Who wouldn't be?"

"I wish I had your confidence in me."

"Seriously, look at all it took to get you down. It wasn't just one problem. It took a lot. When you do what you really like, damn few people can keep up with you."

"I know, I've been doing a lot of thinking about that."

I walked over and introduced myself to Mr. Green. "I'm Dr. Viscott. I'm the psychiatrist on call." I took it for granted that Mr. Green might be suicidal and I wanted to be reassuring, supportive. "I'm just a minute away from the ward if you need me. I'll be back later to make evening rounds. Anything you'd like to talk over with me?" I learned to make that offer during internship. Usually patients' questions were easy to answer. If the doctor on call appeared aloof or disinterested it made patients so angry and frightened that he got called in the middle of the night to come see them, to reassure them.

I'm really not *that* considerate a clinician, I just don't like to be awakened at night by stupid calls. I do like patients to be comfortable. But when I'm woken up in the middle of the night I'm no good to anyone. I'm up, so they tell me, but that's about it. I went back to the nurses' station.

"Gary Goldman, Mrs. Goldman's husband, wants to see you," said Candy. "What a funny-looking guy."

"Funny-looking" did not describe Gary Goldman. He stood six-foot-four, weighed under a hundred sixty. Although he was only twenty-six, he appeared very old. He looked as if he had Marfan's syndrome: he was gangly and had exceptionally long fingers.

We sat down in my office and I waited for him to speak.

He didn't.

"Mr. Goldman," I said after a minute—I didn't find making people anxious by being silent was very helpful—"What can I do for you?"

"Roberta said you had a big conference on her today and that you decided the problem was with her father or something. How does her father have anything to do with her wanting to give up her job and have a baby just when I'm just finishing my last year of grad school? It doesn't make sense."

What am I supposed to tell this man about his wife? I can't tell him any of the details she gave me because they're none of his business. If I did tell him what his wife was thinking or feeling he might use it against her. I could finally appreciate Dr. Gavin's warning to tell relatives little. It was the only way to go.

"Your wife is very upset. She's going through a very difficult period in her life." I caught myself. If I went on like this Mr. Goldman would pick me up on individual points and start to press me for specific answers or explanations. I changed my tack.

"Mr. Goldman, what do *you* think is going on?" I asked, a nice open-ended question which thanks to my cleverness should lead to a broad answer, letting me get a better picture of Mr. Goldman without revealing anything about his wife.

"I don't know," he said and became silent. Very clever, Dr. Viscott. Do I have good psychiatric interviewing technique or do I have good psychiatric interviewing technique?

"Let me put it another way," I said, trying like mad to think of another way to put it. "Can you describe how your wife became upset?"

"She just became upset." Can you believe this?

"When did she become upset?" I tried again.

"I'm not sure."

"I'm trying to find out if you noticed any change in her."

"Yes, she was more upset after the winter."

"*In what way* was she more upset after the winter?"

"Maybe," he answered, confusing the hell out of me. He shrugged and looked at the van Gogh print on my office wall. "That's not a real van Gogh, is it?"

I was flabbergasted. Was this guy an idiot or something? How did he get so far in the demanding study of architecture? He had no idea what was going on with his wife, what she was upset about, and he was asking me if my van Gogh print was real when I had a hole in my rug. What was it with him?

"Mr. Goldman, how do you get along with your wife?"

"For a few hours at a time." He stared at the ceiling.

"Can you tell me about the change in her lately?" I tried that tack again.

"No. Why, did she say there was a change?"

"Look, Mr. Goldman," I said, "I understand you told the admitting doctor there was a question of you getting divorced."

"I guess."

"Now, it seems strange to me that two people would consider divorce unless they aren't getting along." There is a phenomenon in psychiatry called the Ganser Syndrome, in which the patient gives unusually oblique answers to questions and appears to be feigning mental illness. It is most often seen in people awaiting trial or in other situations where it might be to the person's advantage to appear a little disturbed. "Don't you think that it's strange for two people to consider divorce unless something is wrong between them?" I repeated.

"Two people are two people, peas in a pod," he said, standing up and fixing my phony van Gogh. "It looks like an original. You must charge very high rates."

Mr. Goldman had to be a Ganser's Syndrome. He must have felt under a great deal of pressure and didn't want to take any responsibility for his role in his wife's illness. He just didn't want to get involved. He only wanted to get attention for himself and to be free from having to care for her.

Roberta Goldman, it seemed, would have to make her life better on her own because Gary was not about to help her. He didn't want to be a husband or father. He wanted to stay a child. Mrs. Goldman needed someone who could take care of her. I had doubts about that marriage, I reflected sagely.

Mr. Goldman left the ward after spending less than five minutes with his wife, in which time he told her that her hair looked messy, that he couldn't stand her crying, and that he had moved in with his parents while she was in the hospital to keep from being lonely. He did not ask how she felt.

I made a mental note to check every new building I ever went into to be sure that Mr. Goldman was not the architect.

I walked into the lounge where Ernie Stone, the sixteen-year-old boy who felt he was drifting away, was waiting to play Ping-Pong with me.

"OK, folks, the wonder kid from Acton is about to beat Dr. Viscott," Ernie announced to the patients in the day hall. Ernie was bright, animated and introspective, a bit too introspective. He worried. More accurately, he was obsessed about everything that went on in his head. If he felt dizzy he would stop whatever he was doing and think about it and consider the most horrible possibilities.

How should I play Ping-Pong with this kid who happened to be a psychiatric patient? Should I lose all the games so he feels good and his fragile ego is not injured? Should I go halfway or should I go all out and try to beat him, which out of my own vanity I assumed I could.

I decided to let Ernie feel he could beat me. It would be a good feeling for him. It would be therapeutic and would help him overcome some of his self-doubts. He took the first three points on serve. He had a nice spin. Each time I pretended to go after the ball, and hit it into the net. I decided I should return the fourth and make him work for that one. I hit into the net—same with the fifth. He slammed my first serve. He slammed my second serve and my third as well as my fourth. I somehow returned his slam of my fifth serve and he slammed my return.

OK, enough of this therapy, damn it. Ten to nothing. I was ready. No problem, I could handle his serve. Pow!

"Eleven, nothing. A shutout, doc. Want to go again?"

I got three points in the second game, playing like I had my life bet. Betsy Lewis, the fainter, watched intently as Ernie beat me 21–5 in the third game.

"OK, Ernie," I said, trying a little psychology (whatever that means). "I guess I'll have to play you right-handed" (which is what I'd been doing! I'm right-handed and can't even feed myself with my left). I kept the racket in my right hand, hoping rather feebly that Ernie wouldn't notice it had been there all along. We started another game.

Betsy Lewis got up and, without warning, slipped to the floor. Her arms just happened to protect her face as she fell. There she was in the middle of the day hall demanding attention while I was playing with Ernie and, dammit, with the score 4 to 2. I even thought I had a pretty good chance.

"What are you going to do?" asked Ernie, trembling and looking dizzy.

"Wait a minute," I said. I walked over to Betsy and bent down and said very quietly. "If you'd like to talk to me I'd be very pleased to discuss anything you'd like, but I don't think that the middle of the day hall is a very good place."

Betsy's eyes fluttered. Her family had spent a fortune on neurological examinations to determine if she had a physical ailment. All of them were negative. Betsy had had electroencephalograms—brain wave studies—skull X-rays and also a brain scan to make sure she didn't have a tumor. Betsy was a classical hysteric who converted her feelings into physical symptoms. Any second-year medical student could have made the diagnosis. Betsy apparently wanted to consider my offer, but she preferred to lie in the middle of the floor while doing so.

"My serve," I said, and belted one past Ernie, who looked bewildered. It was 4 to 6, my favor, before Ernie realized what had happened. "Hey, aren't you going to do anything?" he said.

"If Betsy wants to lie on the floor it's her business," I said. "Beating you is mine, at the moment."

"I'm getting those funny feelings again," said Ernie.

"Not half as funny as the feeling you're going to get when I beat you."

Ernie started to move away from the table.

"Hey, get back there. I'm winning, you clown. I didn't pull any sick act on you when you were beating me and I've earned the right to try to beat you."

Ernie looked at me angrily and picked up his racket. We played a vicious game. Although I had a lead, Ernie still whipped me, but this time the score was 21–8. At least the doctor was making some progress.

Best of all, Ernie had forgotten about his feeling of dizziness. At least until he saw Betsy still lying on the day hall floor.

"Oh, oh."

"You see, Ernie," I said, "you get frightened and then you expect the absolute worst. Expecting to feel bad makes you feel bad." I bent over Betsy again. "Betsy," I said, "I respect your right to feel and act any way you want, and I've told the nurses to let you stay where you are if you aren't in someone's way or hurting yourself."

Effie Sacks walked by me and gave me a sneer. "You could learn a lot from Andre," she said. Effie moved to help Betsy. I shook my head and Effie backed off, sensing that I had my reasons and knew what I was doing. I hoped she was right . . .

At ten o'clock patients crowded around the nurses' station for cookies, milk, juice, and medications. "I feel like one big udder," said Candy.

"No comment," I said, and went to the doctor's lounge in the dormitory to catch the TV news and to sack out.

CHAPTER EIGHT

THE GROUP

EVERY Monday afternoon at precisely one thirty we met for our group dynamics seminar. Myself, Bert, D.J., Stanley Lovett, M.D., Terry O'Conner, and Marshall Kell, a second-year psychiatric resident who was assigned to the psychiatric outpatient department. Marshall spent his first year of residency at the State Hospital, where I would go next year. Enid Wilson Rust was also in our group. She was a forty-five-year-old divorcee who gave the psychiatric tests to patients on Bamberg 5. She sometimes used as much jargon as Stanley Lovett in interpreting her psychological tests. She was also bitter, nasty, and castrating, and I hated her guts. In my more paranoid moments I even imagined she spent hours going over the tests she'd done on my patients, trying to contradict my diagnoses. Bert and D.J. felt the same way. We were the three musketeers, paranoids together perhaps, but together just the same.

At least that's how we felt when we started the group dynamics seminar. Who's kidding who? It was a form of encounter group. What's an encounter group? It's when a group of people come together in a group to discuss what happens when they come together in a group. If the group is led by a qualified psychologist or psychiatrist it is called group therapy and he charges you ten to fifteen bucks a head and furnishes his den while you furnish your mind with a sense of togetherness and acceptance by the members of the group.

Our group leader was the famous and marvelous, sometimes

inscrutable, always darling, slightly foreign-accented (Hungarian, I think), well-trained, conservatively dressed (with a distinct preference for brown—if you recall what the *Reader's Digest* says about that you may choose to infer something), medium-statured, twenty pounds overweight, Dr. Michael Gabor.

Let's hear it for Dr. Gabor, group (OK, you got me—wiseass covers nervousness).

Since Dr. Gabor our leader was a psychoanalyst we suspected we were in group therapy for treatment rather than to learn about group dynamics. All we knew about Dr. Michael Gabor was the skimpy background I've just given, and because he was silent and apparently unwilling to talk about himself, just like real therapists do, we concluded we were right. Aha!

I almost forgot. There was an eighth member of our group. Her problem was that people either didn't notice her or forgot she was present. Her name: Carol Downs, psychiatric social worker assigned to Bamberg 5. She always appeared to be just on the edge of tears. My grandmother would have called her a nice sensible girl, so she's a *little* quiet! Carol performed her work well, but she was so boring to listen to that when she gave you a report on a patient's relative she had seen, you wouldn't hear a word because your mind would be on something else, almost *anything* else.

We had been in group therapy—whoops, pardon the slip—we had been coming to the group dynamics seminar for almost four months. If you were late, Dr. Gabor would look at you with a benign smile and nod, raising his eyebrows very slightly. Which meant, "Why are you late? Won't you share that with the rest of us?" If you said nothing and sat down and looked around, Gabor would look at you until he caught your eye and say clearly and softly, "Why are you late? Won't you share that with the rest of us?" (It was something to learn. If the line suits, don't fiddle with it.)

The point was that everything we did in group was considered suitable material for group analysis. Being late for a group session was interpreted to mean that you felt negative or at least ambivalent about coming to the group or about someone in the group. It was one of the rules of the game, Gabor told us. Everything we did meant something, so said the rules, and interpreting what it meant was what the seminar was all about.

We were certain of one thing: all of us were ambivalent about the nature of the group. Was it therapeutic or didactic? The circuitous, boring, defensive, angry, tearful, passionate, and childish discussions we held trying to resolve this question were part of each and every session.

"I can't see what difference it makes," Terry said. "Here we are just a lot of very nice people meeting together and talking about whatever we want one afternoon a week. I think it's fun and I think it gives us a chance to get to know each other. It's much better than the other kinds of nursing I've done where you have to work all the time. At least here people are interested in you as a person."

"But I want to learn something about groups," said Stanley Lovett. "I'd like a list of appropriate books to read and I'd like to have a discussion about the best techniques for dealing with group issues and transference. After all, that's what we're here for."

Enid Wilson Rust, the tester, was more direct. "I'd like to have a complete set of projective tests on you, Dr. Gabor, to find out why you're being so hostile to us."

Marshall Kell also felt strongly. "I've got to go through all this shit here and put up with the same shit from my own therapy group in the OPD. Look, Dr. Gabor, I'm a group leader myself. There's nothing wrong with loosening up a little and letting us in on what you're like. You don't need to hide behind your mask. I don't hide behind a mask in my group in the OPD."

D.J. found the group stimulating. "I love watching everyone make a big thing out of whether or not this is a therapy or a didactic group. I think it's all a big defensive game. The only thing I don't understand, Dr. Gabor, is why you let us waste time like this. Why don't you get down to business?" (Whatever that was, I wondered.)

Bert liked sitting around and talking. He often brought candy to share. He felt any verbal or oral activity couldn't be all bad, although (except for smart D.J.) he was usually the one most caught up in the group's confounding question—whether we were in treatment or in class. I think he enjoyed every minute of the group.

I enjoyed the group because I liked sitting around trying to figure myself out and trying to figure out how and why people reacted to me and to others the way they did. I liked Gabor, but I felt he could talk a little more. I mean, it would be nice to know if he liked us. I'll be more honest, it'd be nice to know if he liked me best. . . . Would someone please tell me when I'll really grow up?

Carol Downs said she didn't like groups. I think she said that. As usual, I wasn't really listening to her. Mea culpa. Hers too.

When we first began, we'd agreed not to discuss on the outside what we talked about inside the group. That was called "The Confidentiality Issue" and was quickly settled. Next Dr. Gabor, after very close questioning from Bert, who asked what we could and could not discuss in the group, answered, "Be appropriate." We spent three sessions trying to define what appropriate meant and finally decided it had something to do with not crowing about the number of alleged simultaneous orgasms you had during your last sexual encounter but to respond to each other in the group in a human way. Pretty good definition for a bunch of amateur professionals.

We began to evolve from a guarded collection of strangers to a group of people who believed they saw similarities in each other which probably didn't exist, which they probably invented to keep each other from being strangers. It's similar to a new father's situation when a baby is born. The exhausted father comes up to the hospital nursery window, presses his nose against the glass and thinks, Now that kid looks like a gorilla. I know it's a lousy thing to say because he's my kid but it's the truth. And boy, is this gorilla costing me money! And he'll need clothes and a room of his own. And I'll probably have to sell or trade-in my little two-seat sports car that I saved so hard for and wanted all my life. And we won't be able to make love for a long time. And the next thing you know *she'll* decide he needs a baby sister because *she* wants a little girl. Did I ever make a *mistake*, and for a gorilla, yet. At precisely this time some kindly relative steps up and says, "Charlie, the baby looks just like you." The father looks at the kid again. "He does have my chin and my eyes," he says. "Look, is that the Mulcahey nose or is that the Mulcahey nose?" Father is taken in by his own deception. The stranger has been made more human by the father attributing his own likeness to him. This is one way some fathers keep from going off in a rage at their newborn kids. (Although I'm sure Mr. Goldman would go off in a rage if his baby were born six-feet-four, had spider fingers, and was wearing the old man's army dog tags.)

That's what we did. We projected our self-styled similarities on each other for a couple of months. We formed little cliques, Ivy League cliques, resident vs. nonresident cliques, men vs. women cliques—anything-for-sense-of-identity cliques. We were trying to discover what we were in the eyes of this man, the great and silent Dr. Gabor, who led these magical proceedings like some mystical medium. He said practically nothing and allowed us to pass through this stage; which was characterized by a sense of "exaggerated togetherness," a nice phrase he liked to use. That's just what it was, looking back on it all, exaggerated. We really didn't feel all those things we said we felt for each other. Like:

> D.J.: Terry, I really know just what you mean. God, the same thing happened to me when I was in school—and the humiliation.
> TERRY: Yes (*crying*).
> D.J.: I just felt so awful (*also now crying*).
> TERRY: I know.
>
> (*or*)
>
> LOVETT: You know, I get angry at you a lot because I think you're smarter than I am.
> ME: Really? You know, I think sometimes I act the same way to you because I'm afraid you really do know more than all of us.
> LOVETT: If you only knew . . .

The truth was often quite far removed from these little encounters, which in some way were probably staged to please Dr. Gabor, who happened to be doing research on resident training groups and was a pioneer in that area. We all knew our reactions were exaggerated, but I don't think any of us would have admitted that our feelings were inflated. Thinking back on it, years later, it seems a bit embarrassing. Well, everyone's entitled to be a kid at least once in his life. The question is, how long can you be a kid before people start getting wise to you?

The next phase the group went through was developing a sense of belonging to a group. We began not to feel complete if one of the group members was absent. We would sit around for hours and worry about all the horrible things that could have happened to the absent group member. We discussed the vacations and absences of members as if they had taken a trip to another planet or had died.

During the first few months, everyone established territorial rights. You knew which seat was yours, which wasn't. You knew that any alteration of the seating arrangement would inevitably be discussed. All attempts to alter the seating plan were seen as an effort to attract the interest of the group to you or to distract the group's attention away from something you didn't want to discuss.

Other territorial rights were also established—emotional ones. We got to know what we could and could not do to each other. For instance, people felt rather free in attacking me, because I tended to appear resilient. My glibness sometimes hid the fact that I was as vulnerable as anyone else. We never, well, almost never, attacked

Carol Downs. As much as I may joke about Carol Downs' vulnerability, it upset us, made us uneasy. Carol was depressed much of the time. The rest of us wanted to help her. Carol wanted friendship but didn't know what to do when we offered it. She would push you away, saying in effect, because you can't help me, you are helpless and useless besides. This made me feel lousy because I like to think of myself as helpful, strong, brave, cheerful, etc., if not especially obedient. I wasn't a perfect boy scout. (I got busted out of my troop for smoking in the cellar of the Methodist church where our troop met. The Dreyfus affair again, or so I viewed it in my usual modest perspective, except with Dean Stockwell playing me.)

So the group wouldn't attack Carol even though we got mad as hell at her. The group would attack Stanley or me. Sometimes I would invite others to attack me by setting myself up, especially if I felt it was going too hard against someone else. Only D.J. caught me at it. She'd say something like, "Stop trying to rescue Marshall, David. He's a big boy." I also learned that some people resented my acting protective of them. Marshall and Enid hated it. Marshall agreed with D.J. that he didn't need my help; after all, he was a *second-year resident* and I was only a first-year resident. Enid just felt she could take care of herself, thank you!

Once during a session D.J. suggested, "David, did you ever think that the person you're trying to protect Enid from is probably yourself?"

"Yes, why don't you say what you really feel about me, David?" Enid challenged.

"Really?" I said. I could hear Dr. Gabor thinking, be appropriate. I really wanted to rip into Enid.

"Go ahead. That's what we're here for," said Enid, pushing me.

"Or are we here for something else?" asked Bert, still not sure whether this was a therapy group or a learning group.

"Well," I began, feeling my inhibitions closing in on me and watering down my attack, "I think . . ."

"Go on, and don't be so guarded," snapped Enid.

". . . that you are a miserable, man-eating bitch who'd cut off a guy's balls to test out your knife." I said it with a straight face.

"No, be serious," said Enid, convinced I was joking.

And then we all knew we really couldn't attack Enid.

Everything we said or did was interpreted either by the group or Dr. Gabor. Everything we neglected to say or do was also interpreted.

One drizzly afternoon in October Dr. Gabor was not present when we came into the conference room. We took our usual seats, assuming he would arrive momentarily. We waited. No Dr. Gabor.

"He's never done this before," Terry said.

"Some of the residents said he was sick a few times last year," said Marshall Kell. "I think it was pneumonia."

"Thanks for turning on my fantasy factory," said Bert, who looked worried. "I finally decided—this isn't a teaching group, it's therapy."

"How do you know?" I asked.

"Because I never felt this way when a teacher was absent."

"He'll be around," said Enid. "Don't act so childish!"

"How do you know?" asked Carol, actually getting misty-eyed.

"I *know*. And stop worrying," Enid ordered.

"Did you see him?" asked D.J.

"Huh, did you?" asked Bert, who was getting restless, sweaty.

"Well, no," Enid hedged.

"So you're just making a power play," said Marshall. He liked Enid less than I, but felt more comfortable in letting her know it. Enid, as you saw, didn't feel comfortable knowing.

"I think we're getting angry at Enid because we're angry at Gabor," said D.J., right on top of things as usual. I felt very close to D.J. in the group. Any group.

Besides being very bright, D.J. had a talent for being warm and reassuring. The first time you saw D.J. you would say she was an attractive, well-groomed girl. If she smiled at you, you would think (I at least did) that she wanted to go to bed with you. When she spoke she almost always made sense, and even though she was hardly pretentious, you tended to invest her comments with special significance because she said them. When Larry Danielson gave a picnic for the residents and nurses at his in-laws' summer place at the lake, I expected everyone to be staring at Terry O'Conner, who walked around in a one-piece bathing suit striking poses. D.J. wore an orange bikini, and took the honors going away. She was simply a devastatingly feminine person, self-confident about it and without apologies.

"Good point," said Lovett. "D.J.'s right, we're just displacing our hostile feelings on Enid."

"Maybe it's because you're the same age as Gabor," Marshall said to Enid.

Enid recoiled.

"Hey, Marshall," I said, getting up out of my chair and moving into Gabor's chair. "The way you said 'age' made me think you figure maybe something happened to Gabor. People his age do have medical problems."

"You mean like a heart attack or something?" said Marshall, looking worried. "I guess I *was* thinking something had happened to him." We all were. I suspect it must be written on the wall of a sacred cave somewhere that when a group leader is unexpectedly absent, the group members are supposed to wonder if he is dead or dying. We also felt guilty about thinking that. To a psychiatrist's way of thinking, worrying if an absent leader is hurt is an expression of the group's anger at the leader for abandoning them. We were afraid that our angry thoughts and feelings toward Dr. Gabor might have come true. We felt stressed, angry, and defensive.

A person's defenses under stress are usually consistent. Everyone has his own characteristic pattern of reacting to stress which is determined in part by his experience in growing up in his particular family. When a person is a member of a group he tends to see it as another family. His behavior often resembles the way he acted in his home, and his feelings about the leader often resemble his feelings toward his own parents.

While most people learn to adapt to new situations, they still keep their old pattern of reacting to the world. The world which people perceive is in some way distorted because only part of it, the part which can be tolerated, is allowed to filter in. One views the world subjectively and tends to see only the evidence that supports one's way of thinking. Everyone in the group had his own psychological blind spots. Gabor's absence made us exaggerate our style of acting because it reminded us of our family, the place where our styles developed, where our worlds began. We all acted characteristically.

So when Carol Downs began to realize that Gabor was not coming, she took it personally, feeling he was avoiding something about her he didn't like. She also felt that way about her father. Carol turned her feelings against herself, and felt she was to blame for Gabor's absence. Marshall couldn't express anger at Gabor and attacked whomever was available. He displaced his feelings. Bert was busy suggesting reasons why Gabor was away. "Maybe he had an emergency"—he rationalized his feelings. D.J. was "identifying with the aggressor." By interpreting the actions of the rest of us she was in some way taking over Dr. Gabor's role. Stanley Lovett suggested that Gabor's unannounced absence might just be a test to see how we reacted. He decided he just wasn't going to get upset about it. He was into both denial and intellectualization. And I sat in Gabor's chair, in some way protecting Gabor from further attack by offering myself up as a human sacrifice. That's a little bit of everything. I was in effect saying, "Attack me, not Dr. Gabor."

And everyone did attack. "That's not your chair," whined Carol. "It's not!"

"Grow up," said Enid. "Stop being annoying."

"Why don't we just call Gabor's secretary and find out what happened," said D.J., "instead of attacking David." I swear she smiled at me.

"That bastard could have the decency to call us," said Marshall.

Carol winced at the word "bastard."

"I think it's interesting to see what's happening to our feelings in Gabor's absence," said analyst-to-be Lovett.

"I think it's fun having a group without Gabor for a change," said Terry, doing her thing.

"We should go to the coffee shop and talk about this. It's not the same group without Gabor," said Bert.

"Wait a minute, Bert," D.J. said, as if just remembering something. "You stayed outside in the corridor for almost ten minutes before. Why didn't you come in on time with the rest of us?" It was a question Gabor would have asked.

"I looked in the door and saw there was no one in here. So I waited."

"No one?" said Enid. "We were all here."

"Oh!" said Bert.

"I guess without Gabor, Bert sees the group as no one," said D.J. It was a good point, but it still was a defense on D.J.'s part.

"Will you get out of that seat," said Carol, getting angry.

"Yes, come off it," said Stanley. "The king is not dead."

"How do we know that?" Carol said, actually crying now.

"Boy, this is silly," said Terry. "Gee, he's only late. No one ever cries for me when I'm late for a meeting."

Gabor was indeed the father of the group. He was silent and didn't respond to our efforts to get him to react to us and treat us the way we wanted. Because he didn't react, we each tried harder in our characteristic way to get him to react. And in so doing, our defenses began to show. Each could see better what his pattern was and how he reacted in a group situation. We had the opportunity to examine our feelings and question why we acted the way we did and what it was that we really wanted. We went through a long and confusing cycle of feelings in the group.

To people who have never been in such a group situation, our reactions might seem silly or farfetched. Therapy often seems that way to those who have no personal experience with it. In a sense they're right: it *is* contrived, not real. The relationship of a doctor and his patient doesn't seem as though it should be so emotionally important. But the patient's feelings about his doctor often reflect how he feels about important people in his family as well as the doctor. The feelings are real but to the outsider they seem out of place. They *are;* they're transferred.

In the group we learned something about how we appeared to others and had a chance to be more honest and learn to deal with others when they were being honest with us. We learned that no matter how bright, how well-educated, how pedantic, how irritating, or how groveling we were, we all had our human needs. Each of us had his own pattern of defenses to fill his needs or to cope with his pain when they weren't filled. We learned to tolerate each other's defenses, although some defenses made relating to people rather difficult.

I could not relate to Enid because she was so hostile, so quick to attack, and so castrating. Even when she told how her father used to beat her mother in front of her and how she was put down by her father because she was a woman, even after I understood how and why she was what she was, I still couldn't develop any warm feeling for Enid.

Understanding how and why you are a rat won't change the fact that you're a rat who irritates the hell out of people, unless you do something about it. Some patients who use therapy to get a complete understanding of everything in their life and still don't change can and often do use therapy as a weapon. It's as if they're saying, "I know I hurt you, but try to understand the motivations behind my actions. You have to forgive me." Bullshit! When you hurt someone, you hurt someone. Knowing that your mother and father sold you into white slavery when you were nine and so made you cruel and vindictive doesn't make the person you hurt feel any better. As a matter of fact, it can make him feel worse, because now he may feel that since you've already been punished so much he has no *right* to get angry at you and so feels guilty for his totally legitimate anger.

Gabor walked into the conference room thirty minutes late. We attacked him like a pride of lions having at a wounded antelope. I was, of course, sitting in his seat when he came in.

"Get out of his seat," said Carol, trying to deal with her mixed feelings of intense anger at Gabor for deserting her, and her joy over his return. "Let him sit down, David. Stop acting so angry toward him." Angry? Maybe I was, but I felt Carol was making a big deal about my anger as a way of expressing hers.

"Would you like the loan of a dime?" asked Marshall, throwing a dime onto the conference table. "You could have called, you know."

Dr. Gabor did not say a word. He walked to the end of the table where I was sitting. What if I don't get up, I thought. What if I just sit here and act outrageous. I could say, Dr. Gabor, I decided that since you didn't come on time I would take over the group today. I could, but I didn't. Who'm I kidding? I just *couldn't* have said that.

I got up and took my usual seat.

Terry smiled, said sweetly, "I'm glad to see you," and turned to us. "See, I told you not to worry." When Terry had uncomfortable feelings, such as worrying about Dr. Gabor, she buried them until it was safe to express them. When the danger was over she would say what she felt so histrionically that it was hard to know if she were sincere. She said the right things, but blew them out of proportion. Terry was not in touch with her feelings. She overstated or under- stated them. She seemed to be playing a role, to be acting a part, trying to get the rest of us to feel what she couldn't.

"I really was *so* worried, Dr. Gabor," Terry said. "I couldn't imagine what had happened to you. Marshall and David were talking as if you were sick, and Stanley was being cruel, suggesting you were experimenting with us or something. I knew you wouldn't do that. *I* just missed you." And then Terry started crying. You got the feeling about Terry that she was pretty much full of shit. She impressed me as the sort of girl who would not enjoy making love while she was in bed with you, but later when she was alone thinking about it she would have an orgasm imagining how good it could have been.

Gabor smiled kindly, obviously, I was sure, understanding fully who and what Terry was. But he said nothing.

"OK," I began, "I think it's only fair that you tell us why you were late. You give us the third degree when we're late. Besides, your absence caused a helluva lot of anxiety in everyone here and I think we're entitled to know what happened—something! For Christ sake, Michael . . ." I called Dr. Gabor "Michael."

Carol predictably winced. After all, Gabor was her father figure or some such psychological shit. I didn't care. I was angry.

Gabor smiled in answer. He looked at D.J. and then at Stanley. It was his way of getting us to talk, getting our feelings out in the open, provoking each of us to tell our fantasies about his absence since they provided a valuable clue to understanding each of our individual patterns of defense.

"OK," I said, anticipating his questioning, "everyone did his usual bit." I quickly went through everyone's activities. Stanley visibly cringed when I said he used denial and intellectualization. I didn't care. All of a sudden I was pissed at everyone for being so passive and dopey when this guy was not even going to talk to us, let alone tell us why he was late. I liked Gabor but felt he was again overdoing the silent routine. I finished with Enid's defenses and added, "I am also identifying with the aggressor and intellectualizing by pointing out everyone else's style, but I just want to cut through some of this shit and find out why you were late."

Gabor turned to me, said in a quiet voice, "Sensitive!"

I said, "Always," and then *I* (believe it, please) started to cry. It was a comment with great clout for me. I felt Gabor was, in effect, saying to me, I know you're bright, insightful, and can easily see other people's problems. I know you're angry at me for being late, but in spite of all your talent and brains you're very sensitive to being hurt. All your carrying on, taking my chair, was your way of handling your feelings. And it's all right. I understand.

Of course all Gabor had said was the word "sensitive." Somehow, though, he'd conjured up feelings in me of not being understood, and memories of my playing the buffoon so many times when I was a child when I really wanted to get close to people, and making me remember being afraid of rejection if I exposed my real feelings. I'd used my supposedly clever wit and talent for mimicry to handle difficult situations throughout my life because I wasn't sure how to handle myself and was afraid of being hurt.

I'd always been a rather exceptional student and was frequently called "the brain" by other kids, and I remember resenting and liking the title at the same time. I always wished I had friends to talk with, but mostly I remembered feeling isolated when I was a child. I recalled spending one Fourth of July evening listening to a new recording of Heifetz playing the Brahms violin concerto and my friends thinking I was pretty odd for not watching the fireworks with them. My friends seemed childish and silly to me, but feeling that way only made me feel more lonely.

I found it tough to get involved in their games or sports because they seemed so meaningless to me. I confess—now—that I preferred taking long walks alone in the woods and listening to classical music and playing my clarinet. I never realized how far removed from other children I was until one day when I was ten. I was playing baseball. I liked baseball although I seldom played. I was deep center field. It was a lovely day in late spring. The batter swung. I heard the sweet sound of the crack of the bat. High and towering the ball floated out toward me. I watched the ball soar, come down, bounce and bounce again and roll to my feet, where it finally stopped.

"Throw it, Vissy," yelled the second baseman, now a nameless face in the afternoon sun.

"Throw it," someone else called.

"Throw it, throw it," they chanted.

I picked the ball up and stared at it. I remember actually saying to myself, "What for?" The batter was rounding second and slid into third in a cloud of dust. He got up, looked at me, and walked home, turning his head and looking damn puzzled. I hadn't moved an inch. What am I doing here? I wondered. I couldn't answer the question. I guess—please forgive the heaviness—I've been searching for that answer all my life.

I wanted to belong, to be taken in. I felt that because I was often brighter and more understanding of other kids, no one would be able to understand me or be able to give back what I could give. I was always slow to anger and when I did get angry I tried to understand why other people did what they did. Noblesse oblige—the prince of defenses. I also used my alleged sense of humor to channel my anger into more acceptable paths and win over my enemies. Still, underneath it all, I was still sensitive, still lonely. I still needed to be given to, to be adored and understood. I really disliked having to be the witty and clever one in strange situations in order to avoid being hurt.

With this one-word comment, "sensitive," Dr. Gabor made me think it just might be possible sometime to be understood, although I didn't believe it possible within the framework of this group, didactic or therapeutic or whatever. I needed something more and didn't know where to look for it. The others in the group helped a little by showing me it was possible to be accepted for myself. But the group wasn't enough. Our commitment to the group was academic, our commitment to each other playful, and our commitment to Dr. Gabor tentative.

Gabor *finally* explained that his car had broken down. How could our leader have a car that broke down. Wasn't he supposed to be immune to such things? It's amazing how a little statement like that changed my image of him. I could picture him getting all greasy struggling with his car. It suddenly made him more human to me.

After about thirty minutes' discussion the air was clear again. Marshall became glassy-eyed and stared at Gabor. "I don't really know how to say this," Marshall began. We all fell silent, knowing the onset of an emotional statement when we heard one. "I've got to get into treatment. I'm as mentally ill as my patients."

"Why do you say that?" Gabor asked.

"My anger and hostility leak out all over the place."

"Why are you bringing it up now?"

"I don't know."

There was a silence for about three minutes.

"Well?" said Gabor.

"I guess I want you to treat me," Marshall said.

"Who doesn't?" said Bert, and everyone laughed, even Michael Gabor.

"I see it's time to end the meeting," he said.

What a great statement to end a group meeting, so clear and so simple. "I see it's time to end the meeting." I'd have to use that statement sometime when I was leading my own group. I had learned a great deal in this seminar. Obviously it *had* been didactic, not therapeutic.

Dr. Michael Gabor, wherever you are, there's something I have to tell you—that despite your silence, you're still a very nice man and I think I love you.

CHAPTER NINE

TECHNIQUES

T HERE was a lot I had to learn about becoming a psychotherapist.

Therapy is a relationship between two people the purpose of which is to make one of them more human. The goal of therapy is to make the patient more complete, more adaptable, and more feeling. The humaneness of the therapist is an important factor in the therapeutic process. In fact, the success of therapy depends as much upon the attitudes of the therapist as it does upon his knowledge. Probably more, because the best therapists are parents whose kids grew up without problems.

Patients tend to be lonely and to seek out people who are helpful or kind to them. Because patients are often aimless, sad, or confused, it's easy for those treating them to feel powerful and all-knowing by comparison. This is a potential danger. Unfortunately, some therapists come to believe in their omnipotence; as a result they tend to devalue any comment their patients make about them or their advice and to see those remarks simply as the product of the patient's disease and, therefore, not to be taken seriously, at least not on a par with the therapist's opinions. If a patient does make a comment about such a therapist's style or personality which is true and which deserves a response, it is unlikely that the omnipotent therapist will deal with it as real but will insist upon discussing the comment in terms of the therapeutic process rather than in human, person-to-person terms. Such patients' comments can frequently reflect the healthy side of the patient, and such attitudes of an omnipotent therapist are dehumanizing and therefore antitherapeutic.

Omnipotent therapists don't regard their patients either as equal or as human as themselves. They are often threatened by their patients and need to think of them as patients first and as people second. They tend to be rigid about the rules of therapy, unwilling to get close to their patients, to interact with feelings. They often tend to see all parts of the patient as sick, even though that is rarely the case. This puts the patient in a bind, making him feel that he must not only change what is sick but justify what is not. Patients may get the feeling they have to prove they are big boys or have minds of their own to such a therapist. While this struggle commonly appears and varies in most therapy, it will dominate the therapy of a doctor who, in order to protect himself, needs to believe that his patients are inferior. They waste much valuable time coming to terms with the *therapist's* weakness. The real issue is, why does the therapist make them feel inferior? and usually it's not even discussed.

The omnipotent therapist sees patient after patient appearing to struggle for independence, and then tends to conclude that the frequently appearing struggle for independence he sees in his patients is just a part of all therapeutic processes. I believe this is only partly so. More accurately it tends to reflect a special aspect of the omnipotent therapist's personality, his attitude, and his defensiveness. In all therapy the patient has got to deal with his therapist's particular form of defensiveness as well as his own. Hopefully, the therapist is comfortable discussing his own bias with the patient and thereby can avoid wasting time. I suspect many therapists will object to this statement and claim that a good therapist will not in any way influence the issues the patient brings up for discussion. But the only way to do that is for the therapist not to react at all. And that is being neither human nor helpful.

It's really not so much the amount of involvement of the therapist's personality that influences what the patient discusses as the way the therapist handles his involvement. If a therapist is warm and open, he encourages the patient to deal with his personality as real and helps him sort out what is not. The patient is then freer to discuss what he wants than if the therapist stays hidden, except for an attitude which he would deny was his. The patient then would tend to test the therapist's hidden attitude and try to force him to state his belief openly, which he probably wouldn't do. And this would tend to create issues that are introduced by the therapist even though he would claim he acted anonymously. Fortunately the omnipotent therapist isn't omnipresent in our ranks, and a good thing for us and patients that he isn't.

A therapist must develop some special tools. First, he has to learn the signs and symptoms and classifications of a wide number of emotional diseases. He must understand the basic theories explaining how each of the various syndromes develops. It's useful to have a working knowledge of the organization and function of the mind, although that's only incompletely understood and widely disputed. A therapist must know how to do a competent mental status examination, understand how defenses work, how typical reactions to loss and stress manifest themselves and how thoughts, behavior, and fantasies are interrelated.

One of the lovely things about becoming a psychiatrist is you learn everybody has all kinds of thoughts, fantasies, and wishes and that having them doesn't mean very much—certainly not nearly as much (or awful) as too many people think. You can have sexual thoughts about people of the opposite sex, of your own sex, animals, and trees. You can have aggressive thoughts about nuns, a baby in its mother's arms, even your own baby, especially your own baby, about your parents, especially your parents. You can have hatred for people you are supposed to love and for people who have just died. You can have perverted, twisted, kinky, obnoxious, selfish, stupid, childish, obsessive, and violent thoughts. The presence of all these thoughts in fantasy is only another proof of the fact that you are human and have feelings.

Feelings that are not dealt with at their source and resolved almost always give rise to other fantasies or forms of behavior whose purpose is to discharge the feeling in some way and "clear" the mental apparatus. In the process of therapy these feelings and thoughts are expressed freely by the patient, with the help of the therapist. The goal is to try to understand them and see where they came from; and to determine what they mean and to learn how to deal with the feelings so they no longer intrude on the patient's life and cause symptoms. Symptoms are created by unsettled feelings in the past intruding upon events in a person's present life. They are the ghosts of unresolved past hurts.

Much of the fear Mrs. Goldman felt when her husband threatened to leave her was the unresolved fear she experienced when her father left her. Mrs. Goldman's feelings of being abandoned in the past became less and less particular about what present event they attached themselves to. They became more generalized, more remotely related to the present. As a result, Mrs. Goldman tended to feel abandoned when *anyone* or *anything* left her. She once, for example, described feeling abandoned when a strange car she had been following on a superhighway for some thirty or forty miles turned off at an exit.

The therapist tries to help the patient find the source of his unresolved feelings and to reattach the feelings to the event that originally caused them. Hopefully, the patient will see the original problem more clearly and will be better able to cope with it than before. If he is able to resolve his original problem once and for all, he will be able to go through life without being burdened by ghosts from his past.

Putting the pieces together and seeing the patient suddenly get better may look good in novels, films, or plays, and sound very simple, but it's not all that common. When it does happen, though, it can really be spectacular!

Andrew Wallace was a college student who was admitted to Bamberg 5 during the fall. He was sleepless and anxious and didn't know why. He took a lot of drugs and overdosed himself with barbiturates. He did not appear suicidal but rather like someone trying to hide from his feelings.

He told me that his father died in his sleep of a heart attack almost four years before. He was the only one at home at the time and discovered his father dead in bed. We talked a good deal about his feelings about the death and funeral, but talking about them didn't seem to make any impact on him. Although he could talk about the events surrounding his father's death, he couldn't feel anything about them. His grief was inhibited and discussing the events that caused his symptoms didn't make him better. He needed to feel his father's death. I decided to plug away again.

"Andrew," I said, "I'd like to go through everything that happened the day your father died."

"But we've done it a dozen times already and it never seems to do any good." Andrew was chewing on a pencil.

"I insist."

"I woke up, went to the bathroom, brushed my teeth, and got dressed. I went by my father's room and called to him to get dressed for work. He didn't answer. I called again and went in the kitchen and started breakfast. Then I went back to his bedroom and he was still lying in bed. I walked in and said 'Are you OK?' He didn't answer. I just knew he was dead."

"What did he look like?" I asked, looking for a way to make him feel something.

"Like he was sleeping." Andrew seemed irritated.

"What did you do?" I pressed.

"I called my brother and sister from the phone on the night table."

"Where was the night table?" I asked, trying to get him to re-create the scene.

"On the other side of the bed, near the wall."

"How did you get to it?"

"I reached over the bed and—"

"You reached over your father?" My chair was squeaking.

"Yes, and I called up my sister and then went to class."

"Did you touch him?" A sudden silence. Andrew's face turned white and his eyes dilated. He gasped for breath.

"Oh, God yes, he was cold! I remember he felt cold and horrible!" Andrew started to cry and shake. He couldn't move from my office for almost two hours. I spent the next two weeks burying the father and resurrecting the son.

Whenever we residents heard about such a key remark that significantly changed a patient's life, we all wanted to intone one just like it. It was an old and powerful wish that is seen throughout the history of man. It is the search for the magic word, like Ali Baba's "Open Sesame," that moves the rock in front of the cave of the forty thieves. It is the magic word to cure the patient. It is also a trap to catch the omnipotence of psychiatrists. Even though right after that session I said "Let there be light" a couple of times to see if I still had the power, I had to flick the wall switch in my office to make the darkness go away—just like any damn mortal.

There is a great temptation to try to interpret patients' problems in such a brilliantly illuminating way that they suddenly understand themselves, are able to face reality and cope with their problems and give up their symptoms. Unfortunately, that's rarely possible. My comment to Andrew was not an interpretation. I merely pointed out a detail which brought back buried feelings. And if I'd told him he used barbiturates to hide his feelings, that remark would have been a clarification.

An interpretation is subtler. Some days later when Andrew was discussing his father again, he got up in the middle of the session and said, "Well, I'll see you. I'm late for class."

"The hour isn't over," I said. "You just now got up to leave the same way you ran out of the bedroom and went to class the day you found your father dead. The feelings are the same." That was an interpretation, tying an event in the therapy situation to an event in the past. A good interpretation, joining past and present, is rare, but when it works it too can be breathtakingly effective. The patient has a concrete example of how he really feels and his therapist gets an enormous sense of power. It can be very heady.

Most of the time you don't make real interpretations, just clarifications. What's more, you shouldn't try because they soon lose their impact. As residents we were all occasionally guilty of trying to summarize a patient's life in one neat sentence, stating how his present activity reflected his past feelings and wishes. I used to call these comments "life sentences," because they summarized a patient's life, and they made an impression that sometimes lasted for years. Statements like "You seem to be the sort of person who seeks out figures in authority to attack and then when you destroy them, feels guilty and unprotected," or, "You seem interested in conquering women as a way of feeling masculine, but when you make it you tend to depreciate the woman for accepting you so that you end up getting no satisfaction, you feel as unsure of your masculinity as ever."

When these statements did make a great difference in patients by allowing them to see themselves in a new light, you felt good about yourself and believed very strongly that there was a great deal in psychiatry—even more than you dreamed of. And you believed that you were pretty damn wonderful for intoning the magic words.

There were other times when you struggled with a patient for months trying to get him to understand what was going on, and when finally you succeeded it didn't help the patient. The patient might have said, "I understand it all now, but I still feel crappy." What you do then is what most of therapy is all about. You help patients to cope with what can't be changed, to accept their own limitations and not to shrink from their own humanness.

This requires that the therapist be in touch with his own humanity and be willing to accept and examine his own feelings when they come up while listening to patients. Sometimes, when talking with Mrs. Goldman, I would remember times when I was on my own unexpectedly and felt abandoned, my first year at camp or at school. My feelings were sympathetic vibrations touched off by Mrs. Goldman, sort of like harmonics in tune with her emotions. The analysis of these kinds of harmonics sometimes gave me the greatest insights into patients. I sometimes shared these harmonics with my patients with very helpful results. There is a risk in this, of being exposed and of losing your anonymity. I suspect it's often worth taking.

There always was a great deal of discussion among the residents over the question of anonymity. How much should we tell our patients about ourselves? We differed in our opinions about this question. Lovett, predictably, in the style of his psychoanalytic training, believed a psychiatrist should never tell his patient anything about his feelings and not even respond to questions about his personal life. That seemed a little ridiculous to me because Lovett believed this flatly about all patients regardless of their diagnoses. Being anonymous might be a good rule in dealing with some neurotic patients, but it wasn't always valid and it almost surely wasn't the best plan when you were treating psychotic patients or borderline patients who could benefit from some personal feedback. In order to understand this, you may need a little definition of each.

A neurotic is a person whose actions and thoughts in the present symbolically fulfill unresolved conflicts in his past, usually without his being aware of it. Everyone exhibits some neurotic behavior in his life, such as trying to get accepted to the same sorority as your mother even though you may not like it or even approve of sororities. A neurotic symptom can also be the source of a great deal of positive achievement. The need to please one's father has accounted for many successes in this world. God knows my father was a pharmacist who always wanted to be a physician. If the neurotic behavior doesn't interfere with a person's ability to work, love, or be happy, it is probably unnecessary to change it.

A psychotic is someone who often looks and sounds like anyone else except his sense of reality is defective. He is troubled by feelings from the past just like the neurotic, but he perceives the world differently in order to cope with them. He shuts reality out by denying it and holds his feelings in. He is preoccupied with himself and his personal world. He is ambivalent about practically everything. His feelings do not always seem appropriate to his actions, and his thinking is defective. There are large, gaping holes in his logic that everyone else but him can see.

A borderline sees the world like everyone else except he usually brings along his own storehouse of prefabricated feelings and attaches them to everything he sees. He has a preconceived idea of what he will feel and experience. His feelings in the present seem to be derived from events in the past rather than evoked from something in the present. He misses subtleties. He sees things as either black or white and is constantly looking for limits and is often in trouble because he tends to act on his feelings derived from the past.

The present reminds the neurotic of his past, it awakens the *feelings* of the past for the borderline, and it makes the psychotic crawl back into his own world. A neurotic builds castles in the air; a psychotic lives in them; a psychiatrist collects the rent on them and, I guess, a borderline is just furious with all of them but doesn't know why.

When a patient has a weak sense of reality the object of therapy is to help strengthen it. When a psychotic asks, "Are you married or single, doctor?" he is at least in part asking to know something real about his doctor; and showing an interest in anyone outside himself is helpful to the psychotic because it concerns him with reality. It should be encouraged. A neurotic patient might be interested in knowing about his doctor because he likes to fantasize about him and will use anything his doctor tells him as fuel to feed his fantasy production, which is not helpful to him.

There is nothing inherently wrong with fantasy. Fantasy is the mother of thought; the source of creativity, imagination, and wit, and it provides solutions to the great enigmas of this world. In the best sense, fantasy is a possibility which has not yet been thought of, or a reality which has not yet happened. Fantasy is the hundred or so symphonies that Mozart once told a friend he had written in his head for his own pleasure, and it is the dream for a world at peace. It is only when fantasy supplants reality or is used to escape from reality that it becomes a problem. There's nothing wrong with wanting something or wishing for something, but if you spend all your time wishing you don't get anything.

So it's not useful for some patients to know personal details about their doctor. For them it can be a way of getting the doctor to talk about himself and to avoid the patient's problems. For other patients, it is reassuring to know about their doctor and discover that he's human, that he can get sick, hurt, divorced, or depressed. Discovering that their doctor has feelings like this and still survives is very reassuring to some patients, and makes it possible for them to trust their doctor even more.

Ernie decided he could trust Bert after hearing him urinating in the john while Ernie was sitting in the waiting room in the out-patient department. He apparently figured that any doctor who felt secure enough to piss straight into the middle of the toilet bowl instead of on the side without worrying about who heard the noise must really be sure of himself and able to help him. Mind you, I don't think circulating tape recordings of psychotherapists in the bathroom is going to stamp out mental disease, but this humanizing detail of Bert's life did make Bert more real for Ernie and easier to trust.

As far as my anonymity was concerned, I tried to make common sense my guide. If I was seeing a young woman who doused herself with musk and powdered rhinoceros horn and perfumes, and wore slinky short-short dresses and peekaboo blouses with plunging neck-lines, and spent the hour crossing and uncrossing her legs trying to get me to look up her dress, and who also had a history of many superficial sexual involvements with men, and on top of this was always looking to the external world to find excuses for her internal emotional difficulties, I would be wrong to tell her anything about myself. To do so would only make her fantasize more about me and make me less effective in helping her. To do so would be encouraging an erotic transference, which means the patient falls in love with the doctor. Unless you're really hard up, I mean *really* hard up, you need this like a hole in the head—most psychiatrists have enough personal problems already and don't need to go out of their way to add on to them.

However, it was not wrong to share my interest in sports with Mr. Parker. It was a real interest and a basis for mutual understand-ing. In my view it was not unreasonable to tell my psychotic patients a little about myself. It gave them some reality to hang onto.

Dr. Gelb explained to me in supervision, "The best way to get your bearings when patients ask about your personal life is to tell them that you have no reason to conceal anything from them but you'd like to understand why they want to know. Often this opens up into a discussion of their other feelings. Usually you'll discover that they are not interested in you in particular, but in another problem they didn't know how to bring up, and they'll retract the question about your personal life."

Every therapist has to find his own way through this confusion. One needs to walk a line between too cold and too warm. The object is to be human and reasonable and still be a good therapist. I feel being silent as a general rule is a lousy tactic for a therapist and very much out of touch with the loneliness and emptiness that so many people feel in this large, impersonal, cold society of ours. It seems to reinforce the negative side of life.

Why is the question of anonymity so important in therapy and why is there so much concern about how to avoid publicity? The answer, I think, has to do with the issue of transference (any feeling that a patient has about his doctor).

In the classical psychoanalytic tradition, the analyst is very still, almost silent. The patient does all the talking, the doctor listens. In time the patient develops some feelings about his doctor. If the doctor's been playing the game according to plan, he has not revealed himself. He has remained anonymous. All you know about him is that he wants to help and listens to you. You want to know more about him and when your bank sends you his canceled check for the first time, you run like mad to see how his handwriting looks to analyze his character, and you're dismayed to find he endorsed it with a rubber stamp. According to psychoanalytic theory, if he has remained truly anonymous any feelings you have about your doctor are really your feelings about someone else which you have projected onto him. These feelings are called transference. Sorting them out, finding out where they come from, where they belong, and why they are still around is the concern of psychoanalytic therapy.

It looks good on paper. The therapist interprets the patient's feelings about him, which he assumes are the patient's distortions. They may be and then again, they may not. Patients are wholly capable of making some very astute observations about their doctor even if he's silent. If a doctor is open and doesn't believe that everything a patient says about him is a distortion, he can learn a good deal about himself. In reality a doctor cannot be as anonymous as he can in theory. Just because a doctor is silent and doesn't tell his patients about himself doesn't mean that his patients can't learn a great deal about him. They can. They learn almost as much about how he feels as if he told them. Nonverbal signs, like facial expressions, give a great deal away. Even if the patient is not aware that he is picking up clues to his doctor's behavior, he is. The doctor's emotions give him away. The doctor may twitch, may move around a lot or, if he is like me, he may send out little squeaks from his chair (even if the patient is lying down and facing away from the doctor, he can't miss the noises). The doctor may smile, laugh, cough, or do a hundred other things which tell the patient exactly how he feels. The doctor is not anonymous even when he wants to be. You can tell a bastard from a nice guy in a moment if you have any sense at all. It was always funny to me to hear Dr. Gelb tell how he maintained his anonymity with his analytic patients. First, he saw them in an office in his home, which many analysts do. That told them a great deal about their analyst. Second, his waiting room opened onto the main hall and exposed his house with all of its Afro-Jewish art. The aroma of whatever his wife was cooking hit the patient smack in the kisser the minute he walked in. Gelb's patients knew *all about* Gelb.

It is only reasonable to expect patients to conclude a great deal about their therapist that is true, no matter how hard he tries to conceal himself or how much he denies it. His choice of colors, his style of dressing, his choice of the subject of a picture, his magazine subscriptions, the state of care of his house and lawn also give the therapist away. His personality is really very much in evidence. Shhh! Don't say it too loud. He is sometimes the only one who doesn't know it.

Trying to remain anonymous on the ward was not difficult, it was impossible for residents. The patients compared notes about you. They discussed the way you acted with them. When Ernie Stone wasn't playing Ping-Pong and Betsy Lewis wasn't collapsing in the corridor, they would sit together and discuss Bert Feinstein.

"I don't like his beard," Ernie would say.

"He plays with it a lot," said Betsy.

"He does that with me, too. Does he ever say to you, 'We'll talk about it,' when you ask him a very important question and you think he really doesn't know the answer?"

"Does he? All the time, the rat."

"What do you think that means?" asked Ernie.

"I think he's very nervous and doesn't like talking to people," said Betsy, patting her hair. "Do you have a comb?"

"Yuh, I know he's not too experienced because he's so young."

"Young?" said Betsy, fixing her hair in the mirror. "How do I look?" Ernie just shrugged. "How old is he?" she said, making mental bets.

"Twenty-six," said Ernie. "I saw one of the nurses give him a happy-birthday kiss."

Betsy lit up. "No kidding."

"And he's not married either."

"How do you know?"

"I heard one of the nurses, Terry, I think, talking about him."

"Oh, her!" she said, as if she were a rival. "I could fall for Bert."

Ernie winced as he heard Betsy call *his* doctor by his first name as if she had desecrated an altar. He also got angry. "I think you do enough falling around this place already," he said.

Anonymity is maintained not merely to observe patients' distortions more easily (which seems difficult to defend if what I have just pointed out is true) but also to protect the therapist. Many therapists are passive and retiring and don't like to discuss their feelings either—about their patients' problems or about their own lives—in therapy, at home, anywhere. They prefer anonymity because it fits their particular personality as much as their concept of technique. Some therapists who argue that being anonymous with patients is always the best way are really saying that being anonymous is the way for them to be comfortable.

The way one learns to do therapy is to do therapy and to be supervised by other therapists. In the end each therapist must find his own style of interaction and the final judgment of his technique must be how much his patients improve, how much they learn to cope, how much relief they have from their symptoms, and how much their sense of themselves and self-worth increases.

If there were any magic words that would confer on me the ability to help my patients in this way, I swear I'd climb the highest mountain to lie at the feet of the guru who would reveal them to me. But Guru Gelb was fresh out of magical incantations. Anyhow, he preached the word as revealed to Freud in Vienna.

"OK, Dr. Gelb," I said during one of my many supervisory hours, "maybe maintaining anonymity is important with some patients. Let's forget for the moment that I think it's impossible to attain. I admit that sometimes I let my own feelings creep into my therapy sessions. I identify with what the patient has to say. I put myself in their lives. I try to see what it feels like to be them. And I try to give them a little feedback of what I think and feel."

Gelb reamed out his pipe. See, I could tell he was angry by the way he reamed the damn thing. I'm sure his patients could too. He wanted to get every last crusty charred ash out of there. He didn't like what I was saying.

"I think," I went on, "that the empathetic feeling I generate may sometimes get in the way and make it more difficult for me to tell when the patient is distorting his feelings about me. I admit I miss some details but I also think because patients see me as vulnerable and human they're more likely to develop a trust in me. Dr. Gelb, I do think a therapist who stays anonymous may well understand better when his patient distorts what he tells him. . . ." Gelb looked puzzled.

"But I think the patient will tell him much less because he doesn't trust him, and what he does tell him will be more to win over his therapist than to solve his own problems."

"There's an awful lot of theory that goes against that," said Gelb. "The way a patient tries to win over the therapist is often very revealing. You have to keep your distance so you won't get involved, so you'll be able to be objective."

"I think you can be objective and still get involved."

"You're looking for trouble," Gelb warned.

I found it difficult to practice what I preached. It's just so much safer playing silent, especially when the patient corners you. It's easier not answering when you're under pressure. It's easier not giving a human response.

Sometimes I was unable to respond to a patient I didn't particularly like. I couldn't warm up to Mrs. Sacks even though I tried. All I got from her were pounding headaches. I found myself being nasty to her in quiet, subtle ways. When she got angry at me I sometimes pretended she was displacing anger at me that came from somewhere else and not expressing anger I had provoked in her. I found that when I hid behind the mask of psychiatrist I became a counterfeit therapist, and to the same degree a counterfeit human being. I hated doing that, but when I felt unsure of myself I sometimes found myself acting silent and passive. There were times when being silent and giving the patient the time and space to move freely was indicated, such as when I needed more material to find my direction. I don't object to silence at times like that. I object to the times when one of my patients needed a human response from me and I was too overwhelmed to respond. Perhaps I held back because I needed someone to respond to me in the same way and I couldn't admit it or was afraid of losing control of my feelings. So what if I did? Oh, I can say that easily enough now, but at the time it frightened the hell out of me.

"The way you can tell which one is the therapist," Bert once said, "is that the therapist sits on *that* side of the desk and the patient sits in *this* chair."

"What do you do in an office where there is no desk?" I had asked.

"Oh, my God," said Bert. "I don't know, and I've spent weeks trying to figure out who's who."

All year long Gelb and I discussed what a therapist should do in the best of all possible worlds. Gelb made a lot of valuable comments. "The goal of the therapist is to understand the patient. Everything the therapist says and does should be directed toward that end. If you're ever in doubt about what you're doing, reconsider your questions and try to make them reveal as much as possible about the patient's feelings. And relate their feelings in the present to their feelings in the past.

"Always interpret the style of the patients' behavior before you interpret what they tell you. If someone is acting angry and hostile and telling you about a flower show they went to, point out that they are angry. Don't get tricked into talking about the flower show. When a patient tells you something painful and does it in a way that doesn't show he is feeling pain, point out the discrepancy to him and ask him if he understands it.

"Get the patient to want to understand himself, to spend time thinking about why he does what he does, even when he isn't with you. Always ask patients how they feel about things, but be careful not to lead them into feeling what you think. Let them discover it for themselves, they'll accept it more. It's their job to feel. It's your job to help them.

"One of the most useful statements to make to a patient who tells you a painful story is, 'It must have been very difficult for you.' It makes you the patient's ally. The object of all of this is to open the patient up to himself.

"If you do have an insight about the patient, keep your mouth shut. Let the patient discover it for himself. There's no need to tell patients everything you see and discover about them. It will just overwhelm them and they won't be able to accept it. They have to move at their own pace. If only one person sitting in the room with the therapist has insight into the patient's problems, it should be the therapist. In time, both may. If it's the patient who has the insight and you don't, *you've* got a problem."

Unless things have changed by the time this book gets to print, this is still not the best of all possible worlds and it is not always possible to do and say the exact right thing at the right time with every patient. I used to think it was when I first watched Dr. Gavin, but in the past few months I'd seen him pull a few blunders. And

I've seen Gelb and Karlsson make stupid errors, too. Everyone's human.

You learn a lot doing therapy both about the patient and about yourself. You get to meet a lot of the women you're glad you never married, and you learn that no matter how bad your problems get there's still someone worse off than you. You also learn how to wing it, how to improvise with a patient and still come out smelling like a rose. In fact, some of your best therapeutic moments happen in a flash of insight, just at the point when you think you're hopelessly cornered.

Mr. Hall was a young man I evaluated on the medical service one night when I was on call. He was easily the most boring and pedantic person I'd ever listened to, and I went to an Ivy League school where my professors routinely sent their shirts out to be stuffed. I fell asleep in the chair at his bedside. I just zonked off to sleep.

Mr. Hall said, "Are you asleep?"

I woke with a start, flushing away an image of a trip to the Grand Canyon when I was eight, and a fleeting glimpse of the face of Carla Bellingham, the first girl who ever let me unbutton her blouse. I stared at this man, sitting bolt upright buttoning his hospital Johnny and demanding to know why I had fallen asleep on him.

"The nerve," he began.

"Yes, I did fall asleep," I said, sounding as if I'd planned it this way, "and do you know something, Mr. Hall, that was the first time I ever fell asleep listening to a patient. I must say you have been absolutely the most boring person I have ever listened to." Mr. Hall's mouth fell open. "Mr. Hall"—I took the chance—"I think you wanted me to become bored with what you were talking about so I would get off the track and not ask you revealing questions. Mr. Hall, you've told me absolutely nothing about what is really bothering you or what you really feel. Now please cut the crap with me and start being honest."

Mr. Hall finished buttoning up his hospital gown, looking for something to say. In a while he admitted he was afraid to talk and was using words to push me away. He told me about the problems he'd been having with his wife and acknowledged he was having an affair. He felt relieved to get it all off his chest and thought I was terrific! I got a complete history in half the usual time and wrote one of my clearest, most succinct notes in his chart. I looked at the note and thought about the entire incident.

I also wondered whatever happened to old Carla Bellingham.

I enjoyed improvising with patients. I once saw a deaf mute in therapy on Bamberg 5, a man who became depressed following the loss of his job. I tried to learn sign language, but mostly I would type out my comments. He would talk with his hands and his voice, but he was difficult for me to understand. Although I learned only a few words in sign language, I once noticed when he was talking about taking care of his wife and trying hard that he mistakenly made the sign which meant pushing her away. It was a slip, just like a slip of the tongue, when a person says something he doesn't mean to say but which reveals how he really feels.

When I told Gelb about it he really ate it up, thought it was fascinating. That's the sort of person Gelb was. I found him to be gentle, bright, if a trifle academic and a bit hesitant about taking bold steps with patients, even if such moves seemed clearly indicated. I really liked Gelb. He was warm, appreciative and totally without malice. When he was doubtful about one of my tactics he was totally fairhanded about it. He wasn't interested in putting me down, only in understanding. The world could be in flames, but if he understood why he was happy.

I suppose I really did want to go into therapy or analysis with him during the early months of my training, something specifically forbidden by Dr. M. Austin Noyes, the chairman of the department. No resident could be in treatment with his supervisor. For good reason, I supposed, but that didn't stop me from wanting.

I threw my back out shoveling snow, which came early that year. I was flat on my back for two days. I could do anything but sit in a chair. A nice injury for a psychiatrist! I stood up, talking to my patients. One little gray-haired psychotic man thought I was crazy and refused to stay in the office with me, even after I explained why I was standing. I tried standing during supervision with Gelb but got tired. When I sat down I felt great for the first five minutes and then I started to ache in the small of my back. By the time I stood up I was ready to play the hunchback of Notre Dame. I got sympathy from my patients trying to score points, but the reactions of my fellow residents were mixed. Marty just made fun of me. Bert offered to bring me lunch. Lovett wanted to know what feelings I was secretly repressing. D.J. wanted to know if I had slipped a disc at the fifth lumbosacral intervertebral space. Terry, God bless her hysterical character, wanted to rub my back.

I couldn't sit down in supervision, so without asking Gelb I lay flat down on Gelb's analytic couch. Gelb, of course was sitting in his usual seat behind the couch, reaming out his pipe. He stopped reaming the pipe when I lay down. He stopped the sentence he had begun. I think he stopped breathing.

"Relax, Jerry," I said. "I threw my back out and it just hurts like hell to sit."

I could tell he didn't believe me. He said so.

"I don't believe you," he said. "You want to talk about it?"

"It's true," I said, staring up at that horrible tribal mask on his door. "That's a horrible mask, Jerry," I said.

"That's what all my patients say the first time they lie down on the couch," he said, and then added in typical psychoanalytic style, "So's your mask—now do you want to tell me what's going on?"

I started to laugh and suppressed it, because I got these shooting pains down my legs whenever I laughed or coughed.

The more therapy I did, the more inventive I like to think I became. I liked trying to find ways to put the patients' problems in clearer perspective for them. During the first few months of residency I found myself drawing diagrams that outlined what a patient was feeling, where the feeling came from, where it went, what symptoms it caused and why.

"You see, you, the circle with the X in it, are angry with your husband. That's him in the circle with the H in it. But you can't express it." I drew an arrow going from the circle with an X to the one with the H. "Instead you take it out on yourself." I made the arrow miss the H and turn back to the X.

It was pretty stupid and I feel silly even telling you about it. I did that for about two months. Not all the time. Just when I felt insecure. I never was honest enough to tell Jerry Gelb about it. I was sure he would tell me I was being childish and was afraid he would think I didn't know anything. And I still had these visions of being drummed out of the corps.

About this time I was developing a very ornate system of taking notes while listening to my patients. My notes were terrific. Except there was one thing wrong. I was paying so much attention to taking notes that I sometimes missed valuable clues from my patients. Why was I taking notes? Probably to be sure I had all the answers to the questions Gelb used to ask afterward. I hated not knowing all the answers. Supervisors had a way of asking, "And how did he feel about his sister when he was young?" You probably would never in a million years think to ask some of the questions supervisors asked, so you took notes and said, "We haven't gone into that yet," which freely translated meant, "I forgot to ask." And you did forget to ask about a lot of things. Taking notes was sometimes helpful in organizing your thinking when you were listening to a patient, but it could be a crutch and a way of keeping aloof.

I came to see taking notes as a hindrance and figured that if the patient said something really important I would remember it—that is, if I was tuned into the patient and the sort of person he was. If I wasn't, taking notes wouldn't nearly make up for it. When a patient is suffering from a severe loss, every loss he mentions shows like a bloody wound anyway. You don't need notes to be on the lookout for what concerns him. Sometimes I wrote brief notes after the sessions to record the gist, the direction of the hour. I gave up taking notes when I saw patients, except for writing down statistics such as addresses and the like. In time, I needed less to hide behind than when I began, and came to see notes as a mask.

"So what do you think therapy is all about?" I asked Marty DiAngelo over lunch.

Marty looked very serious and thoughtful and sipped his coffee. Could you believe this, for once I was going to get a serious answer. D.J. smiled her accepting warm smile at him. Marty said, "Therapy is an arrangement in which a patient pays a doctor some money which obligates the doctor to listen and keeps him from going away no matter how badly he is treated or what the patient says to him. After a while the patient gets to feel guilty over the way he's been acting toward this doctor. After all, even if the doctor is paid to listen and takes all the abuse, he still is a person. So the patient begins to look at how he acts and tries to be nicer to the doctor. And then after a while the patient starts being nicer even to people he isn't paying to listen to him. And that's what therapy is."

"You're probably right," D.J. said.

In learning about therapy, I learned a great deal more about myself and about doctors. I was not called by divine inspiration to the practice of medicine. I became a physician because I thought it would be an interesting career and because I thought I would enjoy doing what physicians did. I elected to become a physician by taking the courses required to get into medical school and by doing well enough to get accepted, and finally by working hard enough to get through.

There was no mystery, no great sense of personal sacrifice, no overwhelming self-denial other than having to study on weekends because I had to get a good grade in organic chemistry when my college roommates were off to Skidmore to sample the lovelies in the freshman class. I had to give up a few years to the study of some meaningless details which I would have to know exceedingly well just to get my degree and never have the opportunity or need to use ever again. But that too was no big sacrifice. People who tell you medical school is a struggle are putting you on. It's mostly a bore.

Doctors are only people. They're not saints whose word is the final and absolute end. Their knowledge is often tentative, their understanding empiric and imperfect, and their motivations frequently mixed. The doctors who hid behind the mask of privileged sainthood, who refused to come down from their high horses, were always irritating as hell to me. Doctors who didn't understand they were only human were less likely to admit they made mistakes or that their patients could sometimes be right and they could sometimes be wrong.

When a doctor feels he's been called to the profession, and many really do even though they will strongly deny it, he demands respect for his authority just because he is a doctor and because he feels he has struggled to become what he is. Doctors become doctors for reasons of their own, and patients owe them no reverence.

As I learned to be a therapist, I decided I would much rather a patient felt kindly toward me because I'd helped him than feel in awe of me because I was a physician. Whatever struggle I confronted in becoming a physician was a personal one. I wasn't trying to solve the problems of mankind, I only wanted to fulfill myself and be happy in my work. If mankind were the better for it I would be pleased, but my joy would first have to come from my work itself, from being me, from myself.

As I became more confident, I felt less need to hide behind the mask of being a physician and more willing to give of myself.

The process of becoming a psychiatrist, whatever it was, had apparently begun.

CHAPTER TEN

TWO PATIENTS—OPENING GAMBITS

I WAS nearing the end of my first six months and doing, I felt, surprisingly well. Mr. Parker went home, resigned to letting Edgar, his manager, handle his business. He accepted a position as an athletic adviser to his old prep school and became an honorary director of a camp for underprivileged children. Mrs. Sacks gradually came to understand that being nasty wasn't the way to keep her husband. I had worked with the Sackses for several sessions. They each made promises I personally doubted they would keep, but they left the hospital hand in hand, promising to try. I had seen about twenty patients on Bamberg 5. Most of them stayed three to five weeks and went home and seemed to be better. I wanted to think it was my magic touch, but Marty DiAngelo reminded me that patients sometimes get better on their own. It seemed Roberta Goldman would be one of my long-term patients, and I planned to see her once a week for the next two or three years to try to help her with some of her problems.

Residents saw patients after discharge in follow-up visits in the outpatient clinics instead of on the ward. Dr. Karlsson believed the ward was a magnet to some patients after discharge, especially if they were facing a crisis and were on the edge of trying or giving in to their feelings of helplessness.

I worked out a schedule to use Marshall Kell's office in the OPD to see Roberta Goldman. Patients, somehow, looked physically better outside the hospital. It had been three months since Roberta left the hospital. In that time we didn't seem to make progress.

Dr. Gavin's brilliant advice didn't seem to help. Gary returned home when Roberta left the hospital, and the situation at home was pretty much the same as it had been throughout their marriage. Gary had a new job, Roberta kept her old one. Her motivation to change, to work in therapy, dwindled. Each week we would discuss what she was doing and her plans. To hear her tell it, everything seemed just fine. I became upset with the stalemate in therapy. I felt we were never going to discuss the problem of her father or look at her marriage. I felt maybe I was wasting my time and that therapy, if you could call what we were doing therapy, should be stopped. I decided to talk about cutting down on her sessions.

"Hello," Roberta said, right on time for her appointment. Strange, if she had so little to discuss and everything was going so well, why was she always on time? What did she need me for?

"Hello, Roberta." She sat down. "Well, what would you like to talk about today?" I began, thinking, who knows, maybe she'll talk today.

"I don't know. Everything's going along fine at home," she said, smiling.

"What does 'fine' mean?"

"Gary's happy at his job. They're letting him work on a wing for the town library. You should see his plans. They're really great. Cathedral ceilings and an open court."

"Have you talked to him about wanting to have a baby?"

"Not this week. Gary doesn't like to talk about problems in the middle of the week. He says he works hard and when he comes home he deserves peace and quiet and if I want to talk to him about something serious, it'll have to wait till the weekend."

"And what happens on the weekend?" I thought I already knew the answer, and wasn't happy about it.

"Well, he says we're getting along so well that I'd be ruining our *good* times if I brought up our problems."

"Well, what does that mean?"

"It means I have to find the right time to discuss wanting to have a baby with Gary." Roberta shrugged and smiled.

"And when will that be?"

"I don't know."

"Why are you afraid of bringing it up to him?"

"I'm not afraid of bringing it up to him. The time just isn't right."

"You expect me to believe that in the last three months there hasn't been time to discuss having a baby?" She nodded without looking at me. "It sounds to me like you're afraid to discuss it."

"No, I'm not. I'm sure we'll work it out someday." Roberta stared into space.

"I think you're afraid you'll push him away if you bring the subject up."

"No, I'm not. Last year was just one great big misunderstanding. Everything will work out."

"What will work out, Roberta? In the last three months you've sat in that chair telling me how wonderful your marriage is, how much you want a baby, and yet nothing in your life has changed. As far as I can see you're right where you were before you got upset. I think you're afraid of speaking your mind because you're afraid Gary will take off again."

"No . . ."

"Not 'no,' yes! Yes, you are avoiding the question." I was sick of pretending she'd come to her senses by herself. I was sick and tired of letting her give herself the runaround. What was the sense of my being there if I didn't *do* something? If she understood Gary's limitations and accepted them that was one thing, but she wouldn't even look at him objectively.

"Look, Roberta, you're still afraid of being abandoned by Gary and still refuse to discuss a lot of problems with your past that have never been resolved. If you don't, the next time they come up you'll be in no better position to handle them."

"I think you're trying to put words in my mouth. Everything is going great as far as I'm concerned. You have no right to tell me how I should run my life and how I should deal with my husband. If I want to deal with him like this, it's my business, Dr. Viscott. You don't know *everything*. There's no rule that says a patient has to discuss absolutely everything in her life when she doesn't want to."

"You don't want to discuss anything you might find upsetting, Roberta. I think you're prepared to sit in a little shell and do nothing while your husband does whatever he wants. You'll secretly feel angry and hurt about it. And when you do decide something, he'll get upset and walk out again and you'll be over your head again."

"What the hell is going on here, Dr. Viscott?" said Roberta angrily. "A doctor isn't supposed to knock a patient down. I'm perfectly fine the way I am! You have no right to try and change me. I'm not an idiot, you know."

"That's beside the point, Roberta. You don't want to talk about your problems."

"That's my right." She sat back in her chair and lit a cigarette. I sat back in my chair and *I* lit a cigarette. We blew smoke at each other, expressing our feelings like two Indians using smoke signals.

"You're absolutely right," I said after a minute. "It's your right to refuse to talk about your problems." I took a deep drag of my cigarette and aimed the smoke right at her. I don't know why the hell I was smoking these goddamn things. They probably do cause cancer, warns you right on the pack.

Roberta looked at me, pleased and relieved that I'd come to my senses—that is, to her way of thinking. "Hmmm," she said, purring away gently.

"Well, I guess there's not much point in you continuing to see me on a regular basis," I said quietly, deliberately.

"What!"

"I'll be here if you need me, but I don't think we should have regular appointments, only when you need them."

"Why?" She looked pale and frightened.

"Because as nice a person as you are to talk to, you still aren't really interested in looking at yourself or your feelings. I have only so much time in the week to invest in long-term therapy. I think it's only fair that the patients I work with should be interested in working with me."

"But you can't abandon me just like that." She used the key word "abandon."

"I'm not abandoning you. I said I'd see you if you need me, but this is a waste of time for both of us. Yours because you think you're accomplishing something when you're only putting in the time, not the effort, and mine because I'm not really doing therapy. I'm baby-sitting." Maybe I was too harsh?

"But I *need* to talk to you. Gary won't talk to me. You're the only one I have to talk with."

"But you don't talk to me," I said, making the point for the hundredth time.

"But I could, I mean, it's nice knowing that if I wanted to talk with you, you'd talk with me." Roberta sounded desperate. "What good is it? You haven't done anything for me. You haven't made Gary want to be a father."

"You're playing at being helpless again. You expect something to be done for you without asking for it and without doing anything. For nothing you get nothing. You expect me to give you answers to questions you're afraid to ask."

"I'm afraid to ask because I know you won't stick with me, you'll push me away like you just did."

"Did it ever occur to you, Roberta, that you haven't given me any reason to stick with you in this therapeutic relationship? You won't discuss anything. You just want me to be here like a security blanket."

"Well," she protested, "aren't doctors supposed to help patients? Aren't *you* supposed to help *me?*" Roberta stared at me, angry and sad at the same time.

"By being a security blanket?"

"If that's what I need."

"I said I'd be here for you, if you really needed me. In one breath you tell me everything is just fine. So you obviously don't need me. And next you tell me you can't live without me. I have some feelings about being used, too, I don't like it."

"You're a doctor, you have no choice. You have to do what I want."

"Bullshit! I have a choice, and if you aren't interested in working with me, I have a right to work with someone who is."

"You can't abandon me and leave me all alone." Roberta was crying.

"What do you mean, 'all alone'?"

"You're the only person I have, the only one I feel comfortable talking with. I knew it from the first time you walked into the lounge and were gentle about the books. I can't understand why you're being so cruel to me now."

"Roberta, I very much want to help you, but I can't do it alone. I wouldn't abandon you, but until you're willing to . . . Oh, what the hell, I don't even want to talk about this anymore. I'm sick of repeating this. Look, Roberta, I think that when you have me around you feel secure and that you don't need to face your problems with your husband. When you can't talk to your husband you pretend that it's all right because you talk to me, even though you really don't. It's as if having me as a doctor makes you feel you don't need to get better. Everything's at a standstill here and at home."

"If I got better, I'd lose you." Roberta was almost seductive.

That was a new one for me. I didn't know what to say.

"Dr. Viscott," Roberta continued, "I want you to help me but . . ." She put her cigarette out and lit another one. "I'm afraid if I tell you how I really feel and what I want you'll push me away."

"Look, Roberta, you feel you have to behave a certain way with me or else I'll push you away. You feel you must act a certain way with your husband or else he'll leave you. You see the world as a place where you always risk losing something and never have a chance of winning anything."

"That's right," Roberta said, starting to cry. "I've always felt I had to do what other people wanted me to. Even in here I feel I have to act a certain way to please you."

"I only want you to look at what you feel, to try to be your own person, to do what *you* want, to judge for yourself whether something is good or bad for you. You don't need to ask someone's permission to say something is hurting you when it's you that hurts. I'm interested in the part of you that hurts and understanding why you hurt and trying to help you feel better and what you really want—if you could ever be honest enough with yourself to admit what you really *do* want."

"I'll never be able to do that."

"I think you will," I said, perhaps a little too easily.

"How the hell do you know? You aren't even sure what's wrong with me. What went wrong in my life?" Roberta was almost shouting now. "Come on and tell me what went wrong. You, the big smartass doctor with the crystal ball."

"I have . . ." I began, not really knowing where I was headed.

"You tell me what went wrong." Roberta was pounding the palms of her hands on my desk. "What went wrong with my life? Tell me. You know and you won't tell me. You just want to leave me." She was hysterical now, yelling and screaming.

She seemed very different from the other times when she was angry. Apparently the threat of losing me had somehow shaken her loose from her usual front of complacency. She was angry at me for threatening to leave and the old feelings of abandonment had crept in. From what I knew of Roberta, it was the first time she'd been able to get angry at someone and tell them to their face how she felt.

Roberta took out a handkerchief and started to blow her nose. The office seemed very quiet all of a sudden.

"I think you're afraid of getting angry at people and pushing them away."

"My mother," said Roberta, suddenly reflective, "was always angry at my father. She was always telling me how *we* don't like the way father does this and how *we* don't like the way father does that and how *we* think father is cruel for making us poor. She really did.

She was always fighting with him and trying to make me believe I should feel the way she did. She always said *we* didn't like father and should forget about him because *we* hated him. . . . But"—Roberta started to cry again—"I always liked my father. He really was very good to me. He always gave me presents. My mother always made me give them back.

"He, my God! he was the one who gave me the Raggedy Ann doll when we moved. Wait, it wasn't a Raggedy Ann, it was a Raggedy Andy. He told me he would have to go away and I should pretend he was the Raggedy Andy and . . ." She was crying so hard she could barely talk. "My mother tried to make me give the doll back, but I wouldn't. I kept it! She even insisted I call it Raggedy Ann. Can you imagine that?

"I never hated my father. I used to stay up and wait for him to come home. I remember listening for his car and running to my window with my doll and pretending he'd come home—but of course he never did, but I didn't know why. I really loved my father and I really miss him."

Roberta cried for about ten minutes. I said little. Those tears were many years late as it was.

"Please forgive me for yelling at you," she said, wiping her nose.

"You only said what you felt."

"But I hurt your feelings?"

"No, you didn't. If you did, I'd tell you," although I wasn't sure whether I would or not.

"Really? You're really not upset?"

"There's nothing wrong with getting angry at someone and letting them know it. You've spent most of your life believing that anger drives people away and that's just not true. It doesn't. Not always. It often clears the air and allows warm feelings to come through and sometimes lets people get closer and trust each other. Maybe even in here with me."

"What about not seeing me regularly?"

"That was assuming you didn't want to work in therapy. If you want to talk about your feelings and try to understand them, I want to see you regularly. Why should I see someone who keeps telling me everything in her life is all right?"

"Everything in my life," said Roberta with a big smile, "is shit."

And with that smile Roberta Goldman became involved in the painful process of psychotherapy.

Donald Johnson was a seventeen-year-old high school student who had been on Bamberg 5 for two months. Gavin thought he was schizophrenic. In effect schizophrenia is a form of psychosis in which the part of a person that says I am, I want, and I do becomes submerged, leaving his conscience and his animal impulses to battle it out for control over his mind.

Donald was constantly bothered by wild ideas and theories that intruded on and nearly took over his thinking.

Donald Johnson was also a handsome, dark-haired, fine-featured young man who probably shaved less than once a week. To tell the truth, he was almost a little too good-looking. He was meticulous about his appearance and dressed conservatively, in classic Ivy League style, though most kids his age were no longer dressing that way. Even when he was at his worst, during the first week he was admitted to the hospital, he wore neatly pressed gray flannel slacks, a crew-neck sweater, a clean shirt, and freshly shined brown loafers. His fingernails, which he fussed over all the time, were immaculate and sometimes coated with colorless nail polish.

Donald was aloof, diffident, and haughty all at the same time. He impressed you as considerably older than seventeen, maybe twenty-three or twenty-four. Perhaps it was his height. He was over six feet. Perhaps it was his lean, hungry appearance.

One look into those huge black eyes and you got the feeling he'd never been a baby, yet at the same time wondered if he'd ever grow up. It was his stare that gave him a timeless look. If you took a picture of him standing in a formal garden and told people it was a picture of a famous nineteenth-century poet, they'd probably believe you. Donald's thin, bony face was the kind that probably would look the same ten, twenty, maybe even thirty years from now with perhaps only graying hair giving his real age away. And why shouldn't he always appear the same age? Psychologically, Donald hadn't grown very much over the years and, without help, he would probably not grow very much in the future.

There had been a big debate among Gavin, Gelb, and myself about Donald's diagnosis. Gavin and Gelb both felt Donald was psychotic. I disagreed. How do you like that—Dr. David Viscott, the great clinician, invoking his long and estimable experience, was in dispute with his more learned colleagues—and they sure as hell *were* more learned. But I just felt that Donald's behavior, as wild and crazy as it might seem at times, could also be explained as an adolescent adjustment reaction. It was not uncommon to observe crazy behavior in adolescents and to be certain that they were psychotic and then to see them a few years later and find they weren't.

"Yes," said Jerry Gelb, "that's true, but even in wild 'normal' adolescents one usually sees some fluidity of defenses. I mean, they show one kind of crazy behavior today and another kind tomorrow. They don't stay fixed on one particular form of craziness. It's as if they're trying to find the defenses that work best for them, trying on different suits of armor to protect them from the world, looking for their right size and style. Since most of them don't fit, the troublesome impulses and thoughts aren't kept in place and these kids often look crazy. But to me, when Donald looks crazy he always looks crazy in the same way. He's found a suit of armor too small and too soon. He's trapped in it and can't grow."

Equally as optimistic, Gavin predicted, "Work with him for a few years. I'm sure you can do a great deal for him, but I also think you'll become aware of the presence of a psychotic core of thinking underneath all of his disorganized action. You'll find he's a paranoid schizophrenic who somehow is able to generate a little warmth—just enough to confuse us in making a diagnosis. I'll bet you find much of that warmth is generated by your own need to see him as healthy and by your desire to help him and also because he's attractive and young. One tends to see these people as healthier than they really are."

I suppose there was some truth in what Gavin said. And maybe I refused to see Donald as Gavin did because in some way I was defending the way I thought I was during my own adolescence. Hell, I'd take odds that if I told some psychiatrist everything I thought, wished, or did when I was a kid, he'd have *me* committed.

I suppose there are times during everyone's adolescence when they feel crazy and disorganized and can't find anything to believe in or attach their feelings to. There are times when no one seems to understand you, when you feel no one can be a true friend, or when you believe you and your parents disagree so completely that you'll go out of your mind if you don't get out of the house. Adolescents are often too afraid of failing to go out on their own, so they stay home and endure it all and somehow usually survive.

Some of the craziness lingers on. People who were aloof, inflexible, dogmatic, mean, retiring, silly, or deceitful in adolescence often turn out to be that way later on in life—though not always, fortunately.

People often change in adolescence or just after adolescence because they do get out of the house and away from people who think of them in one way and expect them to react that way. When young people move to another place, or go to school and find new friends and meet new people who don't have the same old prejudices about them as the people in their past, they are freer to try out new roles without being expected to act a certain way. They are free to grow.

All people tend to act the way they are treated and this is even truer for adolescents, who often have little power to change the events in their lives. They spend much of their time reacting to people rather than their own needs and feelings. Their actions rather than their words become the way they express their feelings. A typical adolescent will contradict himself every ten or fifteen minutes. The rule of thumb I used to tell when someone was no longer an adolescent was if he could do something he liked even though doing it pleased or at least might please—God forbid!—his parents.

There is an adolescent in each of us who is demanding, self-interested, selfish, cruel, vindictive, spoiled, easily bruised, and all the other disagreeable things we associate with immature people. The very same adolescent inside us is also idealistic, charming, playful, and has a touch of the romantic.

Most adolescents are ambivalent about everything. They wonder, am I good, am I a man or a woman, am I strong or weak. The negative side of ambivalence is easily reinforced. The positive side is easily undermined. That was the chief problem I found generally in dealing with adolescents. That was also the problem with Donald Johnson.

I wanted to treat Donald because I thought I understood him. I knew what it was like to feel like a recluse when I was a kid, although I always fought against the desire to hide and forced myself to make friends even if I did play the clown a lot. I knew how it felt to be an adolescent. Hell, I remembered very clearly what it felt like being an adolescent. At least I thought I remembered better than Gavin and Gelb, who hadn't been adolescents for a long, long time.

OK, let's face it; in some ways I was still an adolescent.

Donald Johnson was hospitalized following a six-month period in which his parents thought his behavior was distinctly strange. He would stay out late at night. Although he never came in drunk, he appeared out of it, as if he were sleepwalking, confused, preoccupied when he returned from God knows where.

Donald was generally very bright in school, and in mathematics in particular he was gifted. Besides getting A's in math, he was interested in algebraic geometry and involved forms of calculus. He read a great deal about them, alone in his room.

The fact that he played no sports did not just upset his father; it offended him. "I don't want a queer growing up in my house," he said. Donald's father used to beat up homosexuals when he was on leave in New York when he was in the Marines. A respectable bit of common, garden-variety overreacting. His mother said, "He's a good boy." That was her only description of Donald. What made that limited description remarkable was that mother graduated from Vassar and yet sounded as flat and bland as some mental defectives. There was definitely something wrong with mother. Depressed, perhaps. I wasn't sure. In all, it was a very unpromising family grouping. Both Donald's mother and father were driving him crazy and he was afraid to open his mouth about it.

"Well," Donald said in his usual quiet, cool way, explaining why he got in trouble with the law, "my father wanted me to act tough, so I acted tough!" The month prior to Donald's admission had indeed been very hectic. He had stolen twenty-one automobiles. Actually, he had taken them for joyrides. He crossed the ignition wires with his alligator clamps and just drove away.

He preferred to drive out into the country in the late fall evenings. When he started to run low on gas he would look for another car to expropriate. Sometimes when he couldn't find one he would walk alone for miles. He said he liked to stand in the middle of an open field and look up at the stars and the moon in the clear October sky. When he did he would feel he was drifting across the sky, merging into the stars. Perspective became flattened for him. He felt as if he were standing in front of a painting. He didn't feel real.

Sometimes he would also talk to the constellations. He knew them all by name. He liked Orion, the Hunter, because he felt a bit like a hunter himself, stalking all those late-model cars. "Oldsmobiles are best," he said. "Sometimes Orion and I would discuss the other constellations and how they got their names." This seemed to me a little like the way some younger children talk to their dolls. Maybe the things Donald did weren't so crazy. Maybe they were a little immature. Perhaps Donald wasn't a delayed adolescent, perhaps he was a delayed *child*.

"Orion," I began, "the constellation Orion, did he talk back to you?"

"You don't need to be so hesitant," Donald said. "Of course he did!"

Correction! Some of the things Donald did were pretty crazy, and not merely his talking to the heavenly bodies but his frantic, frenetic actions. One evening he kidnapped a large English sheepdog. "For company," he said. He pushed it into the front seat of a stolen pickup truck "which I hated but it was the only thing I could get started." He drove across Connecticut into the Berkshires. He and the dog got out of the car in the center of Pittsfield, Massachusetts, and walked into a coffee shop. He insisted on feeding the dog an entire blueberry pie right off the table. He was thrown out, but the blue-bearded sheepdog refused to move. A cop asked him to call the animal out, but since he stole it, he didn't know the dog's name.

"Come on, Orion," he yelled, improvising. Donald was a great ad-libber.

The cop just stood there, apparently disarmed by the news that Donald owned a dog with an Irish name. He even helped Donald get the dog out.

"Where you going, son?" the cop asked.

"Just walking my dog."

"Well, it's one A.M. I'd better give you a lift home."

"Thank you, but Orion and I would prefer to walk. We both love long walks and he's been cooped up for a long time with my aunt who's been taking care of him since my folks got killed in a car accident a few weeks ago."

"Oh, I'm sorry to hear that," said the cop, who was a little embarrassed and now even less anxious to bug Donald, and pleased to let him go on his way. (It's strange how accurately Donald could sense what made other people uncomfortable and either use it to his advantage to push them away or to manipulate them as he sometimes tried to manipulate me. If that kid ever got straightened out he could become president or a good psychiatrist or even an encyclopedia salesman.)

Donald next rang a false alarm to create a diversion while he looked for another car. (He told me he didn't like ringing alarms unless it was absolutely necessary because he felt someone might need the apparatus, if there was a real fire—a considerate kid in his fashion.) He found a late-model Mustang with the keys in it and a full tank of gas as well. He and Orion were off over the backroads to New York State.

He arrived at Lake Placid at three in the morning and tried to get into the Marcy Hotel. "I remember going there once when I was a kid," he said. "I loved the pinball machines. I used to play them by the hour." He pounded on the door and the night clerk called the police. He called in a false alarm in Lake Placid, one in Lake George, one in Troy, and another in Albany, where he stole another car and drove to Schenectady, where he and Orion were finally found sleeping in the middle of a park. Donald was out of false alarms.

No one pressed charges because Donald's parents convinced the police in each town that he was troubled. Donald was deposited on Bamberg 5 by his father with the instructions, "Fix him, doc." Donald's parents were like people doing an imitation of ineffectual parents, and a lousy imitation at that. I always had the feeling in talking with Donald's father that Mr. Johnson should stop trying to imitate whomever he was trying to imitate and try doing something else for a change, like W. C. Fields. ("Ah, yes . . . the boy's daffy—out of his skull.") But Mr. Johnson just kept on trying to imitate Donald's father, not *being* him.

My problem with Donald was to try and figure out what the problem with Donald was. Self-evident, but not so simple. I would spend hours listening to him and hear his side of the situation and began to forget about the fact that there was another side of the story. Friends and relatives of patients are always worried that the patient is giving the doctor a distorted, make-believe story and want to intrude, just to set the facts straight. But unless the patient is a con man, the facts are not the main issue. Psychiatrists are more concerned with the patient's style and his feelings. A scorecard or referee in grievance collecting isn't in order.

Donald continued to do well in school, so I knew his concentration was good. His schoolwork was a bit weird though, and once he showed me some of the poetry he had written and I almost wished he hadn't.

Bright Star

First out again
If you find the empty sky so lonely
Why don't you go back in?
No one cares when a bright star fades.
They love another sun best.

That was Donald. Sometimes he gave me gooseflesh just talking to him. He would tell of his long walks alone in winter by the sea, standing alone on some isolated promontory, imagining voices in the crashing of the waves, handling the seaweed and calling it the matted hair of the rock princess. He would throw stones in the water and listen to the ocean cry out in pain and then apologize to it.

"Everything has feelings," he said. "This chair, your wristwatch, the windowpanes, the sidewalk, everything has feelings."

"Do you always know what they are?"

"Oh, yes," he said, stroking his chair. "This chair is happy being together with me again."

"Did you ever think, Donald, that these objects don't really feel, but you might be seeing your feelings in the world around you? For instance, today I know you're glad to be here because you wanted to share the good news about getting into college with me. You said the chair was happy to be together with you. Maybe it was your feelings about being in here with me, being happy telling me."

"Maybe."

"Look," I said, "there's nothing wrong with thinking like that. It's very poetic and I personally find it charming. It's like in the musical *Fanny* when Ezio Pinza sings, 'Welcome home, says the door, good to feel your hand once more.' You see, it's a way of thinking that's very common. It's called anthropomorphizing."

"Oh," Donald laughed. He seemed relieved. "You mean, just because I feel that way doesn't mean I'm—"

"Doesn't mean you're crazy."

"Great," he said, and slouched in his chair with a big grin to keep him company.

"If you're crazy it has to be for other reasons," I said, "but not for anthropomorphizing." I wanted to make light of something that was really troubling him. He did worry about this all the time. Donald laughed. He seemed to believe me. I was beginning to use my alleged sense of humor in therapy in a way that finally was helpful. At first, I used it to relieve my anxiety and the patient's anxiety, but I was learning to develop it as a tool—to discuss painful feelings or make a point.

Donald once asked, "Do you think I'm queer?"

"You mean a homosexual?" I knew what he meant. I just wanted to keep the conversation open-ended.

Donald looked down at the floor. He wasn't homosexual. He was just worried about being homosexual. Anyhow, why should I sit there and upset him with a long and involved explanation telling him that being a man means sometimes having tender feelings toward other men. After all, we normally learn at some point to love our fathers and mothers, so everyone usually learns to love someone of the same sex. The feelings of goodwill, philanthropy, and brotherhood all have some homosexual connotation to them, but are basically good and beneficial. Should I sit and waste my time telling Donald this and making him more anxious? No, I decided.

"You've got to be kidding." I laughed. "You're about the least homosexual sort of person I know. You may spend a lot of time worrying about being homosexual, but that doesn't make you homosexual. It's not worth worrying about . . ." I tried to make his concern seem farfetched. "You know what I think your concern about homosexuality is really all about?"

"What?" Donald looked up.

"I think you're worried about your father liking you. He's always making a big deal about you being a big he-man. It's not so much that you're worried about being homosexual as you are about him really liking you for what you are. You want to please him and you're angry at him at the same time."

"Interesting," said Donald. "You don't think I'm a queer?"

"Sorry, I can't pin that one on you."

"Even if I told you that I once jerked a guy off at camp and let him jerk me off?"

"Sounds like the camp I went to."

"Really?"

"Really!"

"But this was an older guy. Everyone said he was queer. He said I had some homo in me. He said everyone does."

"Real homosexuals use that line over and over, Donald."

"Is it true?" he asked anxiously.

"No, not in the way you're thinking." I went into the routine about everyone learns to love their mother and father. "Donald, having warm feelings toward another person of the same sex doesn't mean they're basic sexual feelings and doesn't mean they're bad. Homosexuals generally are very friendly and flattering toward young boys. If you have warm feelings back it only means you're appreciative of being treated nicely. Everyone likes to be flattered. It doesn't usually mean anything sexual. If this guy at camp was trying to seduce you, it's not surprising he would try to get you to focus on your positive feelings about him and try and convince you they were really sexual."

"He was a pretty slick operator!" said Donald, relaxing in his chair. "I knew I wasn't queer all the time."

If you believe that last statement, you'll believe anything.

Donald did do strange things, nonetheless. Once when he was looking for sympathy, he stole a small tricycle and put blocks on one of the pedals. He took the tricycle to a playground and sat on a bench waiting for someone to come by.

A large lady wheeling a carriage sat down beside him.

"I remember," he began telling the lady, "when I was a kid I used to come here with my tricycle and play, but none of the kids would play with me because one of my legs was shorter." He held up the tricycle and pointed to the blocks on the pedal.

The lady looked at him with a very sad look and said, "Oh, you poor dear," and tried to keep her eyes from staring impolitely at his leg to see what had happened to it over the years. Donald had covered it with a newspaper.

"She really made me feel good," said Donald. "I talked to her for almost an hour. She made me feel the way I wanted my mother to make me feel when I got sick as a kid. And so did the lady who sat down after her when she left."

"You really must have been hurting to need sympathy that badly," I said. "I wish you had called me. I would have met you and talked about it."

"You mean I can call you?"

"That's what I'm here for. We could have talked over what was bothering you."

"Really?"

"Really, dammit, Donald." I wrote down my telephone number and handed it to him. "If you're in trouble I'd like to know. You can always call, but just make sure you really want to call. It's better to handle your problems on your own. If you find yourself wanting to play little boy again and really start to get into it, you're not helping yourself. Try calling and we'll decide together whether or not you could have done it on your own."

I wanted Donald to feel he could lean on me if he needed to, but to know I wasn't going to let him become dependent on me. I'd prefer he put the telephone number on his wall, just feel very comfortable that it was there, and never use it.

"By the way, what were you so upset about?" I asked.

"Oh, it was nothing."

"Come on, Donald, you wouldn't have done all that if you weren't upset."

"I wasn't that upset. I was just a little hurt with the way things went at home that afternoon. My mother yelled at me. So I decided to make other people feel sorry for me."

"What did she yell at you for?"

"For having a messy room. She wanted me to clean it up. I told her I was too tired."

"What did she do then?"

"She yelled at me and called my father in to yell at me too."

"What did they say?"

"What difference does it make? It just made me angry. I'm entitled to keep some feelings to myself."

Does *every* patient have to say this at one time or another? What do they have, a script that they pass along to each other in the waiting room? I felt like I was a panelist on *I've Got a Secret.*

"Look, Donald, you have such time-consuming fantasies and activities when you get hurt and angry that it would be nice if we could understand what you felt and how it related to what you think and do. That way you could be more direct about your feelings and spend less time and energy involved in fantasy and useless action. What did your mother yell at you?"

"Oh, for Christsake." He started laughing, as if he'd just understood something. "She said, ha ha"—he could barely talk—"stop acting like a helpless cripple."

Will the real mental patient please stand up?

CHAPTER ELEVEN

TAKING STOCK: SIX DOWN, SIX TO GO

IT HAD finally happened. Larry Danielson had rubbed the top of his head so much that it now was shiny as an apple. As I said, when Larry talked, he rubbed his head; when Larry thought, he rubbed his head; when Larry worried, he rubbed his head. It seemed as though he rested his hand on the top of his head in order to support his body, and once when he stood up at grand rounds to make a comment, I fantasized pouring epoxy glue on his hand and imagined him spending the rest of his life with his arm permanently attached to his head.

"OK, you guys, knock it off. There's some important business this morning," said Larry.

Marty was needling Lovett about something.

"Knock it off." Larry was irritated. "Marty, did you ever think of going into therapy to find out why you keep making jokes?" Some groans from Bert and Jackie Rose.

"Did you ever think of going into therapy to find out why you can't?" retorted Marty. The wit was really flashing.

D. J. applauded. Bert ate. Lovett sat in the corner competing with Amanda Little to see who could say the least. I stared at Terry's blouse, which she had forgotten to button again. Nothing much had changed.

"Fact is, I thought of going to your therapist," said Marty —a sensitive area; Danielson had been in analysis for three years— "but he told me I had too much hair."

Even Larry laughed. "Today," said Larry, "is an anniversary. You've completed a half year of residency. And," he continued, "Jackie and I have two surprises for you."

They were, in order, a dozen fresh doughnuts (one for each of us and four for Bert) and news that Dr. Noyes had assigned a bigger on-call room for us in place of the box we'd suffered to date.

"You'll be sleeping in a new room. The resident in it is going off service today. Room 403."

"Hey, that's my room!" said D.J., who also lived in the residents' dorm.

"I can't imagine what I was thinking," said Larry.

"I have your analyst's telephone number here somewhere," said Marty, looking through his pockets.

"The new on-call room will be 407," said Larry, correcting himself.

"And that's right across from me," said D.J., but even the feeble if good-natured rejoinders were exhausted and it was back to work.

It was a routine day. I spent the next hour with Mrs. Rifkin, a new patient. She had a nameless fear of almost anything you could name, including cats, trolleys, subways, elevators, tall men, snakes, medicines, hospitals, penises, bridges, ladders, rugs, germs, and sewers. Cats might scratch her. Trolleys might run over her. Elevator cables might snap. Tall men might crush her. Snakes might bite her. Medicines might make her think about taking an overdose. Hospitals might infect her. Penises might impregnate her. Ladders might fall on her. And she feared rugs, sewers, and gutters because they contained germs. Mrs. Rifkin was concerned that she would somehow get involved with a man and he might force her to do something that wasn't nice, although she couldn't say what that might be. She was interesting but difficult for me to reach.

Later that morning I had to present another patient, Mr. McCord. He had recently become manic and had been running himself to the point of exhaustion. He was not sleeping. He started a hundred different projects all at the same time. He was dating three women, and had just become engaged to two of them. Both proposals were made on the anniversary of his mother's death. He took both girls to visit his mother's grave—one in the morning and the other in the afternoon—and he went out with the third woman that evening. All that night he telephoned his friends and neighbors as well as some perfect strangers to tell them the good news. When he called some of his friends for the fifth time, they came over and brought him into the hospital.

We discussed giving Mr. McCord lithium carbonate, a new drug which until recently had been used mostly in research. "Well," our supervisor said, running his hand over his gray military crewcut, "why don't we give the lithium a try?" Why? Why not? A little casual? . . .

In the afternoon I saw my other patient, Charlie Freeman, a thirty-five-year-old stock broker who had been on the ward for two weeks. A few years ago Charlie had been a hotshot, one of those *wunderkinder* in the money management field. He had become threatened by his own power and overwhelmed by his customers' trust in him to manage their fortunes. They believed he really knew what he was doing when he himself felt that he really didn't, that he made up most of what he told his clients from the skimpy, vague reports that his company issued.

"Christ," he said, "half of the research reports came down to 'If you invest in this stock, it can either go up or down.'"

Charlie Freeman sadly reported, "I was lucky until the bottom of the Kennedy market, when the losses I took for my customers made them forget I bought Syntex for them at twenty-five." Charlie had taken huge personal losses in his own portfolio and was beginning to hear the wolves at the door. He had never been in a squeeze like this before and was starting to crack under the pressure.

"Someone could write a book about all the crap I've gone through," Charlie said.

"Perhaps you'll have to cut down on some of your living expenses for a while, just until you get back on your feet," I suggested. "It won't be too hard after a while."

"You don't know the stock market, doc," he said, patting his fancy embroidered vest. "It's hard, I mean it's tough!"

"I know the market a little," I said. "I sold mutual funds for a while between college and medical school. I know that at least half of the brokers I've ever met know less than you. To survive as a stockbroker, Charlie, you have to learn to live with a constant sense of uncertainty and to accept the idea that much of the time you won't know what's going on. Instead of panicking, try to find out what's happening. When you're not sure of what you're doing, wait, don't panic." That sounded just like Gelb supervising me.

Charlie looked at me as if I were the reincarnation of Sigmund Freud. I thought he was really soaking up all my sound advice.

"Oh, yeah? And what fund were you selling?"he asked. He sounded as though he were trying for some inside information. He even called my psychiatric advice "tips."

(Charlie would make it back to work, feeling more confident about not feeling confident all the time, an irony he could learn to live with, an occupational hazard.)

Charlie had many shortcomings as a broker, but one was especially fascinating. He had repeatedly lost money on Anaconda Copper. He referred to Anaconda Copper as "Anna." Charlie's mother's name was Anna and Charlie felt he had to keep some Anaconda Copper shares in each of his clients' portfolios at all times. Otherwise, he felt he was dishonoring her sainted memory (or more accurately, not compensating her for the disappointment he'd caused her).

From what I could gather from Charlie, his mother had been a rejecting, hard woman. She disowned him when he failed to get into either medical, law, dental, engineering, or architectural school (he had applied to all of them at the same time), and she was made to bear the burden of being the only mother she knew whose son had graduated from Harvard and hadn't made it to graduate school. When a customer demanded that Charlie divest his portfolio of old Anna, Charlie became unreasonable and angry and fought with the customer, as a result losing the account.

My obvious solution to this problem struck Charlie like a thunderbolt. "Why not," I suggested, "buy ten shares of Anaconda Copper for yourself and keep it permanently in your folder as a remembrance to your mother. Then you wouldn't have to worry about your clients."

"My God, doc," he said, "I really *do* believe you must have been a mutual fund salesman. I bet a regular shrink who didn't know about the stock market would *never* have thought about that."

In this business I'd already learned to take my compliments where I got them, also not to look a gift horse in the mouth.

It had indeed been exactly six months since we'd started. Each resident was at a different stage of becoming whatever it was he wanted to become. Over coffee we compared notes about how well we thought we were doing. "I'm not sure exactly what it is I'm doing all the time," said Bert, "but it doesn't worry me as much as it used

to. Before, when I was totally inexperienced and didn't know anything, I would sit with patients and get anxious worrying whether or
not I was the one who was crazy. Now, I don't worry about it."

"Why?" asked D.J.

"Because now I'm sure I'm crazy." Bert was one of the sanest
residents in the department. He was reasonable, affable, and willing
to compromise. His patients liked and respected him. He was especially good in setting limits with adolescents. He had several younger
patients who needed to know just how far they could go before he
would slam the lid right down on them. He showed them. He made
Ernie go to school when Ernie wanted to play schizophrenic, which
he was lousy at. He was very effective with Betsy Lewis—he made
her see how childish she'd been and how primitive and demanding
she'd acted. He also had great success with Miss Marsh, a spinster
schoolteacher who felt worthless and who had been in therapy with
two other psychiatrists for several years with no results, by making
what I thought was a brilliant improvisation. One day he announced
he was going to take a look at the world she felt so miserable and
irrelevant in and pretend she had never been born. He was able to
show her some good and positive things about herself she had never
seen or believed before. She even began to feel worthwhile enough
to get better in therapy.

"Where did you hear about a technique like that?" Stanley
Lovett asked. "It sounds like some kind of psychodrama, but it's not
role reversal. What exactly were you following?"

"Well, Stanley," Bert said, "I don't think you'd be very recep-
tive to this kind of idea."

"Why not?" asked Stanley, threatened and indignant.

"It's just too esoteric, too far removed from the usual channels
of psychiatric theory. It's a form of Clarencism."

"Clarencism?"

"Well, what is it, boy?" coaxed D.J. Everyone looked puzzled.

"Does it have to do with Theodor Reik?" Stanley asked, reaching.

"No, it has to do with Jimmy Stewart. I saw him in *It's a Great
Life* on television. He plays this nice guy who does all these great
self-sacrificing things for people but gets depressed and is about
to drown himself when his guardian angel appears and leaps off the
bridge. Well, you know Jimmy Stewart can't let someone drown,
even if he's going to kill himself in a minute. It's not his personality
profile. So Stewart rescues the guardian angel, whose name happens
to be Clarence. And Clarence decides that the only way to make

Stewart see that he really has led a good life is to show him how things would have been if he were never born."

"Watch out with that kind of reasoning," said D.J. "There's slack in the universe, my boy. One life doesn't always have that much impact. It could be the reverse, too. The world might be better off without some people."

"Shh," said Bert, "don't tell Miss Marsh."

"I won't," said D.J.

D.J., as I've said before, was a marvelous person. She was of course very bright, but not the austere kind of bright I imagined her to be the first day I met her. She had a great deal of feeling for other people. She had been independent since high school and gone through college and medical school on scholarship. She's had a horrible home life—including a drunken father and a promiscuous mother. Somehow she survived to become a sturdy, engaging human being who had a special ability to reach other people. In many ways I adored her. She didn't like Stanley Lovett. "Not just because he's a pedant," she said, "but because he reminds me so much of a man I was engaged to. Not very professional, I know. But I'd bet someday Stanley will feel trapped by his feelings toward Terry and run away from her—and I'm sure she's the best thing that's ever happened to him." By now it was generally known (and reluctantly accepted by some of us more jealous types) that the five-foot-four wonder from Brooklyn Heights had captured the heart and body of Terry O'Conner, the hysteric Irish nurse with the X-rated body.

D.J. was a very good therapist. She was usually two or three steps ahead of her patients, even though she often said, "I never feel I'm in control of the situation." If she had a fault, it was the image she projected to male patients when they first met her. She just couldn't be fully aware of the overwhelming impact, which threatened some of them at first. They were sometimes afraid of her. D.J. had managed extremely well with Jud Cain, the psychopathic phony ski instructor. She kept him running rather than the other way around, which was more typical of psychiatrists' dealings with psychopaths.

Psychopaths always mess up a hospital ward. They play one person against another and are able to read their doctors' and nurses' personalities like a book. They seem to know just what you're afraid of or feel guilty about, and often can trap you.

Cain greeted D.J. when she first came on the ward with "I'm Jud Cain. I'd like a chance to speak with you. Don't rush. It's not important." Innocuous enough? When D.J. sat down with Cain, it was an altogether different story. He was out to snare and manipulate her. Cain rehearsed everything he said to D.J. to make sure he came off smooth and suave. D.J. once found a list of comments he'd just made to her which he left behind after an extremely rough session in which he unsuccessfully attacked her professionalism. One of the notes read, "You and I both know, Dr. Marley, that you don't have enough background and experience to make the decisions you are faced with. You know that I have to return to court to face charges of stealing a car when I get out of here. Everything I tell you is in confidence. Well, I understand you have told your supervisor what we discuss. That's a violation of my confidence because you didn't ask me first."

"And Cain said it just like that!" D.J. reported. "I mean, I was really frightened. I didn't know the law, and Cain was quoting it, telling me I wasn't being professional and possibly violating it. And then suddenly I realized he was using my own fear of not being a good psychiatrist to manipulate me. So I said, 'Look, you have confidentiality in here, but part of the ground rules are that I discuss everything we talk about with Dr. Karlsson. We'll make our decisions together.'"

Practically any other first-year resident would have fallen into Cain's trap and become defensive about his professional status. Jud Cain impressed Enid Rust, the psychologist, as a warm and sensitive young man who scored the highest on any IQ test she'd ever administered until she found out that he'd studied the test beforehand. If you can learn to read people as well as a psychopath and are a warm, giving person who wants to help others, you would be an unrivaled therapist.

Stanley Lovett, you may remember, felt very aloof when he began his psychiatric training. He was defensive whenever any of us asked him questions and was intellectual and cool when talking to his patients. He had seen enough of psychiatrists in his life to know how some of them acted, and he tried to act the same way. He had been in therapy himself for three years during college and for four years during medical school. And now, after six months of his present psychoanalysis, he said, with previously unaccustomed humanity, "The analysis is not going well." (Which may have meant that it finally was.)

Lovett did fine with some patients; with others, like Bobby

Jacklin, the schizophrenic usher, quite poorly. Lynn, the student nurse, used to call him every name in the book, that is in our book—"insensitive, callous, unfeeling, intellectualized, timid, and afraid of people," was how Lynn put it to Lovett. Admittedly student nurses can get a bit idealistic. Lynn got hold of Lovett and wouldn't let go. During one of their fights she told him that he was afraid of dealing with patients just like the rest of us, and that he'd better start admitting it to himself before he made Bobby Jacklin even crazier. Lovett confided in me—why he picked me to confide in, I don't understand—"I went to my analyst and just tore into that little bitch for almost half an hour. And do you know what he told me? He said, 'Perhaps you're really angry with yourself for not being able to relate to patients the way Lynn does. You mentioned she was warm and friendly.'" That was the beginning of Lovett trying harder to be human and not insisting that all of his patients be analyzed.

"I realized," Lovett said, "that I was putting my patients under the same pressure I felt when I was in my doctor's office." (Which may lead you to some thoughts about Lovett's doctor.)

Lovett in a funny way was slowly becoming one of the guys. Being one of the guys for us meant that your faults were no longer pointed out as reasons for avoiding you and you were accepted just the way you were. Well, Lovett was *almost* one of the guys . . .

"Hey," Bert said, "we've missed grand rounds. I understand there was supposed to be a fabulous presentation of the role of the hypothalamus in affective disorders based on studies of cat brain. Larry better've signed us in."

"Fascinating," said D.J., "too bad we missed it."

"Pity," I sighed, "George Frederick Handel—that's the way I signed old Noyes' attendance sheet—really wanted to hear this one."

"And you know what," said Lovett, "I had a great question all written out to ask. It would really have made me look bright as hell."

"You aren't related to the famous Jud Cain, are you?" asked D.J.

Stanley Lovett had made light of himself. (Damn near incredible!)

Marty DiAngelo had been unusually silent all this time—staring at us, listening.

"How about your year, Marty?" asked D.J. "How's it going? How are *your* patients going?"

"I don't think about it," said Marty. "After spending a year at the state hospital you learn not to measure how well you're doing by your patients' reactions."

"But you have to," I said.

"Relax, David. Wait until you get to the state hospital next July. You'll change your tune. No one there *ever* gets better."

CHAPTER TWELVE

SUICIDES AND OTHER EMERGENCIES

BELLA Grable, the ward secretary, was waiting for me when I returned to the ward. "Dr. Viscott, your wife called. She sounded upset and wants to talk with you."

I walked down to my office. Judy had developed varicose veins during her last pregnancy and lately was having a good deal of pain and getting pretty upset about it. In the past few weeks she'd consulted two doctors. Neither thought her legs looked bad enough to do anything special about them. The fact that she could barely walk because of the pain didn't seem to impress them. "Keep your legs elevated and stay off your feet." (Good, doc. And who makes the meals and the beds?)

"Hi, honey, you call?"

"Oh, David, I don't know what I'm going to do." Judy was crying.

"What happened?"

"I'm pregnant! I have pain so much of the time and now with the added pressure on my veins from a baby I'll be a wreck. I can't go through with it."

What could I say? What should we do?

"I can't even think straight," Judy said. "I'm putting the kids to bed in a while. We'll talk about it when you get home."

Judy was always very active in sports and loved figure skating and tennis. Being in pain was not her style. It was getting her down and making her feel old. I felt terribly helpless about it. I asked other doctors for advice about her legs and they just said "rest and heat" or asked if she was overreacting to something.

I couldn't stop thinking about Judy. I met D.J. for dinner in the hospital cafeteria but couldn't eat. We talked about the indifference of some people in the medical profession and their tendency to brush off any patient who seems to have a problem that won't respond readily to their medicine. Here I was, a physician, getting the layman's runaround (poetic justice? not yet, please). I knew that a problem was still a problem, even if our doctor didn't want to admit it, and that it wouldn't go away by wishing it would. What did ordinary mortals do? They believed in their doctors without realizing that their physician's firmness was sometimes a reflection more of his pride than his knowledge.

Helen Doran and Candy Bourke were on duty again and they expected me to make rounds with them. "Look, David," said Candy, "just sit down with us for ten minutes. I know you've got a lot on your mind. We'll just hit the high spots."

How does a psychiatrist keep his mind on his patients and his work when he has problems of his own? I don't know. It's hard to do. You just try to get your work done as quickly and thoroughly as possible, but you're not as good as you should be. I decided I wouldn't see any patients unless absolutely necessary. The ward was quiet. I changed sleeping medications for two patients who'd been restless the night before. I didn't want to be disturbed, and a good night's sleep wouldn't hurt them. I felt anxious and empty inside. I wanted to call Judy but it was only seven and I figured she was just putting the kids to bed.

I called her at seven thirty.

"How are you feeling?"

"Better."

"I'm glad. Are you resting?"

"Yes. The kids were really sweet tonight."

"That's good." Funny how kids can sense when their mother isn't feeling well. Judy did sound better.

"I really would like to have another baby. I'll try to get through this somehow."

I went to the doctors' lounge, signed in to the hospital switchboard, and turned on the television. It was my audiovisual tranquilizer. Only quiz shows on.

Even though I hate the show, I'm still watching the tube. I'm really worried about Judy. The picture's jumping and fuzzy. The television sets in residents' quarters are always lousy. So are the pool tables. They usually have torn felt, or broken cue tips, or no chalk.

I have walked miles around pool tables in residents' quarters in a dozen different hospitals, and I still can't put a ball into a pocket unless I drop it in with my hand. Look at this table; it's terrible.

Telephone!

"Dr. Viscott?"

"Yes."

"It's me, Candy. They want you on the emergency unit."

Emergency calls and I didn't get along under the best of conditions. I just hated the uncertainty, not knowing what I would find at the other end of the line. I told myself I could handle anything, well, almost anything. All of a sudden, I wasn't so sure. I just felt powerless about Judy.

The emergency room at Union Hospital was like all the other emergency rooms I'd ever known. Lots of medical and surgical equipment everywhere, surgical trays, oxygen tanks, operating tables, airways, and medicine cabinets. There were nurses running around who seemed urgent about everything they did, even about having a cigarette. God, I hoped it wasn't a serious problem, one I'd have to admit to the hospital. That meant spending an hour and a half with the patient, writing a long note, racking my brain to make sure I hadn't left anything out and then writing orders in the order book.

"Your patient is ready for you, doctor," said Miss Bordeleaux, the nurse on duty. "Your patient is ready for you" was a phrase I hadn't heard since internship. It meant that the patient who'd been prepped with antiseptics, draped with sterile towels was ready for you to begin your spinal tap, or that the patient was in stirrups ready for a pelvic examination, or any one of a dozen other uncomfortable, often unnecessary procedures that we often performed just for the sake of completeness. The theory was that the patient was in the hospital anyway and it was a good opportunity that shouldn't be missed.

Besides sound medical indications, there were other factors that determined whether or not a particular procedure was to be carried out on a patient. Sometimes it depended on the doctor's individual preference for the procedure, sometimes on his desire to become proficient and to master the technique of the procedure. Sometimes it depended more on the doctors' needs than the patients'. So many sigmoidoscopes and proctoscopes were used merely to give experience to the user that it often became ridiculous. During my internship we began to define a proctoscope as a "long tube with an asshole at both ends."

My patient was ready, and I was anxious!

Crumpled in a chair, looking drunk but probably sober, was a tall, skinny-legged black girl about twenty. Her hand was hanging limply over the back of her chair. Her eyes were open, staring at the ceiling and fluttering. Clear symptoms of a hysteric, I was fairly sure. Hysterics *did* tend to look alike, by God! Her boy friend was with her, a handsome, tall, well-dressed man about thirty-five. He had a thin mustache and was balding.

"We were leaving North Carolina together for New England. We'd planned to work and live together. Everything looked good. We both had jobs waiting here. We stopped in Baltimore this morning to see her aunt on the way up. They had a few words and we left. She started acting funny while we were driving. When we got to Philadelphia, she said she couldn't walk, that she was paralyzed."

An acute hysterical conversion reaction? In a conversion reaction, the patient usually converts an emotional problem into a physical illness which symbolizes the problem.

"Would you mind waiting outside while I speak to her?" I asked. I read her admission data sheet: "Charlotte Washington, 18, born Mobile, Alabama."

"Charlotte, what's wrong?"

"It's my feet, doc. I can't move my feet." Charlotte looked very calm. She stared at the ceiling. "I have to be at work tomorrow . . ."

"You don't seem very worried about your feet," I said.

"Why should I, doc? You're the doctor. It's your problem. I don't know nothing about no feet. You know about feet." This detached attitude of a hysteric toward her symptoms is typical. The instructors in medical school called it *la belle indifférence*. They loved to pronounce it and give us a little class.

"What happened at your aunt's? I understand you had words."

"Nothing, nothing."

"Maybe we should talk about it. What did your aunt say?"

"She didn't say nothing. She just talked to my mother on the telephone." Aha! It's her mother. When a female hysteric is in a crisis, find out what's going on between her and her mother. It's almost always a fight and it often involves sexual acting-out.

"What did your mother have to say about your coming north?"

"That's my business," said Charlotte, moving one leg.

"It's important."

"It may be important, but it ain't none of your business."

"Mothers sometimes see situations very differently from their daughters." (I hope you can appreciate that that was a very nice therapeutic statement to help the patient open up. Anyway, I *hoped* it was.)

"We sure do." Charlotte looked angry. "She thinks just because I'm going north with a man means I'm a tramp. She says I should marry Warren first, but I say I don't have to. I'm gonna live with him. I can't see getting into something too deep. I got lots of time. She wants me to get married."

"And?"

"She says if I didn't get married I should consider myself a slut and never come back to her house or speak her name and that Glory, Jesus, Hallelujah she was going down to pray for my black soul. And that I was damned in the eyes of God and in every man or woman who would ever set eyes on me."

"I bet you wanted to say something to her." (Another great therapeutic comment.)

"Well—I didn't. I couldn't."

"If you could say what you wanted, what would you have said? Go on, pretend I'm your mother. What would you say to me? Go ahead, let me have it, I can take it."

Charlotte turned out to be very suggestible and got right into it. "You have no right telling me what to do with my life. I went to high school. I didn't get pregnant like half my girl friends did. You can't tell me I got to spend my life in this place."

"But, Charlotte, your father and I have plans for you—"

"You're always talking about you and your plans," she yelled at me. "You keep telling me I gotta do this and I gotta do that because Jesus is watching me. Well, I'm watching me too and I don't like what I see. I'm sick and tired of North Carolina and I got plans of my own."

"You're going to stay right here if I have anything to say about it," I said, slipping into a makeshift Southern accent without really intending to.

"You shut your big fat motherfucking mouth," she said, and stood up. "I'm old enough to do what I want and go where I want, and I don't need to ask your permission."

Charlotte was standing in front of me, glaring and making a fist.

"You sure sound like you've got a lot of good reasons to be angry," I said.

"Yes, I do," she snapped.

"I think maybe you were afraid of getting angry and weren't

as sure of yourself as you sounded. Your mother obviously made you angry and you seem to have felt guilty about something."

I gave Charlotte an appointment for the outpatient clinic, to be seen by one of the second-year residents in follow-up, and led her into the waiting room. Her friend, Warren, couldn't believe it. Neither could Miss Bordeleaux, the nurse on call.

"*Your* patient's ready," I said, feeling almost pleased with myself. "She'll be coming back to clinic just to make sure things are working out."

"Thank you, doc. I mean, really, thank you," Warren said. "Come on, honey."

Charlotte turned to me. "You gonna be at the clinic? I'd like that." (Nothing personal, a typical seductive move of a hysteric, I reminded myself.)

"No, someone else will."

"Too bad," she said as she left. "You sure know how to fix a girl's legs."

If only Judy's legs could be fixed like that.

I resumed my position in front of the TV. Victor Mature was starring in *The Robe,* looking intense as hell. Someone placed Christ's robe on him and he sort of crumbled.

"That's a slipped disc," said Frank Howland, the surgical resident, commenting on the posture that Mature had taken. He lit a cigar. "See how he lists to one side. I'd tell him to report to the centurion and get off his feet for a couple of days before he gets muscle atrophy."

"Boy, you guys are really sacrilegious," said Julian Pell, a third-year medical student who was rotating through Howland's service. He actually seemed to take the movies seriously.

"Will you get the fuck out of here," Howland told him. I loved the directness of surgeons. Julian shook his head. He was really upset by Howland's irreverent diagnosis of Victor Mature. God help him, and his future patients. . . .

Les Ahearn, the medical resident, came in, proud of himself. "Guess what I found on Collins 8? A pheochromocytoma! You hear that? Pretty good, huh? We had Larry Danielson evaluate the patient this morning. He said the patient was probably suffering from anxiety attacks. But the tests came back from the lab, a VMA of seventeen and catachols of six hundred and fifty. He's got the real thing."

A pheochromocytoma is a tumor of the adrenal gland that sporadically secretes substances into the blood, which causes a rapid heart rate, feelings of anxiety, and makes patients very uncomfortable. It's also difficult to diagnose because the same symptoms are shown by people with intense anxiety reactions. In fact, attacks can be triggered off by emotional stress. Ahearn was looking for applause. "When do you send him to me so I can cut the damn thing out?" asked Frank.

"It's a tough diagnosis to make," I said, "and very confusing for psychiatrists."

"You guys," Frank Howland began, "don't really make diagnoses, do you? I mean, you sort of guess what's wrong and try to find a parent to pin it all on."

"Psychiatry," I intoned, "is a discipline which—"

"Psychiatry," interrupted Howland, "is not my idea of a discipline." I laughed with Ahearn. I was just glad to be with people.

"You coming skiing with us to Killington, David?" Les asked. "When are you leaving?"

"Saturday A.M., early."

"I wouldn't ski for anything," said Howland. "Most dangerous sport invented. You have to be a masochist to ski. I can tell you that and I'm not a psychiatrist."

The phone rang. "It's for you," Les said, handing me the receiver. "Sorry, love, it's Candy. They need you in ER again. A suicide."

Miss Bordeleaux was waiting in the hall for me. "There's something wrong with this girl, Dr. Viscott. I mean, really wrong. She has a funny look. She says she slashed her wrist, but there's a big bandage over it and she won't let me look at it."

Nurses like Miss Bordeleaux, with little training in psychiatry, often seemed to think of psychiatric patients as having "something wrong" with them, as if what ailed them didn't fit within the boundaries of any known, respectable medical specialty. Maybe Miss Bordeleaux thought psychiatric patients were under a witch's spell. Meaning, whatever was wrong with them she didn't much like.

Miss Bordeleaux pointed to one of the examining rooms and shook her head. Louise Riley was a very pretty girl, about twenty-one. She was sitting quietly in a chair in the examining room, an oversize army jacket wrapped around her. She had long dirty blonde hair that hung straight down, practically to her waist. She had enormous black eyes fringed with lush, long eyelashes.

"I tried to kill myself," Louise blurted out and went silent. She stared at me.

"Can you tell me more about it?"

"I just did. I tried to kill myself. I took a razor and slashed my wrist."

That's what I call concrete thinking. Usually in response to a question like that you expect a patient to tell you something about what led up to feeling like killing herself.

"What made you want to kill yourself?" I tried again.

"Nothing, I just felt like killing myself." Louise was staring right at me.

"Nothing was going on and you just felt like killing yourself?"

"Yes," she said, smiling the brief tense smile that people smile when they're frightened.

(This is very strange.) "Why did you come here?" (Maybe she's faking, maybe she's psychotic. I don't know.)

"Because I was afraid of hurting myself." She pushed her hair out of her eyes.

"Had you ever felt like this before?"

"Sometimes, but I never did anything about it."

"Can I take a look at your wrist?"

"No!" She pulled her arm off the desk and put it in her lap.

"Why?"

"I—I'm ashamed." Louise was still staring at me. People who feel ashamed don't usually look you in the eye. Very peculiar.

"Nothing to be ashamed about. I'd just like to see if it needs fixing up." After about ten minutes of coaxing she put her arm back on the desk and I took off the bandage. I couldn't see any wound.

"Where did you cut yourself?"

"There," she said, pointing to a scratch. "I could've gone much deeper."

With a fingernail, I thought. "OK," I said, "you did the right thing by coming into the hospital." I wanted her to feel comfortable about being in the emergency room and tell her that her "suicidal attempt" was being taken seriously. I didn't want her to feel she had to take a bread knife and open a major artery just to talk to someone. "Maybe you're worried about really losing all control of your feelings? Maybe that's why you're here?"

"I dunno." Louise just stared at me blankly.

She was puzzling. Although I questioned her about home, work, and friends I still didn't know enough to make up my mind about what to do with her.

When a suicidal patient came to the emergency room he created a special threat because he represented the unknown. When any patient claimed he was suicidal the residents on call had to determine whether or not he really was. That was our first duty. Each potentially suicidal patient had to be taken seriously even if his story was ridiculous, and some of the stories were, like the drunks who stumbled through the door threatening to kill themselves if we didn't let them in or give them a drink.

We had to show the patient we believed him, that we understood how difficult it was to come to the hospital to admit he was desperate. We had to respond to that desperateness, not reject it. It's possible that if you reject a patient you feel is not really suicidal you will make him so angry that he decides to prove you were wrong, and does it. Most patients who claim they are suicidal are asking for help. You have to help them. That may mean hospitalizing them, listening to them, reassuring them, or arranging for follow-up visits to the clinic. Sometimes you send them to a clinic even if they don't really need it, to show that you take them seriously. They need to to be taken seriously.

Residents tend to be frightened of suicidal patients. The thought of one of your patients committing suicide is dreaded. A suicide implies that you have failed in some way. You certainly won't have the chance to redeem yourself.

As I mentioned before in the case of Mr. Parker, there was no standard check list of questions to determine whether a patient was suicidal. Each of us developed his own method. I tried to see how the patient's attitude about suicide changed during the interview while I tried to give him support, told him I was interested in helping and understanding him. If the patient responded to my offer to help by calming down and talking about his problems, he was less likely to kill himself than the patient whose sense of hopelessness only got worse when we talked. Some manipulative patients tried to make you think they were suicidal and almost seemed to be playing games with you. They were always difficult and made everyone anxious. They were uncooperative and threated to kill themselves the moment they hit the street.

I also tried to find out where and with whom the patient lived and what was happening at home. I tried to learn how depressed he was and how long he'd been depressed. A patient who's been severely depressed for a long time may want to kill himself but just doesn't have the energy to act. The time when he begins to feel a little better is the most dangerous, because he's still depressed but now has the energy to kill himself. Such patients need protection until they feel better *and* no longer want to kill themselves, and can use their new energy for something besides self-destruction. Depressed patients who're given antidepressant-drug therapy and are beginning to come out of a deep depression may also become real suicidal risks as they start to improve.

Listening to the way potentially suicidal patients think about the future seems to me another way of discovering if they really are suicidal. Knowing how realistically a patient talks about plans, hopes, and events far away in time is very helpful. Even though a student may take an overdose of sleeping pills and claim he wants to die, he may be talking about an exam he has to take next week or an appointment he has to keep next month. You get the feeling he won't like much of the future, but he'll be there to face it. At least you know he sees himself in the future.

When a patient unrealistically refers to the future as better than now, with every problem finally being almost magically resolved, that's the time to worry about him. People who've been depressed for years often feel hopeless about everything. Sometimes they feel *better* when they are seriously considering suicide. Their friends tell them they look "better than they've looked in years." Friends and family are so pleased that they don't question the sudden improvement, they just enjoy the patient's signs of apparent recovery. At last, the patient is better. He may indeed appear radiant, imperturbable, or joyous right up until the time of the final act. People who suddenly seem to get better from a deep depression have often found their answer to their problems—suicide. (If a patient is unable to decide between killing himself or killing a person he hates, he may become psychotic, which is a whole new problem.)

Louise did not talk of the future. She did not talk of her past. She mentioned not a word of her home. She refused to accept an appointment at the clinic. She didn't want to come into the hospital. She refused to talk to me in any detail, but she really enjoyed sitting there staring at me.

"I'd like to see you again. Let's try to find out what's troubling you," I said.

"OK. Sometime," she said brightly.

Wait—the thought just crossed my mind—this girl possibly *is* psychotic. How do I know her judgment is good enough to keep her from killing herself accidentally, even though she really doesn't appear suicidal? I couldn't be sure. Should I hospitalize her just for that? Her judgment probably has been poor all her life. I took a deep breath and decided to let Louise go home.

Actually, it was not such a difficult decision to make. I gambled that she mostly just wanted to touch bases. During the rest of the year Louise called the hospital at least twice a week to say "I just tried to kill myself." She eventually ended up in therapy with Marshall Kell, whose moment of triumph came one night when she called up the hospital and said, "I'm feeling uncomfortable and I just wanted to hear a friendly voice." See, people sometimes *do* get better in our hands. I only wish Surgeon Frank Howland could have been there to see it.

In the practice of psychiatry there are, to put it mildly, many uncertainties. I treated some patients who were so manipulative I would worry before they arrived at the beginning of every session whether they would show up or if they'd killed themselves. You just can't hospitalize everyone who *might* be suicidal. You often can help a patient a great deal more by showing him he can overcome his fears himself *without* hospitalization, but I learned you should never withhold protection in a hospital setting if you believe a patient needs it. Most patients who say they are suicidal won't kill themselves, and yet those patients who *do* kill themselves generally tell someone about their plans or make a cry for help at least once. It's then that they need help the most. When patients really want to kill themselves they usually do it right, by jumping out of windows, by taking massive overdoses of drugs or poison when no one is home, or by swimming miles out from shore on a lonely beach to the point of exhaustion. When a patient who really is suicidal calls for help and you miss the clues and let him go back on the street, the chances, even then, are that he will not kill himself right away. Every patient who presents himself as suicidal needs to be closely followed the first time, just to ensure yourself another chance to pick up clues you might have missed.

When a patient made a suicidal gesture, as Louise did, it was more asking for help than wanting to commit suicide. Suicidal gestures are usually obvious, and are planned so that someone will discover the patient before it's too late. Often there is a great deal of anger symbolized in the suicidal gesture that is directed at someone important to the patient. It's almost as if the patient is saying through the gesture, "See what you have driven me to. You'll be sorry." Suicidal gestures can also be more punitive than self-destructive. Once you are reasonably sure the patient is not going to kill himself you should ally yourself with him and help him without being diverted by the suicidal gestures. Simply discharging the patient to the street will not do—even though it's done a lot.

A suicide note is a good clue to understanding someone's intent. A suicidal patient is unlikely to write an angry or vindictive note. Usually too much of his energy is directed inward to get that angry at other people. The patient who writes the angry note turns against himself only as a way of getting at others. He wants to be around to hear his relatives crying at his funeral. The time to worry most is when a patient leaves a note simply listing the numbers of bank accounts and insurance policies and closes with, "Don't blame yourself, I'm much better off this way." He's probably dead by the time the letter is discovered. If he's not, he needs immediate protective action because he'll probably kill himself. And sometimes people who only intend to make a suicidal gesture kill themselves by mistake. There are no sure things either way in this business.

Should a psychiatrist, should anyone, have the right to prevent someone from taking his own life? I have seen some lives so full of pain and darkness for such a long time that I felt like an oppressor just by asking the patient to endure more of what was horrible to him. Who has the right to tell someone he must live a life of pain and hell? What in my training gave me the right to tell someone to suffer?

I believe that under certain circumstances it may not make very much more sense to be alive than to be dead. We'll all be dead sooner or later anyway. But being alive is all I know. Although one person's life may not always make sense, I believe there is still a meaning to life itself, even if we don't always understand it. Because we are alive and we are part of life, it makes sense to me to find the part of each of us that has meaning and is worth living for.

I dropped by Bamberg 5 on the way back to the residents' lounge. The ward was quiet. I got back to the lounge just in time to catch the end of The Robe and watch Victor Mature and Jean Seberg walking out into the sunset, all converted.

"Well, you've been busy tonight," said Howland. "I mean, for a psychiatrist. You should try managing someone with a bleeding ulcer." Howland puffed on his cigar.

"Suicide?" asked Les Ahearn.

"No, just a confused girl wanting to talk but afraid to."

"Boy, is that a lot of crap," said Frank Howland. "You guys listen to people tell you their problems and you call it work. I work like a dog all day and then go home to hear my wife tell me about her problems. Do you guys ever have any *real* problems?"

"Well," I said, "once I went to the emergency room and had a wild-looking hippie waiting for me."

"Yes?" said Howland, blowing smoke in my face, "I can hardly stand the suspense."

"I asked her what was wrong and she said, 'I have the sun in Saggitarius, the moon in the *I Ching*, Mercury in Deuteronomy and Saturn in the hanged man of the Tarot.'"

"Now *that's* a real problem," said Les, answering the phone. It was for him. "Be there in a minute," he said and hung up. "Toxic lady in the ER."

CHAPTER THIRTEEN

STRANGERS IN THE NIGHT

Twenty minutes later the phone rang again. It was Les, wanting to speak with me. "Look," he said. "I have the most unusual case I've ever seen down here. I don't think this lady is toxic but I can't figure her at all. I tried to interview her and I got disjointed answers like the Ganser Syndrome, but crazier and more delusional. David, I just don't know what the hell is going on. I've never seen anything like her!"

I left for the emergency room again. Les knew more about psychiatry than most of the medical residents. If he didn't know what was going on, I wasn't all that sure I would.

Miss Bordeleaux said, "She belongs in a state hospital and fast! I don't want her in *my* emergency room."

"David," Les said, "she's talking about some psychiatrist across the river her husband is going to kill for what this guy did to her. She says there's a conspiracy going on. And yet she doesn't really look as paranoid as she sounds. See what you think."

Bessie Gore was a light-complexioned black woman about thirty-five to forty. She was almost six feet tall and must have weighed about a hundred and eighty pounds. Her forehead was deeply furrowed and she looked frightened and preoccupied. Her eyes were darting around. Was she looking at the walls or what she thought she saw on them? Sometimes you can tell when a patient is hallucinating, but I wasn't sure with Bessie.

"I'm Dr. Viscott, I'd like to talk with you."

"You find Dr. Clift. He has the pills. He has the way for me to get Henry back. You know what I mean. See, you're *getting* the idea now! That's a fact. There's no way back for either of us now. He'll murder that man. I know. He's threatened for a long time. I can't take any more responsibilities for these things. You have a turn. I have a headache. I need an Anacin."

What the hell was this lady talking about? Who was Henry? Who was Dr. Clift? Who'd kill whom?

"Who's Henry?" I asked.

"Henry? I don't know any Henry." Bessie started laughing hilariously. Then, just as abruptly, she started to cry. "Dr. Clift got Henry mad because he wrote him there was something wrong with my mind." More laughter, breaking right through her tears. I was bewildered.

"Henry?" I asked again.

"Henry who?" she answered. (Just like the old Abbott and Costello "Who's On First" routine. Except this one wasn't funny, it was scary.) "You getting my aspirin or do I have to send out for some?" Tears were streaming down Bessie Gore's face. She pulled anxiously at her yellow print dress. She was restless and looked like she would burst. "I'm being held prisoner by my brothers. They're going to turn me in. I can tell."

"What've you done that I should turn you in?"

"Oh, don't play cute with me. Don't play so cute. You're not cute at all. You know *all about* it."

"Mrs. Gore, I don't have any idea what's going on."

"I'll show you. They're after both of us." Bessie jumped up and started to knock to the floor whatever she could lay her hands on; an ash tray, prescription blanks, my pen, her glasses. She moved toward some medical instruments; a blood-pressure cuff was her next victim.

"OK, cut it out," I said. "I'm not about to let you wreck this office, Mrs. Gore. Sit down and tell me what I can do to help you."

"Let me out. Let me out." Bessie ran for the door, opened it and knocked Miss Bordeleaux off balance.

I ran after Mrs. Gore. Two men, apparently her brothers, appeared from nowhere and grabbed her.

I had to hospitalize Bessie Gore for observation. I took a commitment form from the desk and filled it out, describing Bessie Gore's strange, uncontrollable behavior. Bessie could not be admitted to Bamberg 5 because there was no way to hold a patient there against her will. There wasn't a single locked door on Bamberg 5. According to Bessie's brothers, she had threatened to kill herself. Bessie was delusional and psychotic. She could be suicidal.

I wasn't sure about her diagnosis. She looked like a paranoid schizophrenic one moment, like a manic-depressive the next. There seemed little question she was psychotic.

"What are you going to do?" Les asked. "Commit her to the state hospital?"

"Yes, I don't have a choice. I'll speak to the doctor on call over there and arrange transportation."

"I can't understand it," said Leroy, one of Bessie's brothers who had been holding her. "She's such a calm person most of the time. Maybe it's her husband getting out of jail today. He was in for attempted murder but they let him out because of some irregularities with the trial."

"Had she ever been like this before?" I asked Leroy.

"The only time she's ever upset is when Henry is around. Then they both go off looking for people who they think have done something wrong to them."

I spoke with Dr. Frogner, the resident on call at the state hospital, who said he would be pleased to accept Bessie.

Leroy had a car and assured me he could take Bessie to State, so I gave him an envelope containing the commitment paper and sent Bessie on her way, telling her I thought she'd feel more comfortable knowing she'd have people looking after her while she was so upset. It was a dumb little speech I made, a little insincere even. Maybe I felt guilty committing her.

"I have my rights," said Bessie. "I'm gonna tell Henry."

Bessie and her brothers left. Les and I walked back to the on-call room, relieved. "I never saw anything like that," he said.

"I have," I said. "It's like breakfast time at my house."

I'd learned never to go to bed early when I was on call; you only get wakened up. That was true last year when I was an intern, the year before when I was a medical student, and it was proving true again this year. It was too late to call Judy. She'd hopefully be asleep by now and I didn't want to disturb her. I collapsed in the plastic chair that was farthest from the TV. Candy Bourke walked into the lounge. She had just finished her evening duty on Bamberg 5. Several other nurses also dropped in. A crowd was forming. Some of the doctors were wearing surgical scrub suits, fresh from the operating room.

The phone rang. It was for Les. "Bessie Gore is *back*," he said. "She overdosed with one hundred Carbrital capsules she had in her pocketbook."

Les and I ran down to the emergency room. Mrs. Gore was comatose. I started an intravenous with isotonic mannitol, which would cause an increased urine output. Les Ahearn put a tube into Mrs. Gore's stomach. Very little came back. The capsules had dissolved.

"That's enough barbiturates to kill a horse," I said. Each Carbrital contained one hundred milligrams of pentobarbital and a bromide salt. The prescription bottle in her purse had contained one hundred pills. It was now empty. According to her brothers, Bessie had just picked it up from the drugstore when they came over to get her. So she probably swallowed all of them. Les was checking to make sure she had unobstructed airway. The emergency room nurse inserted a catheter into Mrs. Gore's bladder so we could monitor her urine output and be sure that the mannitol was washing out the drug.

"I think we're going to have to put her on the artificial kidney," Les said. I checked Bessie's reflexes. They were either diminished or absent. She gave no reaction to pain.

"We may lose her if we don't," I said.

"I need a surgeon," said Les. Howland was only a blade to us now.

At a time like this you don't think of blaming yourself for what you should or shouldn't have done. Your only concern is to get the patient out of danger and do it as quickly as possible. The nurse called Howland.

We wheeled Bessie to the procedure room on Collins 8, Les' floor. Frank was waiting for us. In a half hour he had inserted tubes in blood vessels in Bessie's arm all ready to attach to the kidney machine. Luckily we were able to type and cross-match enough blood to work the machine. Mrs. Gore was plugged into the kidney. All we could do was wait.

"One good thing," I said, "the mannitol drip is working. She's put out over two liters of urine. I've written I.V. orders to cover her for the next few hours." In the excitement I had reverted back to my medical intern ways, the old language and attitude. In a strange way it was even a relief. Probably because I knew I wouldn't have to do it for more than an hour and by playing medical doctor I could avoid thinking about my role in causing all this.

I sat down to write another brief note in Mrs. Gore's chart. I spoke with her brothers. They told me Dr. Frogner at the state hospital had

refused to admit her as a patient. Bessie had excused herself to go
to the bathroom and later became groggy in the waiting room.

Although I had signed Bessie's commitment paper, it was up to
the discretion of the resident in charge whether or not to accept a
patient for hospitalization. Even if he'd agreed to do so beforehand,
he could change his mind. It was still a rotten thing to do, I thought,
especially without even calling. I made a mental note of his name.
Dr. Frogner. Someday, Frogner, I'll get you. Melodramatic, no doubt.
But I meant it and still do.

It was the nurse's duty in our emergency room to look for drugs
and to go through Bessie Gore's clothes. No, it wasn't! Why am I saying that? If I'd admitted Bessie to Union Hospital it would have been
the emergency room nurse's duty to search her for drugs, but I hadn't.
I should have asked about drugs. She did look toxic to Les. It was so
damn confusing that I didn't think of it. She didn't look toxic to me
at all. Still, asking the patient about drugs was supposed to be a routine part of almost every interview. I felt guilty about all this. I could
have asked Leroy for a more detailed history. I could have asked him
about drugs. After all, Leroy knew she had drugs with her. Why
didn't they say something? Perhaps I wanted to get Bessie off my
hands as soon as possible, avoid the problems of admitting her because
I was too tired, too upset over Judy. I wasn't as alert as usual. But if
the same situation occurred tomorrow, my main concern would be to
put Bessie into a state hospital. I'd probably do the same thing. I
couldn't send Bessie to Bamberg 5. Bamberg 5 just wasn't equipped to
handle people in her condition. All this heavy self-review wasn't very
reassuring to me. I still felt unsure and guilty.

I finished writing my note and stared bleary-eyed at the chart. It
was almost one A.M. The page in the chart suddenly seemed darker.
I really must be getting exhausted, I thought. No, someone was
standing in my light.

I looked up to see an enormous man standing next to me, in sil-
houette against the hall light, his bulk blotting out everything in my
field of vision. He towered over me. He must have been six-foot-eight
or nine, over three hundred pounds. His arms reached down and
touched the desk.

"Where's Mrs. Gore?"

"She's in the intensive-care unit," I said, checking to make sure
I knew where the exits were.

"Why?"

"She was upset and was sent to the state hospital. She took an overdose of pills." You'll notice I didn't say, "I sent her." I said, "She was sent."

"Why? There's nothing wrong with her mind! All these people are against us. What room is she in?"

I pointed. . . . He walked to her room and took one brief look inside. He stood at her door, clenched his fists, and groaned. He pressed the elevator call button. When the elevator came, he put his hand over the electric eye and held the elevator on the floor. He waited for a minute, stared at me menacingly, and finally pulled his hand back, allowing the elevator door to close and take him away.

I waited for my heart to slow down and then wrote a few more sentences in the chart, briefly describing Bessie's husband and suggesting that this case may be a *folie à deux*—a rare paranoid psychosis shared by two people in which the weaker usually adopts the delusional system of the stronger. Actually I wrote the additional note to make me feel a little better. A nice intellectual defense, but I was trembling.

"Who was *that* staring in at the door?" asked Les, coming out of the intensive care unit.

"Mr. Gore, I guess."

"No wonder Bessie's paranoid," Les said, trying to smile. I didn't see what was even remotely funny.

I found room 407, our new on-call room. I was so tired I forgot to pick up a surgical scrub suit, the baggy green pants and shirt that I usually wore in place of PJs when I was on call. This way, if I were called to the ward for an emergency I wouldn't need to get dressed, just throw a white lab coat on over the scrub suit and run—an old trick from my medical days. I took off my clothes and got into bed. I located the phone, a pad of paper, and a pencil—the essentials for being on call. I looked around the room to get my bearings. It looked lived in. There were more artifacts around than usual—a few books, a box with some linen, not much else. I shut off the light.

At two thirty the telephone rang. It was Mrs. Gore's brother, Leroy. "Dr. Viscott? We don't know what to do!"

"What's wrong?" I asked, half asleep.

"Henry has been calling us and says he's going to kill us."

"Why don't you and your brother bring your families together in one house tonight?"

"He won't come for us tonight. Tonight, he said he was going to get Dr. Clift, you know, the doctor who gave her the pills, and slit his throat. I never saw Henry this worked up before, and I've seen him bad. He says he'll kill Dr. Clift for causing this."

"Well," I said, rubbing my eyes, "you could call the police if you feel you need protection."

"That's a joke, doctor. We don't get any police protection in our neighborhood, but doubling up our families is a good idea. He won't come for us until he's through with Dr. Clift. And then you."

"How can you be sure?"

"Because he asked who the doctor was who sent Bessie to the state hospital and I just sort of blurted out your name. I told him you signed the papers."

"Well, I don't think I'm going to worry about it," I said, lying through my teeth.

"He had a butcher knife with him."

"You people double up," I repeated, and hung up.

The guilt I already felt could make me a good candidate for a paranoid imagination, I realized. But why should I worry? The resident quarters were locked. Mr. Gore wouldn't know how to find his way to my room anyway. . . .

I went back to sleep remembering Louis Fry, a medical resident who trained with me in Saint Louis. He left his psychiatric residency after a man had come onto the ward following his wife's suicide and had shot and killed his wife's doctor. . . .

The door of my room suddenly began to move. I could see a crack of light growing wider. Someone was pushing the door to see if it were locked. I could hear a key fumbling in the lock. I was standing up on the bed. The door unlocked, started to open. I was standing up on my bed listening to myself scream. It was as if I was dreaming, it seemed so unreal.

The door slammed shut.

I caught my breath. I was definitely awake, trying to remember what had just happened. *Had* I screamed or had I dreamed it? Had Mr. Gore really been there?

Before I had a chance to decide, the door opened again and a hand covered with blood reached in and turned the light on. I opened up again, louder than ever. The bloody hand pulled back, slamming the door behind. I was terrified. It was as if all the punishments I'd ever thought I deserved were being visited upon me. I felt as if I were about to be executed, and not feeling very brave about it. I still questioned whether I had imagined it all, but on the floor were several drops of bright red blood.

Outside the door there was a commotion. Someone was talking loudly in Chinese. I could hear the footsteps of people running. Someone shouted, "What's happening?"

The door was suddenly kicked open. There I was, still standing naked on my bed, staring at Les, Frank, D.J., Candy, and Julian Pell, the third-year medical student, and Dr. Lung, a Chinese resident who was bleeding from his arm. He'd been living in room 407 until today, and was supposed to go to another hospital on rotation. But he had been away for a few days and had forgotten that someone else would be moving into his room. When he heard me yell he pulled his arm back so rapidly that he tore open a vein in his forearm.

"What he doing in my bed?" Lung demanded, holding up his bloody arm for me to see.

"Having a rough night?" Frank asked.

"You apparently thought Lung was Mr. Gore," Les said, walking into the room to throw me a towel, which I put around myself, too glad to be alive to be embarrassed.

Dr. Lung was calling me names which my father had taught me as a kid, so I knew they were not complimentary. "What you doing in my bed, *Mucka hai?*"

"This not your bed. I take over room 407 now. You go rotate someplace else."

"How about rotating down to the emergency room?" Frank suggested to Dr. Lung. "I think you could use a few stitches in that arm." Frank pulled the Chinese resident away.

"Come on," Frank said to a wide-eyed Julian. "You want to learn how to put in stitches?"

"What's wrong with him?" Julian asked, pointing to me.

"Nothing," said Frank, putting one arm around Julian, shepherding him to the emergency room. "He's a psychiatric resident . . . they *all* scream in their sleep!"

D.J. gave me a smile and shook her head. I was grateful for her silence.

In the morning Les told me Mrs. Gore was out of coma.

"Great," I said.

"Yeah. By the way, Mrs. Gore's brothers warned the police and they arrested her husband trying to break into Dr. Clift's home. He had a butcher knife."

I didn't say a word.

CHAPTER FOURTEEN

SPRING MADNESS

SUDDENLY it was spring! Not one of those New England springs that was the delayed departure of a hard winter, leaving black muddy snow right into April, but a scented spring with magnolias blooming early along the wooded mall. Lunchtimes we lay on the hospital roof, basking in the sun fourteen stories above the traffic, and looked out over a budding city, breathing in the fragrant smell of the earth as it floated up above the exhaust fumes of the traffic. The days seemed to be moving more quickly. When you're frightened time seems to slow down, but I was getting to feel more at ease with the routine. I knew what to expect when I came in from the cool air and brilliant sun of an early spring morning and walked onto the ward.

April on the ward. A lovely spring with fine days could be a cruel tormentor to patients. All through the long unhappy winter they had looked forward to the time when the sun would melt away the wornout snow and gild the trees with their first green. The despair of many dark winter nights had been brightened by the hope that the spring would take away their sadness with the snow.

If winter had left behind the sad memory of a merry Christmas that never materialized, its dreariness at least gave patients reason to think that its short dark days and overcast skies were the external cause of all their troubles. Naked April was crueler. Its loveliness and glistening warmth ended the masquerade and made patients realize that while everyone around them was rejoicing in the blossoming of spring, they were feeling no better. Treacherous April tended to make patients doubly sad because for some there seemed nothing left to blame for the way they felt but themselves. More patients tried to kill themselves in April than in any other month.

Because Bamberg 5 was an open ward, it was not really suitable for suicidal patients. Its only form of built-in security was the heavy-duty metal screens that covered the windows, and any patient who wanted to get through them could do so if he really set his mind to it.

Cynthia Papas was more actress than suicidal. She was "looking for controls," as Larry Danielson put it, and the ward personnel were enlisted to help her control herself. Cynthia Papas was also the only patient to get through a window on the ward that year.

Since we did not have the mechanical resources to restrain patients, the work had to be done by people—more accurately, since we couldn't lock a patient up, the patient had to be looked after by the nurses. It was very easy for me to sit down with Cynthia Papas in my office and set limits by saying, "You may not leave the ward today. You must swallow your medication in front of the nurses. I'm not going to let you store up pills like a squirrel and take them all at once," but it would be the nurses' responsibility to make sure that Cynthia followed my instructions. After all, I was not around the ward as much as they were. I was with patients, or in conference.

We were at the conference table when Bella Grable opened the door and said, "Dr. Viscott, they need you."

Amanda Little had run after Cynthia Papas, who had managed to unscrew the protective screen from the window in another patient's room and climb through to a ledge five stories above the sidewalk. She was staring straight ahead, afraid to look down.

Cynthia Papas was a very tiny woman, barely ninety pounds. At twenty-seven she still looked like a teen-ager, and still dressed like one. Her problem was closely related to her looks. She refused to grow up, or to take any responsibility for anything in her life, and she expected other people to do everything for her. When she didn't get what she wanted, she acted in extreme ways to force people into giving in, or doing *something*. Usually you had no choice but to act because the situations she created were always suicidal emergencies or at least appeared that way. Even if you were sure she would eventually back down, there was, of course, always the remote chance she wouldn't. The staff decided to resist giving in to Cynthia's demands, to tolerate her behavior without responding so she would learn that her childishness didn't work in getting her what she wanted. It was to be a kind of retraining.

Great, I thought. I'll tell the brilliant plan to the hospital death committee when they meet next Thursday. I could imagine appearing before the grand inquisitor, Dr. Scarpia, Union Hospital's administrator.

I moved closer toward the window and looked down at the ledge, which was about three feet wide. There was Cynthia, child-like, almost lovely, outlined against a building across the street that was glaring in the warm spring sun. I pulled myself up onto the windowsill and sat there. I jammed my foot between the wall and the radiator pipe behind me to anchor myself.

"Cynthia," I said, in my high school principal's voice, "what are you doing out there?"

"I'm going to—"

"You know that patients aren't allowed out on the ledges," I said authoritatively, cutting her off. I didn't want her to finish her statement "I'm going to jump" because I didn't want her to feel obligated to follow it through. By taking a strong stand, indirectly I could at least give her a chance to save face. And I wasn't challenging her by directly telling her not to commit suicide. I was just telling her she'd broken the rules and was off-limits.

Cynthia turned and looked at me. She appeared confused by my approach. Her long red hair had fallen in her eyes. She brushed it away.

"And besides," I continued, "your room's a mess! You didn't make your bed this morning!" I'd seen her room before and knew that she had.

"I did too," she said, puzzled. She leaned toward me. She looked down to see where her feet were.

I leaned out the window and threw both arms around her. We were back in the room before you could say "foolhardy psychiatrist."

"Leave me *alone.*"

"Go back to your room for the rest of the morning," I said, rigid disciplinarian that I was. "When you decide to behave like a mature grown-up you'll be treated like one."

Cynthia marched off to her room, followed by Amanda, who turned to me, smiling, and said, "Someone around here is finally showing some sense." She knew how to make a fellow feel good.

Nurses were your right arm. Sometimes they were both arms. They often gave you the feedback you needed to make a diagnosis or design a treatment plan. Patients tended to see nurses as friends more than they did doctors. Often they would tell the doctors what they *thought* the doctors wanted to hear. Stanley Lovett's patients told him a lot about their dreams because at the time he was all involved in discussing his own dreams with his psychoanalyst and must have inadvertently revealed his interest.

Sometimes the only decent therapeutic relationship established was the one between the nurse and the patient. Jackie Rose could sit down with a patient for a few hours and at the end of the session you would feel that something important had taken place. The nurses saw patients for as long as they felt necessary. They seemed more flexible than the doctors.

I came to believe the concept of the fifty-minute hour was confining and constricting. Some patients had all they could stand of me in less than fifteen minutes, especially if they were psychotic. I thought a few patients had overstayed their welcome after five minutes, and there was little more that could or should be accomplished by seeing them for any longer. With other patients I felt I was only warming up after an hour, that the ice had just been broken and the good stuff was just beginning.

The nurses had less need to follow the rigid structure of the fifty-minute hour. According to Jerry Gelb, the rationale for maintaining a rigid hour was the simple practicality of being able to keep appointments. It also gave the doctor a tidy way to end each session. He could say, "Well, I see our time is up. We'll have to continue next time."

When a doctor makes a mistake, and we frequently do, there are so many checks built into the routine that we usually catch it ourselves before we need admit it. If you follow the standard procedure, you'll eventually catch your mistakes. The trouble comes when you're wrong and don't follow procedure. If you stay out of trouble and don't follow standard procedure, no one seems to care; but make a mistake while deviating from the accepted ways, even if the accepted ways were in error, and the Dr. Scarpias will land on you and cut you up good. Sometimes doctors also get into trouble because they don't read the nurses' notes carefully enough.

Mrs. Tuoey, the wife of an elderly physician, was complaining of pain in the hip for several weeks. Bert felt she'd been depressed—she had refused to go outside her house to eat, and she'd been unable to sleep. Dr. Tuoey was in his seventies and had little patience with his wife. He only had patience with his *real* patients, the ones with *real* disease. He gave his wife some medication, which didn't seem to help her. Finally, he called in a friend, an internist, to see her. All Mrs. Tuoey would talk about to the internist was how much pain she had and how hopeless and sad she felt about it. "Where's the pain?" the internist had asked. "Everywhere," she had told him, "everywhere and nowhere." The internist, who knew something about psychiatry, decided she was a classic example of somatizing, using the language of the body to communicate feelings, in her case, depressive feelings.

Bert presented Mrs. Tuoey to Dr. Gavin. Dr. Gavin decided that Mrs. Tuoey should walk into the conference room with Amanda Little's help. He wanted to show her that we were interested in her real feelings, not her hip pain. She was rather vague about the pain during the interview.

"How do you feel?" asked Dr. Gavin.

"I'd feel better if I could get one of you doctors to help me."

"Did you have anyone special in mind?" asked Dr. Gavin, thinking she really meant her husband.

"Just someone who could help." She looked at Bert. "Ow." She winced as she shifted her position in the chair. "I just think I need someone a little more experienced than Dr. Feinstein, even though he's a lovely boy. He reminds me of my husband when he was in medical school—Oh, excuse me," she apologized, pulling the dagger out of Bert. "You're not in medical school anymore, are you?"

"How much more experienced a doctor do you think you need?" asked Gavin. "Ten years? Twenty?"

"I don't know." Mrs. Tuoey was puzzled by the question.

"What about a doctor in his seventies? Would *he* have enough experience for you?"

"I don't follow you. It's hard for me to stand." Mrs. Tuoey revealed her feelings again by talking about her somatic illness.

"I think you'd like to get another doctor interested in the way you feel. Maybe you'd like your husband to show *he* cares more?" Gavin, sharp as ever, was really hammering away.

"Yes," said Mrs. Tuoey, and began to cry.

Gavin could get to a patient's feelings instantly. I really envied that guy. What technique!

Unfortunately, Mrs. Tuoey limped out of the conference room uncured, wincing with each step. "I have to lie down," she said as she hobbled out, clinging to Amanda.

"That was a great job of interpreting the secondary gain of her illness, Dr. Gavin," said Stanley Lovett in unrestrained admiration, not to mention jargon. "Secondary gain" means benefits accruing to a patient for being sick—attention; caring; decreased responsibilities —often the reason some patients prefer illness to health.

"What should we do with this woman?" asked Larry. "She's a nuisance on the ward. She really won't cooperate."

"Getting her out of bed is a full-time job for Amanda," Bert said.

"Well, she's tough," said Gavin. "But I wouldn't let that get me down." Amanda returned to the conference room. "She needs to be encouraged to walk, and she needs *our* encouragement that she can do it. I would talk about her hip pain as if it were a metaphor for her emotional pain." By "our" Gavin meant "Amanda's." I couldn't picture Bert trying to get Mrs. Tuoey to walk.

"Where's her pain located?" I asked Bert.

"Everywhere and nowhere," he said, repeating the phrase that hypochondriacs are supposed to use and that Mrs. Tuoey had used with the internist. I read the chart briefly and noticed that Amanda had made extensive comments on it. Amanda seldom wrote long notes. Most of them referred to Mrs. Tuoey's pain. I guessed that Amanda didn't feel comfortable about Mrs. Tuoey. She felt Mrs. Tuoey needed more attention and wanted to be sure her protests were in writing.

On the way back from lunch Bert and I met Amanda, who had just finished walking Mrs. Tuoey as per Dr. Gavin's orders.

"She really has a lot of pain in that leg," said Amanda. "Why don't you people X ray it?"

"Hasn't she been X rayed?" I asked.

"I'm sure she has," said Bert, picking up her chart, "with all the doctors who've seen her."

The only X ray done was one of Mrs. Tuoey's chest. Her chest was fine!

We looked at Mrs. Tuoey. She was lying flat on her back, her eyes closed in pain. Her right leg was bent at the knee. It turned outward and it appeared shortened.

"I don't know how to tell you this," Bert began, "but I think that lady has a broken hip."

"Couldn't be. Dr. Gavin said—" I caught myself.

"I know Gavin's got insight," Bert said, "but he doesn't have X-ray eyes. And no one's ever X rayed that hip. Everyone's been guessing. Even if Gavin were right about the dynamics of her depression, she still could have a broken hip." I nodded. Amanda pulled back Mrs. Tuoey's nightgown, revealing a large red swelling in the area of her right hip.

"I'm going to get sick," said Bert, looking very upset.

The operation on Mrs. Tuoey's fractured hip took the better part of the next morning.

She was lucky.

I thought about Amanda trying to force Mrs. Tuoey to walk, and writing long notes in the chart to cover her actions, while nobody looked at the woman's hip. I also thought of us giving Amanda encouragement, telling her to interpret the metaphor of Mrs. Tuoey's pain by mentioning how she "couldn't get along" or how she "couldn't stand it" and relating those feelings to her husband. I could hear us making mental bets about where Mrs. Tuoey would really like to have gone if she could have walked, since one of the pet theories about psychosomatic illness is that a disabling symptom involves a forbidden wish or feeling. Perhaps Mrs. Tuoey actually wanted to leave her husband and needed the symptom of a painful leg to keep her at home. I could hear all of us inventing explanations for her pain.

We were so accustomed to the logic of our own discipline, and had learned so well how to use it to explain what we saw and to interpret patients' symptoms, that it was possible for us to follow all standard and accepted procedures and still be completely wrong and not realize we'd made a mistake.

I learned something very important from Mrs. Tuoey. I learned that no matter how well the logic of my discipline explained the emotional meaning of a patient's symptom, I could not be sure that what I understood so well was everything there was to know. I could still be missing something—perhaps the most important thing.

Mrs. Tuoey did in fact use her leg to express her feelings about her husband, and she would probably continue to do so after she left the hospital. Gavin was right about that. But it was also true that she had a real injury. Because we saw through her emotional symptoms so easily, no one thought to investigate further to see if there were anything physically wrong with her. It was only Amanda's reluctance to comply that broke through the barriers our system of thinking had raised.

The next time we had a conference with Dr. Gavin, Bert brought up Mrs. Tuoey's operation. "Is that so?" said Dr. Gavin. There really wasn't anything anyone could say. We were all guilty in our own way. Mrs. Tuoey's internist, Dr. Gavin, and all us residents. It was an obvious diagnosis. We had jumped on the psychiatric bandwagon to win Gavin's approval and to avoid appearing stupid— the usual reasons people abandon their own common sense and make mistakes.

As the weather grew warmer, the pace on the ward became hectic. There were several college students hospitalized on Bamberg 5. Spring was a difficult time for students. They worried about not getting into the college of their choice, or their family's choice, or were afraid of flunking out second semester for good. It was also tax time, the season when accountants became upset and the season when many of their clients also became upset.

There were usually more women than men on the ward because women seemed to express their feelings more and give in to them more. Men tended to hold their feelings in and were more likely to develop arteriosclerosis and suffer heart attacks as their reactions to stress. The medical wards of Union Hospital held many patients who had been admitted in disguise, who should have been psychiatric patients.

A flood of patients was admitted that spring and patients seemed to move in and out of the hospital more quickly than at other times. Two of my patients did get well astoundingly fast.

Susan Morris was a middle-aged ex-nun. In the convent she'd spent all her time worrying whether or not she had said a certain word in a prayer and, doubting herself, she would start the prayer again at the beginning, as obsessive-compulsives characteristically behave. She confided to me in a whisper that she must have been a year or two behind the others because she rarely finished any prayer. Suddenly, within one week after hospitalization, Susan became almost completely free of her obsessional thinking and was able to concentrate on other thoughts. She bought some new clothes, read a book, called up old friends, and left the hospital. In the month after her discharge she started to date for the first time and seemed to enjoy it. She seemed like a new person.

Mrs. Carr had also been a severe obsessive-compulsive most of her life. She worried about everything, including whether or not any object she saw floating in the water was the head of someone drowning. She tortured herself and her husband by worrying if she should go back and rescue the person, if it were a person. Often, at two in the morning, the two of them would go back to make sure. She also upset her husband because she hadn't had sexual relations with him in over a decade, and also because she would continually prowl around their house at night to check the windows, the doors, the lights, and to make sure the gas was off. In less than two weeks after hospitalization she also suddenly stopped having troublesome obsessive thoughts. She even had sexual relations with her husband again. Mr. Carr thought I should be elected to the psychiatric hall of fame.

"What did you say to these women?" asked Jerry Gelb, looking intently at me.

"Nothing really unusual, just the standard questions—'What did you feel about this? what did you feel about that?' You know." I was a little embarrassed.

"David, you *had* to say more than that. What was your focus?" He *had* to understand what happened.

"Well, I really felt a bit overwhelmed by Susan Morris and Mrs. Carr. You know how touchy some obsessive-compulsive patients are to work with. Well, with two in the hospital at the same time I felt I was really in for some frustrating hours."

"I advised you not to set unrealistically high goals with them," Gelb reminded me.

"Yes, and I told myself that with these two patients I was not going to try to be a miracle worker. I just wanted to put the lid on the situation and get them out of the hospital."

"Right," said Gelb, reaming his pipe. "Well?"

"I considered the possible ways of dealing with them and I decided to concentrate on the feeling that was easiest to reach."

"Yes, what feeling was that?" asked Jerry, smiling now. "You know how isolated obsessive-compulsives are from their feelings. Isolating feelings is one of their strongest defenses. They can talk about a feeling intellectually, but they don't feel what they talk about."

"I was aware of that, so I made a list of every feeling I ever heard of. It was a huge list." Jerry laughed. "Then I studied the list to see which feelings would be most difficult for an obsessive-compulsive to isolate."

"That's a new approach! What did you decide?" Jerry was very curious.

"That the feeling most difficult to isolate was the feeling of isolation, of loneliness itself. So all I talked about with Carr and Morris was their lonely feelings and how difficult it must be to feel lonely. Anytime I heard something that sounded like a lonely feeling I would comment on it. When Susan Morris told me how she'd fallen behind in her prayers, I said it must have felt very lonely being in such a difficult struggle with none of the other nuns knowing about it, and that she must have felt different and apart all the time. She seemed to respond to that with a lot of feeling."

"What about other feelings?" Jerry asked.

"We talked about other feelings, but in a special way. When I pointed out something like the jealousy Miss Morris felt toward the nuns who seemed to be so comfortably adjusted to the convent, I stayed focused on the lonely aspects of being jealous, like not being able to share her feelings of jealousy. I always talked about her loneliness first, the feeling she could not isolate, and then I attached that loneliness to the other feelings, like lonely resentment."

"And with Mrs. Carr?" Jerry asked.

"I just did the same thing. I really wasn't interested in knocking myself out with these two obsessive patients. It takes too much out of me. I hate struggling with their logic for hours to extract a minute of feeling."

"Specifically, *what* did you say to Mrs. Carr?"

"Remember what you told me when I discussed her with you the first time? You said Mrs. Carr was a very angry lady below the surface and that this anger was the source of many of her problems. You said I should tell her . . ." I thought for a moment, trying to remember Jerry's advice. "What did you say? I'm sorry, it slipped my mind."

"Something like, 'Mrs. Carr, I know you're not the sort of person who likes to be angry,'" said Jerry, restating his therapeutic remark.

"Well, I told Mrs. Carr that and she agreed with me. And when I pointed out how lonely I suspected she was when she felt angry, it made more sense to her. We talked about her loneliness going around the house at night checking to make sure the stove was turned off. I always focused on the loneliness instead of the anger beneath, like her unconscious wish to turn the gas on and asphyxiate her husband. I also pointed out how hard it must be to feel anger alone. I just followed the same pattern with about everything she brought up."

"Well," said Jerry, "that *is* interesting! You know, this probably represents a transference cure. These patients somehow adopted your superego and put their own superego aside. I think your technique of dealing with the feelings that can't be isolated is a good one, but I doubt it's responsible for either of these two patients improving like this. It seems a typical transference cure in which the patient identifies himself with the nonthreatening part of the therapist." Jerry was happy. He had decided what was going on and had managed to fit it into his system.

"Do you think pointing out the loneliness and sharing it made that more possible?" I asked.

"Maybe, you made them feel you understood them. I think the major point, David, is that you tend to be open and accept people as they are. I know you sometimes think your patients' antics are silly, even laughable, and sometimes you do retell them here in pretty funny ways, but you don't really make fun of them. You come across to your patients as genuinely interested. I talked with Cynthia Papas after you pulled her off the ledge and then went after her, telling her to pick up her room. She said she knew you didn't care about the room and was glad you didn't lean on how stupid she'd been. You let her save face. It was as if you were saying, 'Don't give me any of this suicide crap, you're just trying to get out of cleaning your room.' Cynthia knew you were very serious about helping her."

This was damn nice to hear, and encouraged me to open up more. "Jerry, would you think I was crazy if I told you I'd worked out a treatment plan based on the same theory for other kinds of problems? Why can't therapy focus on the feelings that can't be defended against by each patient? You'd make a list of the defenses in each disease and try to figure out which feelings could get through and work on them."

"Interesting," said Gelb, noncommittal. "By the way, don't be too disappointed when Mrs. Carr and Miss Morris both lapse back. Transference cures are frequently short-lived."

"Oh," I said. As it turned out, Miss Morris got a job and eventually married; after two years I never heard from her again. Mrs. Carr went back to her suburban psychiatrist after three weeks in the hospital. For a while she saw him once a month, then stopped. Some of the symptoms returned from time to time, but in much milder form. She did well for five years at least, when I lost contact with her. Who *really* knows what was going on?

Having a patient who is suddenly "cured" can be very embarrassing for a resident. First of all, you have to disown any role in the patient's sudden improvement because it would be ridiculous to claim responsibility for results and then discover you might have nothing to do with them, although you might secretly want to have a magic power to cure patients. Secretly? What am I talking about? You openly wished you had the power. Second, because the patient's outcome was uncertain you didn't want to set yourself up for a lot of "I told you so's" when the patient fell apart (which Jerry had implicitly warned me about).

Because I had two transference cures on the ward at the same time, my problems were multiplied. My worst problem was that I could almost believe it was really me who did it. I took a lot of ribbing.

"It's a typical flight into health," said Stanley Lovett, translated roughly as sudden improvement in a patient's symptoms. "That's really just another defense. The patients don't seem to have any more insight than before."

"Who said it was solely a matter of insight?" D.J. said. "Maybe they're *feeling* more." D.J., as you've seen, liked to put Stanley down.

"It sure is interesting, David," Bert remarked. "Maybe you'd like to put your hand on one of my patients. You know Fred Donovan, the manic. How about curing him for me, and laying your hands on Mrs. Craven, too, while you're at it."

"Two of my patients have already requested a transfer," Marty said. "It's really funny to hear them all talking about you in the lounge at night. I can't believe all the nice things they say."

"How are you at making hair grow?" asked Larry.

They were reminding me that you win one, you lose one. Same goes for two.

CHAPTER FIFTEEN

CONSPIRACY AGAINST THE WEAK

$\mathcal{S}$OME of the admissions to Bamberg 5 were ridiculous. They often resulted from people losing control and picking on the most vulnerable member of their family, labeling him sick and sending him to the hospital as a human sacrifice to solve everyone else's problems.

Anyhow that was the way it seemed with Peter Atkins. Peter was seventeen and had growing pains. He was continually arguing with his mother over the proper length of his hair, fighting with his father over the use of the family car, and battling with his younger brother over anything at all. His brother also fought with his parents, just about as frequently.

One evening, all the other members of the family formally declared war on Peter. Peter and his brother were fighting over the ownership of a particular sports jacket Peter planned to wear on a date that night. Father wasn't sure Peter should have the car since he hadn't cut the lawn as he had promised. Nor had he cut his hair, so mother also joined the fun.

Understandably Peter felt outnumbered. Father called in a next-door neighbor, Dr. Blade, a local surgeon who knew Peter well. Dr. Blade came over and tried to calm Peter down. He gave him advice based on what Peter's father, never one for objectivity, told him on the phone. Peter told the good doctor to "fuck off" because Peter had a date.

Dr. Blade told the family, "That's not like the Peter I know. Something has changed. He may be having an emotional break."

Another reason why I love surgeons—at times like this they all seem to act like a Back Passage.

Peter grabbed the disputed sports jacket and headed for the door. Dr. Blade shouted, "Don't let him out." Father and brother pounced on him and held him down. While he was being held down on the Oriental rug in the entrance hall, he started to cry, something he hadn't done in years. That stopped them. At Dr. Blade's suggestion (prompted by his guilt?) Peter was taken by ambulance to Bamberg 5. By ambulance! Can you believe that? I wanted to ask Mr. Atkins when Peter arrived why he didn't have a police escort. I'm sure Atkins would have told me that Dr. Blade didn't think of it. Would someone please check to see if Blue Cross covers police escorts?

I had no choice but to admit Peter overnight because the situation at home was so overheated. I opened our session by saying, "I've already heard your father's, your mother's, and your brother's side of the story—all at once. If you've been through what they put me through you probably could use a vacation from them." Peter looked clobbered but he managed to smile. After Peter told me his story I said, "Well, this is the mistake of the century. When do you want to go home? How's tomorrow morning?"

"Home?" he said, startled. "I can go home?"

"Sure, there's nothing wrong with you," I said, getting up from my chair. "Want a pizza?"

Peter stared at me disbelievingly, but eventually managed to put away two pizzas at Primo's Pizza down the street. He liked them large, with extra cheese and without anchovies. Peter, after all, was a growing boy. We talked and cleared the air. By the time we got back to the ward Peter at least felt someone understood him. He was completely relaxed, although somewhat thirsty. Helen Doran, who adored adolescents, gave him a quart of milk, which he gulped down from the cardboard container in one swig, in classic locker-room-after-winning-the-big-game style. Peter asked for some cookies to wash down the milk.

"It's great to see a normal kid on the ward for a change," said Helen, loud enough for Peter to hear, and handed him a box of cookies. "Leave at least one for someone else," she added. Peter left two. "Besides being normal, he's also generous," said Helen pursing her lips.

Carol Downs, the psychiatric social worker, appeared on the ward. It was nine thirty. Why is she here? I wondered. "I was asked to speak with you about the Atkins family," said Carol. "I would like to see the Atkinses and evaluate each family member individually and then together as a family unit later. It's a new program in the social service department. We'll be seeing the family of each new patient as well as the patient from the time of admission. We'll follow them through the hospitalization all the way to discharge and in follow-up visits after discharge."

"Sure, but you'd better hurry, Carol, because this kid is going to be discharged tomorrow so he can make Saturday morning baseball practice."

"You can't do that without a formal presentation!" Carol protested. "This is a new program. My supervisor and the head of the psychiatric social worker training program will be at the presentation. It's important. I've been assigned to the case. We need a minimum of fifteen case studies to meet the requirements of the grant."

"Well, you'll just have to evaluate the Atkinses on an outpatient basis."

"No, I can't. We need at least one week in the hospital to determine an emotional baseline."

"Well, this patient isn't going to be here a week. So he isn't suitable. And I think your study is unscientific." (I shouldn't have said that.)

"Well, he can't be discharged without a workup," Carol said. "That's *standard operating procedure*." Carol was pulling protocol and at a loose end in her cardigan. Here it was a warm May night and she was still wearing a sweater!

"This kid shouldn't have been admitted." I practically shouted. "I won't compound one error by making another. I'm writing an order to discharge him tomorrow."

I did.

The next morning I told Bert what was going on and left the hospital at nine. Tough luck, Bert, having duty on a weekend as beautiful as this.

When I came in on Monday I found Peter Atkins waiting for me at the nurses' station.

"What the hell are you doing here?" I asked.

"They changed your order."

"Can I see you?" said Bert, who apparently was also waiting for me to appear. "It's about this case."

"Come on, Peter, you're going to sit in on this."

"Good for you, David," called out Jackie Rose as we walked to my office. "Let the kid know what's happening."

Bert sat in my chair. I sat on the desk. Peter sat in the patient's chair.

"Carol Downs," Bert began, his chair squeaking like crazy, "called her supervisor, who called Dr. Noyes, and Dr. Noyes rescinded your order."

"On what authority?" I demanded, forgetting Bert was on my side.

"He made up some bullshit about it being too impulsive a decision and that an adequate evaluation was not possible in that short a time."

"Maybe not enough time for Noyes to evaluate an adolescent, because no adolescent I know would talk to that authoritarian sonofabitch."

"We got along just great," Peter said. "You guys have the same bullshit here that I get at home."

"The kid's got a point," Bert said. "Did you have breakfast?" he asked, inviting Peter to join him in the coffee shop. *Everyone* could tell Peter was OK.

I walked by Dr. Noyes' office and asked to see him. Field Marshall von Noyes happened to be free. As a matter of fact, his secretary said he *wanted* to see me.

"Ah, yes," Dr. Noyes began, "I hear there was some sort of misunderstanding this weekend. You know Dr. Michael Blade, the surgeon, don't you? A fine man. A fine surgeon, and one of the most respected people on the medical school staff. An excellent teacher— excellent. Well, when one of our own, so to speak, sends us a patient, I think we owe it to him to give the patient as professional a workup as we know how, don't you? We must not act impulsively. It's not only bad practice, but it gives the department a bad name. Also, there is a departmental study for which, according to the descriptions of the case I have received, this boy and his family would be excellent candidates. I'd like to see that we get a good baseline of family-patient interaction for the study. You do agree, don't you?"

"No! I—"

"Are you so confident of what you casually observed about this young man during a time of crisis, when his entire family was confused and he was in turmoil, that you would discharge him after so short a time? In my opinion that is very poor judgment. Very poor indeed. We don't discharge patients unless they've been properly evaluated."

"He was evaluated," I said.

"By you." Noyes stated.

"Yes, by me. This boy was—"

"I am quite familiar with his story. I spoke with the head of social service."

"But she didn't see the patient!"

"No, but Miss Downs saw the family."

"Do you mean that a decision based on the firsthand experience of a resident trained in your program with a patient is going to be overruled by people who never saw the patient? That's the craziest thing I ever heard of."

"That patient must be evaluated before discharge," Noyes said, restating his position. "And Dr. Viscott, if you have any comments or opinions you will keep them to yourself. We don't want to appear anti-research."

I called Jerry Gelb as soon as I got out of Noyes' office. You can't win an argument against Noyes, and I was afraid that if I tried he'd hold it against me and be vindictive enough to ruin my references.

Jerry was sympathetic to my argument. He saw Peter Atkins, agreed with me, and was willing to sign a discharge order. Peter Atkins left; Carol Downs called her supervisor; and M. Austin Noyes called Jerry and me in on the carpet.

"What do you have to say, Dr. Viscott?"

"I don't think he needs to say anything," said Jerry. "I saw the Atkins boy. I read the admission note. I know Dr. Viscott, and I trust his judgment. The standard I used, Austin, was simple. I asked myself, if the boy were my private patient would I keep him in the hospital. The answer was I would not. I didn't think the boy even needed an appointment for a follow-up visit. To keep him in the hospital unjustifiably would only have given him more ammunition to use against his parents and make it more difficult for him to come to terms with them later on."

"I think the boy should stay here, Jerry," Noyes repeated. "I said as much."

"But you didn't talk with him," Jerry pointed out.

"I'm planning to see him on Wednesday. I have a meeting with the Planning Committee for the new mental health center on Mondays."

Noyes had not been terribly active treating patients for several years. He rarely saw patients as far as I could tell. He was an administrative psychiatrist, a political. He wrote a lot of articles, enjoyed an excellent reputation and was involved in a lot of departmental in-fighting. He arranged university appointments for the people he liked and was active in the politics and planning of community mental health facilities. He often carried blueprints with him to conferences. It got to the point where I felt I was taking a graduate course in architecture. I suspected he saw the Governor more frequently than he saw any patient, especially an adolescent patient like Peter.

No one in the department really seemed to like Dr. Noyes, and many psychiatrists, supposedly even some grown-up psychoanalysts, were afraid of him. Amazing. Or maybe not, if you had certain ambitions.

M. Austin Noyes stopped and looked at both of us, as if he expected us to understand how much more important his appointment was than this trivial matter.

"Wednesday's a long time for a kid who wants to be out playing baseball," I said.

"Young people are remarkably resilient, Dr. Viscott. A few days in the hospital will not be as upsetting to him as you think. And certainly not as disruptive as the rebellion I'd have between this department and social services and the department of surgery. You've made Dr. Blade appear like an ass."

I kept my big mouth shut for a change, and walked out with Jerry. Jerry sighed. "I was sure you were going to say something." He was almost right.

One nice thing that happened that month was meeting Fern Woods. Fern had just been hired as the occupational therapist for Bamberg 5. During my internship I used to refer to OTs as basket weavers. OTs seemed to be very normal, nonscrewed-up types. I guess what they did was really therapeutic, even for them. Fern was a special kind of OT. She had a sixth, or maybe even a seventh, sense of what to do with a patient, and she did it instinctively. It was no big deal to her. One of my patients, Mr. Brodner, was deeply depressed and he got absolutely nothing out of therapy with me. He seemed to get much more out of OT than anything else. OT, apparently, was the one area where Mr. Brodner could function, and function well.

Mr. Brodner became depressed at his son's birthday party just as he opened his presents. At that moment when his presents were all about, he felt a strong surge of hatred for the boy and a powerful wish to stick a knife through his heart. Mr. Brodner loved his son very much and was terrified by his feelings. Having been in therapy many

years, he knew all the ropes. He was very verbal, but talking about
his feelings didn't seem to help. When he was admitted, his therapist,
Dr. Clarkson, relinquished treatment to me, as was customary during
a patient's stay on Bamberg 5. He had no suggestions. After some
weeks of deepening depression, Jerry Gelb said, "I know Bud Clarkson
pretty well. He may be a dull guy, but he's a good therapist. If he's in
a corner and you're in a corner, and all the drugs that this man has
been swallowing aren't helping, we should consider electroshock
therapy." From a psychoanalyst's mouth!

"Did you just read an article last night on how psychoanalytically
oriented psychiatrists neglect electroshock when it's indicated, or do
you really believe that?" I asked.

"Don't be such a wiseass," said Jerry, puffing away on his pipe.
"I can't see that we're doing anything for him, and it might help."

"But he has all the wrong signs. He had a long history of neurotic symptoms as a child. He doesn't have any psychomotor retarda-
tion. He has insomnia but doesn't wake early in the morning. He's
had his disease for years. There are some acute precipitating events
which caused the present problem, and he tends to be a hypochondriac." I was reeling off the points which supposedly indicated
a poor response to electroshock, and which I read in some journal
somewhere.

Jerry said, "Did you just make those up or do you really know
they're the negative prognostic signs?"

"I read it in a journal," I said. "I'll find it for you."

"Don't bother. Look, nothing else we're doing is working. Let's
give it a try."

I gave in. I was still grateful to Jerry for sticking up for me
with Peter Atkins and I was also curious about EST. I had never
seen a patient receive shock therapy. After all, I wasn't that sure that
shock therapy wouldn't help, and to tell the truth, Mr. Brodner was
not getting any better with me or with anyone else.

Fern Woods objejcted. "He seems to be making real progress in
OT. I have him making all the toys for himself that he wanted but
didn't have when he was a child. When he sighed and told me, 'But
there were so many,' I told him to start anyway."

Fern was wonderful. She was symbolically showing Mr. Brodner that he could have everything he wanted, but he would have to
do it himself. A brilliant attack, I felt.

In shock therapy the patient undergoes a grand mal seizure induced either by an electrical current administered to the patient's temples by means of an electrode or by inhaling a convulsion-producing gas. Sometimes insulin is used to induce a coma. How these shock therapies work is not entirely known, but they all stimulate the brain, altering temporarily its electrical and hormonal activity. Shock therapy has been shown to be beneficial in some forms of depression and in certain other emotional diseases.

Mr. Brodner was terrified. "I don't think it's going to help," he said. He was brought into the conference room on a litter. Jerry, Amanda, and I were there, waiting for the anesthesiologist to get ready. "Haven't done one of these in years up here," the anesthesiologist said. Jerry put his finger over his mouth to say, "Shh." Mr. Brodner was put to sleep with pentothal and given a muscle relaxant to soften the seizure so he wouldn't move or break any bones as a result. Electroshock properly administered is fairly safe today. Amanda held the electrodes on tight.

I reached over to the electroshock console. It was a little black machine with dials, levers, and buttons. It had been preset to give a precise amount of electricity.

"Throw the switch," Gelb said. My mind was someplace else.

"Excuse me, Dr. Gelb." I hadn't gotten to the point where I could call him "Jerry" in front of other members of the staff. "I didn't hear you."

"Throw the switch," Jerry repeated.

"You press a button," I corrected. "Read the manual." I pressed the button and a current of electricity caused Mr. Brodner to grimace. He quivered a bit, but that's all. In five minutes he was awake. Awake, but confused.

He stayed confused for five weeks. We gave him sixteen shocks. That's right, folks, sixteen, count 'em, sixteen. After number eight, when I could see nothing was happening, I mentioned my impression to Jerry.

I was very upset about giving shock treatments to Mr. Brodner. I was almost sure at the beginning that they wouldn't help. As the treatments progressed what we were doing seemed useless, and finally it felt barbaric. I began to complain more and more to Jerry, but he was intent on giving electroshock a fair chance. In looking back on this now, I'm a little ashamed of myself for not making a bigger stink about it because I had good reasons to believe I was right and that the outcome would not be beneficial. But Gelb *was* my supervisor and I did look up to him, and I was not *that* sure of myself in spite of the way I might have sounded. And that is an example of rationalization if I ever heard one.

At treatment number sixteen, we stopped. Mr. Brodner was not much better.

Fern Woods had taken over therapy during the time that Mr. Brodner was receiving shock. Mr. Brodner was just too vague and too confused for me to work with effectively. At least I couldn't make any headway. I think I actually felt too guilty to work with him.

In June, three weeks after we stopped therapy, Mr. Brodner suddenly and dramatically began to improve. It was remarkable. Jerry and I were sure it had nothing to do with anything I was discussing in therapy, and we attributed Mr. Brodner's improvement to the EST, a delayed reaction.

We were both wrong. Dear, charming, unassuming twenty-three-year-old Fern Woods had been at work like the shoemaker's elves. Mr. Brodner had just finished making all the toys he wanted to have as a child and began to cry bitterly over them all. "He just sat there and cried," said Fern. "He said a lot of things about his mother, but they were so garbled I couldn't make them out. He wouldn't talk about what he'd thought or done, and then I got an idea. Instead of my writing reports on each patient each day in OT, I decided that after each session everyone would write a report on themselves and then discuss it with the group. The group would decide whether or not it was acceptable, and what should be changed and why."

Smart. What Fern had done was to give each patient a chance to observe himself from another point of view, a sort of makeshift, unofficial group therapy. Each patient would have to put himself in the place of the occupational therapist and also consider what each of the other patients in the group would say about his or her self-opinions. It was a marvelous way of providing insight quickly.

Mr. Brodner was able to see himself as someone who had finally proved he could get what he wanted for himself. He now felt he could give to his children without feeling competitive with them, the way he had felt at his son's birthday party, watching him get toys and feeling cheated. Now he was making new toys for his children, and was even considering giving away the toys he made for himself, not to his own children but to children in an orphanage who'd had even less than he did as a child. In other words, he began to see his own past as better, and to see himself as stronger. And he did get better and stronger, and went home. Fern had a great deal to teach, but she didn't know what it was that she knew. She just did what came naturally.

Speaking of doing what came naturally, as my first year of residency was drawing to a close, my wife Judy was beginning to show. She was either in her fifth or sixth month. Her obstetrician wasn't sure. And they call psychiatry an inexact science! It was a rough pregnancy for her and for me, watching her suffer through it.

June was a time for fond good-byes to the people we liked, and a time for saying good-bye to the patients and preparing them for our departure. I sometimes found myself secretly hoping that some patients would miss me as much as Effie Sacks had missed Dr. Jabers. It was a time for cleaning out desks, for dictating final notes on patients, for getting charts up to date, and for writing off-service notes that made you sound, if not brilliant, at least moderately helpful.

It was also a time of sadness and panic. I'd heard stories about the state hospital where I would be for my second year that gave me nightmares. I saw wild men screaming and attacking me, throwing feces at me, stepping on me. But why should I worry? I felt I could get through anything.

I got through this first year, didn't I?

CHAPTER SIXTEEN

THE STATE HOSPITAL

‖MAGINE a kaleidoscope containing vague-shaped pieces, peeling grays, waterstained browns, and fading greens; indefinite edges that seem to change when you try to get close to them. To the psychotic the real objects of his world are not important, only the patterns that form in his mirrors. It is a world turned in on itself, a world so self-dependent that even without any real objects to distort, the mirrors would still form a pattern. They would form a pattern even when there was no more light. It is a world where the patients have become lost in the pattern of their own symptoms.

There is no color in this world; color comes from the world outside the state hospital, from my world. When I arrived at the state hospital I was not even seen as an intruder by the patients, merely as another object that had to be fitted into their pattern. The state hospital was a place I knew well because I used to live in the neighborhood when I was a kid. I remembered playing ball on one of the streets that ran alongside the fenced-in hospital grounds. Once I hit a ball over the fence and had to retrieve it. None of the other kids would get it because they said there were crazy people, lying on the grass and walking around, waiting to grab you.

I walked down the wide sidewalk, trying to pretend that I did not notice all of the sad-looking and strange-acting people who bumped into me.

"That's a nice little boy," an old lady in a housedress cackled.

"Him?" said another lady, tapping my shoulder to get a look at my face. Apparently deciding she didn't like what she saw, she made a grimace, "Naw," and pushed me away.

I ran past people who were motionless and pretended they were playing "statues," I guess so their odd behavior wouldn't frighten me as much. I ran across the grass to where the ball was. There was an old man lying next to it. I got very brave, walked over to it, and picked up the ball. The old man said, "Who are you?" I suddenly turned around and ran for the gate, for the walk, for the street, for my friends. I never wanted to go in there again! Those peculiar people in such strange postures, with strange expressions, wearing strange clothes. They didn't seem real. They just seemed terrifying, and they also looked so sad. Sadness can be very terrifying when you're small.

I felt a chill the first time I drove through the large iron gates, past the crowd of patients who milled around on the sidewalk. They hadn't moved one inch in twenty years, I thought. Glaciers move more quickly.

The state hospital grounds were huge. They covered a couple of hundred acres, at least, and contained many large red brick buildings. There were expanses of green lawn which were dotted in the summer with patients lying in the sun, and were crossed by the tracks that patients made in the snow in the winter. Psychotics made very strange pattens when they walked in the snow. In the summer, you would never notice the way patients walked on the grass, but in the snow, some of them left tracings as intricate as a figure-skater's ovals, eights, and loops. Each well-traced figure recorded their anxiety and reflected the hopelessness of their routine. They waited for the sun and time to melt them both away. In time, both the designs and their makers would be gone, neither leaving any traces.

Besides the remembered fears of my childhood, the fear of everything that is different or unknown, I had other feelings about the state hospital. I felt a strange kinship to the patients, a gnawing sense of familiarity. I felt as if I were in touch with a reservoir of half-forgotten sadness all my own.

My grandfather had been a quiet man all his life, a gentle sort of man who rarely raised his voice. He was content to take things as he found them and was very easily satisfied. He enjoyed taking life at his pace. I remember spending hours at a time driving around in his car with him on business. Sometimes he didn't shift into third gear because he felt that second was good enough for him, or that shifting into third was just too much trouble since eventually he would just have to shift back. I used to watch him burn leaves in the gutter, pick cherries from the two cherry trees in his back yard, and play pinochle with his cronies on the kitchen table Tuesday nights.

I loved him very much.

When I was thirteen my grandfather started to lose his memory and was unable to care for himself. He became too difficult for my grandmother to handle because he had developed a frightening temper. He moved in with my parents and stayed in the bedroom across the hall from me. At night I would help him get undressed. Sometimes he forgot my name. I pretended that I was very businesslike about helping him, but inside I felt sick about it. Finally he started to wander and became so confused he could not be managed at home. I don't know all the details, I never asked how, but he was admitted to this state hospital, and soon after, he died here.

I was assigned to the Dutton Building, to the chronic male service. I had ward D and Bert had ward C. D.J. had a woman's ward on the acute service, and Stanley Lovett was assigned to an acute male ward. When a patient was admitted to the hospital for the first time, he would be sent to the acute service. If he had not improved after six months, he was transferred to the chronic service.

Ward D seemed like the other side of the world from Bamberg 5. Instead of spending an hour a day with three or four patients who would all eventually leave the hospital, I found myself with seventy patients whom I would hardly ever see and who had been on D ward an average of over twenty-five years. Most of them would probably die there.

Dr. Jim Sellers was the psychiatrist in charge of the Dutton Building. He was a muscular, spirited man who had played halfback at Penn State in his senior year and had scored the winning touchdown against Boston College. He kept the ball on the mantle in his office. Jim Sellers was a man interested in progress—with a capital P, please!

"You will find this rotation to be an opportunity limited only by your inventiveness and by your determination," he announced to Bert and me the first day. "You have many patients. You have the opportunity to confront their disease, to challenge it and to win over it! I can't tell you how much I would've liked the opportunity that you two young men have; to treat patients the way you want.

"It's a great opportunity for you to grow. You have the chance to learn more in a short space of time than you will ever get again in your life. It's an opportunity for the patients of Dutton Building. The patients have a chance to be treated by *real* psychiatrists, not just to be seen occasionally by a medical doctor and to be told that physically they are all right, but to see a *real* psychiatrist. Only a year or two ago, residents weren't even assigned to the back wards because we didn't have enough doctors, but now anything is possible. It really is. And it's also a great opportunity for me, to teach you whatever I know and to help you wherever I can, and to prove to Dr. Benjamin Fazio, the director of this hospital, that he wasn't mistaken in allowing me to treat the patients on the chronic wards in the same way we treat patients on the acute wards." Sellers looked very proud.

There was a difference between the chronic and the acute patients which Jim Sellers had failed to mention. Patients on the acute wards generally talked. I had heard that there were chronic patients on my wards who hadn't said a single word for years.

"I know the job is tough," Sellers continued. "I know the conditions here are not the best. But our team is a good team. The nurses are willing and able. The aides are sometimes weak but they can be strengthened and there are some good ones. You'll learn who they are soon enough. Be cautious, but be bold at the same time. I want you guys to know that I'm behind you all the way!"

OK now, let's hear it! I could suddenly see it . . . the stadium filled to capacity with mental patients dressed in dull hospital-gray pants and shirts or housedresses, obese and braless, toothless and sweaty, with matted or stringy hair, and splotches of lipstick put on crooked. On the sidelines, thirteen nurses dressed in freshly starched whites, each of them with a different letter sewn on the back, spelling out S-C-H-I-Z-O-P-H-R-E-N-I-A, waiting for the cry, "Give me an S!" and for the doctors to break out of the huddle to face the amorphous foe. Pacing back and forth, Coach Jim Sellers. . . .

"By the way, Dr. Viscott," said Sellers, "you have a new ward nurse, Sue Corwin. She just started. She's a little frightened but she's a nice girl and really interested in helping the patients. Sue's quite a looker." Jim Sellers winked.

I started on my way up to D ward. In the central corridor was Frank, one of Bert's patients. He used to be an aide at the hospital twenty years ago. He continually paced back and forth in the corridor saying, "Goddamn fucking psychiatrists" over and over. If you said "Hello, Frank," he'd stop and say, "Hello, doctor. How are you today?" and then go on pacing and repeating "Goddamn fucking psychiatrists." Frank ran errands for the nurses.

The dingy stairs were furnished with people. Each landing "belonged" to someone who had spent every day for years there hallucinating his life away. A fat man in his fifties, always wearing a heavy winter coat regardless of the season, kept watch at the first landing. (Many chronic schizophrenics wear winter clothes all year round. A patient once told me, "If I put my coat away, I could lose it and then I would have to go without one next winter.")

Climbing the stairs was eerie, like being on an escalator in slow motion. It was crowded. The patients did not talk to each other or even acknowledge each other's presence. They just shuffled by, staring blankly. Each person seemed to be a world apart from everyone else. Each person was the center of a singular reality, a reality which could not be verified by anyone else.

It was very quiet. In the very center of bedlam, it was still.

Ward D was the top floor of the Dutton Building. Its large day hall was crowded. It seemed like a bus terminal filled wtih stranded passengers who were living in a makeshift purgatory until transportation arrived to take them to their final destination.

Along the walls were chairs where the patients sat. All sat silently. A catatonic patient clutched his arms close to his chest, clenching his fists as if he were trying to resist an angry wish to strike. A man dressed in whites was playing cards with some patients. It was the only activity on the ward. He looked over at me, stood up, and asked, "Can I help you?" with a thick Spanish accent.

"I'm Dr. Viscott," I said. The patients had stopped playing cards and were just staring across the table at each other.

"I'm Rudy Garcia," said the man in white. "I'm the ward attendant. You want to find the office and Miss Corwin?" Rudy had a big smile and a thin mustache. He led me through the day hall like a museum guide leading a visitor through a sculpture garden. "This is the place where most of the patients stay most of the time," Rudy said, pointing around. "Some of them work in the greenhouse. Some hang out in the cellar. Higgins is always in the cellar. Merrill is usually in this hall." We stepped into a hallway. I heard a peculiar noise but couldn't place it.

A short, gray-haired man with a railroad engineer's cap suddenly rushed by me going "Dum, dum, dum, dum."

"He used to be a railroad engineer," said Rudy, smiling. "He still thinks he's on the train. Never says nothing else."

Merrill came by again and stopped. He held out his hand as if he were asking me to shake. So I took his hand and shook it. He pulled away abruptly and went "Dum, dum, dum" again and disappeared down a hallway. Merrill would greet me the same way several times each day. Merrill made the way Harold Parker occasionally touched me seem ordinary.

We walked into the dormitory. It was a hollow, cavernous room with fifty beds arranged in rows, with night tables between. One wall of the room was lined with windows which were covered with heavy iron grillwork. I walked over to them and looked out. For the first time since I had been in the Dutton Building, I remembered that it was summer. Even though the windows were almost opaque with years' accumulation of dust, I could see trees moving slowly in the light morning wind, and flowers, I think they were flowers, on a knoll a short distance away. The cold gray of the ward made me feel it was November, but this room felt like summer. Perhaps because there were no patients here, only sunlight. The patients lived in a world where it was always November—where the longest span of time was a single day.

Rudy led me to the nurses' office and introduced me to Sue Corwin.

Sue Corwin looked as if she'd just stepped out of a painting by Botticelli. She was so delicate and beautiful, the impact heightened no doubt by the contrast with the patients on the ward, who looked like they'd just stepped out of a painting by Hieronymous Bosch. Sue Corwin had enormous blue eyes, long black hair, and a shapely figure, although none of the patients seemed to notice.

Rudy waved and left. "I'm new here," I began. "I don't know anything about the routine on the ward or about the patients, so I'm going to have to depend on you."

"Well, I've only been here six months myself. So I'm still learning. What do you mean by 'routine'?"

"What the patients do, the ward schedule."

"Is there supposed to be a ward schedule?"

"I don't know." I really didn't.

She looked worried. "I just make sure all the patients get up in the morning and then get them all to breakfast. We march them in a line."

"March?"

"They don't march, actually. They just sort of drag their feet. After breakfast there's occupational therapy for some of them, the ones that want to. They make things like rugs. The rest just sit in their chairs until lunchtime. The afternoons are usually quiet. I try to get the medicines ready. We give medicines at nine and at six thirty."

"Just twice a day?"

"Yes, Dr. Sellers' orders, to save time! It takes two hours each time to get the medicines ready. If someone's on a special antibiotic, you can have them get it four times a day.

"Then there's gym, at the top of the stairs. It has everything, Ping-Pong and pool tables. We use it in the mornings sometimes and do calisthenics with the patients. The patients really don't use it very much."

"That's understandable," I said. "They're all old men."

"That's the biggest problem with most of them," Sue said. "Rudy spends most of his time washing them and helping them shower or getting them dressed. Most of these men are more old than sick."

More old than sick!

More old than sick! That's the same way I used to think of my grandfather.

"That's the schedule?" I tried to stay focused on my work.

"Yes. Is there supposed to be more? We go for walks, but it takes the whole afternoon to get people moving. They're so slow because the medications make them sleepy."

"Well, I guess I have a lot of work to do here to get acquainted. Let's go over the patients one by one and talk about them."

"OK," said Sue, pushing her chair next to mine so we were both sitting at her desk. Sue had a large looseleaf notebook containing the patients' orders. Each patient had a page all his own. In this hospital the only thing a patient could be sure of having all to himself was his hospital record. "Are you going to have ward meetings like Dr. Jabers?"

Hell, do I always have to follow that guy in rotation? "When did he have meetings?" I asked sheepishly.

"Once a week. Usually Thursday, today."

"I guess so," I said. "What am I supposed to do?"

"Sit and lecture to them. That's what Dr. Jabers did."

"Don't the patients talk?"

Sue seemed confused. "These patients don't talk," she said.

What the hell was I supposed to do here? How do you treat patients who don't talk?

Sue and I began to review the list of patients. Out of my seventy patients, all but a few were chronic schizophrenics. One patient, Richard, who had been brain-damaged at birth, would come up to me each day when I arrived on the ward, would stutter my name, and ask for praise that he remembered it. There were few deeper conversations on D ward. Another patient, Denny O'Dell, was a manic-depressive. He was the busiest patient on D ward and spent his time continually sweeping up after the others.

Most of the patients had been in the hospital for so many years that by now they suffered more from being hospitalized than they did from the disease which originally brought them in. At least half my patients no longer showed signs of active psychosis. They were just burned-out shells of people. They had been forgotten, uncared for, or lost in the shuffle.

When the newscaster on the radio spoke of "certain necessary cutbacks in spending in the state mental health program this year" these patients were the people who would be affected by them. There would be less money for aides, nurses, doctors, equipment, and medication. The catatonic patient, unable to wash himself because he was so rigid from sitting in the same position for twenty years, would now be given a bath once a week instead of twice. A necessary cutback. Of course the people who feel the effects of the cutbacks don't speak out. They don't vote. Vote! Half the time they don't even know what day, month, year, or century it is. The only span of time these patients understand is now. And *now* means something different for each of them. Now may mean yesterday, now may mean tomorrow. Now may not mean any time at all. Now may be nothingness—the absence of time.

Sue and I spent ten minutes discussing the first patient, who was only a name to me when we began and still only a name when we finished. We took about two or three minutes discussing each of the rest. It was lunchtime. Three hours were gone and we hadn't really done anything.

One thing was clear; all of these patients were taking a great deal of medication. Without exception, *every* patient on that ward was taking medication—and the doses! I never saw such high doses of medication. 400 mg. of Thorazine twice a day! 800 mg. of Thorazine twice a day! 300 mg. of Mellaril twice a day! Whatever medication these patients received was in elephantine amounts. Why, I'd take on a caged tiger who'd been given doses as high as some of my patients—armed only with a featherduster. Let me give you an idea of what I'm talking about. Let's assume that you have been under great business and family stress and can't seem to manage because you're so anxious. Your family doctor decides to give you a fairly stiff dose of tranquilizer, and prescribes 50 mg. of Thorazine four times a day. The chances are you will be drowsy and your activity will slow down considerably. If you had no symptoms and took the same dose of medication, you would probably be falling asleep all the time. Well, some of my patients were taking five to ten times that amount of medicine. No wonder they were just sitting around staring into space. Who the hell wouldn't be?

A great change occurred in mental hospitals when tranquilizers were first introduced. The hospitals seemed quieter, less chaotic, almost respectable. Why? Was it the tranquilizers? To some extent, yes, but at least as much of the improvement resulted from the new interest that was shown in the patients being studied. For some patients, being included in the study marked the first time that anyone had talked to them in years. Some patients did respond very well to the tranquilizers, but some responded to the attention. Eventually, the effectiveness of tranquilizers found its own level, and although hospitals are still pretty quiet, not very much has really changed.

Often patients were placed on large doses of medication because it was simpler for the staff to manage them this way than to try and reason with them. While giving medication frequently did make it possible to reason with a difficult patient, it was just as frequently abused. Often when a patient presented a difficult problem, such as refusing to take a bath, talking back to an authoritarian nurse, taking a swing at a homosexual aide for making an advance at him, or complaining when the television was abruptly shut off during his favorite program, the doctor in charge was called and asked to help out, to control this patient who was "upsetting the ward." (That's the phrase nurses love to use on the phone to get the doctor on call all stirred up.) Chances were that the doctor on call was already busy and knew how little good could be gained by going over and talking to the patient. After all, the patient probably wouldn't even talk with him if he did come up to the ward. So the doctor would probably ask the nurse about the patient's medication, and increase the dosage. This was most likely to happen at the state hospital at night when the doctor on call was responsibile for almost two thousand patients and knew almost none of them personally. Hell, many doctors didn't even know all of *their own* patients personally.

"If you know the names of all the patients on your ward by the end of six months at the state hospital," Marty DiAngelo had told me, "you'll be one hell of a doctor." At night the doctor on call had the choice of seeing some twenty or thirty patients individually or of giving orders over the telephone, usually for increased medication. In time, patients' medication levels rose and the noise level of the ward decreased, although at very high drug dosages the sound on the ward tended to rise again because patients couldn't pick up their feet and scuffled more.

I asked Sue Corwin to lunch. We ate at the employees' cafeteria, not at the doctors' cafeteria in the administration building. Usually only doctors ate there. Although I could take Sue there and no one would say anything, I wanted her to feel comfortable. Also I liked the idea of having her all to myself to stare at. Suzanne—you'll forgive me, I hope—was spring, a form in silk moving through the morning mist. You had to see her to understand. She was so good-looking that she could almost be used as a diagnostic test for mental disease. If a male didn't look up when she spoke to him, or walked by, he just had to be sick. That's all there was to it.

"Are you going to have a ward meeting today?" Sue asked again.

"Why not?" I said. I had no idea what one would be like. Beauty makes you brave.

"You'll find out," Gracie Obermeyer said, sitting down. She was another nurse from the chronic service. "Dr. Feinstein had his first ward meeting today."

"How'd it go?" I asked, always interested in checking up on the competition.

"Wonderful, he's very nice," said Gracie, putting four sugars in her tea. I guessed she needed them to soothe her throat—she had an extraordinary, rough, hoarse voice.

"Gracie's ward," Sue explained, "has much younger patients than D ward and even some acute patients. Well, they're patients fresh from the acute service. They seem like acute patients to me. They'd be a welcome change on D."

"You can have 'em, honey," coughed Gracie, stirring her tea. "All they are is a pain in the neck—the carryings-on I have to put up with. What's this I hear about your getting student nurses?"

"Only a rumor," said Sue. "Dr. Sellers just asked me if I'd like to have student nurses on D. I really wouldn't know what to tell student nurses to do."

"You just tell them what nurses used to tell you when you were a student in training," Gracie said. "Like, pass out these meds, or take this patient for a walk. If you play it right, you could have all your scut work cleaned up by early morning and be free for the rest of the day. Hell, give me a couple of student nurses and I'll be a liberated woman, let me tell you." Gracie lit up a cigarette, although I had visions of her pulling out a cigar. "I wish I had your looks, honey, Dr. Sellers would take good care of me."

Sue blushed. "He's married," she explained, as if that was all the protection from him she would ever need.

"I hope Dr. Viscott here is a decent sort, honey," Gracie said, "because you don't know a wolf at the door from an Avon lady."

"Ding dong. All right, ladies, let's go back to the ward and have a ward meeting."

Rudy and Sue pulled the patients from all their various corners and hiding places and arranged them in neat rows in the day hall. Denny O'Dell's assistance had also been enlisted to make sure no one was hiding anywhere.

"OK, doc," shouted Denny from the back of the day hall. "You can begin anytime now." Who was running this place anyhow?

"Isn't he something?" Sue said to me. "He's so energetic and helpful!"

Good God! Was it possible this angel-like creature sitting next to me didn't understand that Denny O'Dell, in his six-foot-four of restless talking, pacing, housecleaning, busybodying, and perpetual motion was a manic patient? All manic patients are energetic. That's their problem. Their energies are directed outside themselves, away from their fear. They keep moving just to ward off the fear of dying.

"Let's get going, doc," shouted Denny impatiently.

"I'm your new doctor, Dr. Viscott," I began, "and I'm taking over from Dr. Jabers. I hope to get to know all of you personally and later on to discuss your problems with you. If you have any questions, please ask." (Pretty please?)

How's that for an opening? I looked around the day hall. I know it's foolish but I wanted to reassure myself that Dr. Michael Gabor wasn't around watching me screw up.

Sitting in front of me were almost sixty patients. The others were unaccounted for. I could hear Merrill dum-dumming away in the corridor behind me; he refused to come in when Rudy asked.

From there on it was all downhill. Richard kept telling me proudly that he knew my name. Another man broke the deadening silence by blowing his noise, for which I was thankful. But the silence returned to make me uneasy again.

CHAPTER SEVENTEEN

"RUNNING" THE CHRONIC WARD

‖ BEGAN to read each of my seventy patients' charts. I tried to find something new about them, some clue that would unlock the mystery of their disease. Perhaps, armed with the newest in drugs and instruction in techniques that weren't available to my predecessors, *I* might be able to cure them. And you thought I'd given up all my childish wishes to be omnipotent long ago, like last Friday when I was only a first-year resident. Flourish of trumpets! Start spinning those windmills. Cue Sancho Panza. Enter stage left, Don Quixote.

Some advice for those of you who would attack windmills: wear a crash helmet!

I had a great deal of work ahead of me. I calculated that with only two hours a day left over from my schedule of meetings and seminars, it would take me three months just to see each of my patients once and read his chart. So I decided to cut most of the less important seminars. I could hear my father saying, "You're so smart, you know everything already? I'm surprised you even bothered to go to medical school."

At the state hospital there were seminars scheduled for every hour of the working day. I suppose I could have convinced myself that I was learning about patients by attending, but tell me, what do you learn about patients by avoiding the ward? It was possible for a resident to spend almost no time on his ward and, by putting in an appearance at every conference, to give other people the impression he was really interested in learning. Of course he might not have any idea of what to do with a real live patient, but he could fake it good.

The first problem was to find charts in the record room. That could take hours. When a patient has been in the hospital as long as some of these patients, his chart grows; it wasn't unusual for a chart covering twenty-five years' hospitalization to have a *thousand* pages in it. Just to uncover the circumstances that brought a patient into the hospital years ago was like solving a mystery.

The very first record I picked up had an admission note written by Dr. Gavin when he was a resident. It was a good note, clearly thought out. His follow-up notes were also excellent. So were the notes that Dr. Michael Gabor wrote in the same chart four years later, when he was a resident. I read notes written by Jerome Gelb, by Alex Karlsson, and by M. Austin Noyes, when he was in clinical training. He was a damn good resident. I also read notes by Bud Clarkson, Noyes' protégé, and even a few written by Stanley Lovett's psychoanalyst. The very best psychiatrists in town had trained at this hospital.

What an honor to follow in their shoes!

What am I talking about? If with all their collective intelligence and skill they were unsuccessful with these patients, what did that say about my chances?

"It says," said Bert, "that you are going to leave great notes for some future resident to read."

"How's it going with you?" I asked Bert.

"OK, I notice that you don't go to many conferences. Neither does D.J. She said one year of listening to Stanley tell how much he knew was enough. Some of the other residents really think Stanley is sharp. Stanley is superb at discussing *other people's* ideas."

"I do go to Dr. Rutberg's seminars," I said. Rutberg was a brilliant clinician. "Rutberg's fantastic." Rutberg seemed to understand everything even the craziest patients told him. It was as if he had a special pipeline to a patient's unconscious. Dr. Rutberg once told us, "You will all work very hard and expend a great deal of energy this year, and you will believe that you have helped patients and changed them. But if you return in six months or a year you'll find them exactly the way you left them."

I couldn't accept that.

The state hospital was affiliated with Union Hospital and with St. Mark's Hospital, each of which had a psychiatric training program, but neither had facilities for caring for seriously ill psychotic patients. Residents from Union and St. Mark's spent a year at the state hospital. The state hospital also had a residency program of its own. The question which had nagged at the back of my mind for years—what happens to the guys at the bottom of the class in medical school—was answered. They become residents at state hospitals. There were some losers among the residents from Union and St. Mark's Hospital to be sure; some were terrible. And there were some excellent psychiatric residents in the state hospital residency program, but both of these groups were in the minority.

In a field of a hundred losing residents, Karl Frogner would come in last. Frogner was a foreign-trained resident. Now don't get me wrong, I have nothing against foreign-trained residents. It happened that the best residents in the state hospital training program were also foreign. Tanya Milhady, for example, a Hungarian refugee, was bright as hell and related beautifully to patients. There were two excellent Egyptian physicians, man and wife, who had practiced general medicine in Cairo and had come to the States and were studying psychiatry. Frogner never revealed exactly where he had trained, although he became a physician years ago in Nazi Germany and he probably was rushed through medical school to meet the demand on the front lines. He practiced medicine after the war on the Swiss-German border because he was a skiing fanatic. He made a living setting fractures. "Perhaps," he said, "they were not set as well as a specialist might, but I do the best I can." If you see some skier skiing a crooked mile in Switzerland, you know who to blame.

Frogner emigrated to the United States and decided to go into psychiatry. There were many former general practictioners now going through their residency in psychiatry at the state hospital. The government had a program for general practitioners paying them $12,000 a year to go through psychiatric residency. I even bumped into my old family physician, Dr. George Irving, walking across the state hospital grounds. He had given up an $80,000-a-year practice at age fifty to begin a psychiatric residency.

Frogner somehow got into the state hospital residency program. He was simply inept. He had preconceived ideas about how his patients should act and what they should do, and he demanded respect from them for his years and expertise. He refused to learn anything from his patients. Like I said when he refused Mrs. Gore admission, I had a score to settle with that bastard. One day I sat next to him at lunch.

"Tell me, Karl," I asked, using his first name because I knew it irritated him, "do you remember Bessie Gore? She was probably a schizo-affective, a black lady. You saw her six months ago. I sent her over from Union."

"Ah, I am not certain," Frogner said, with his mouth full. "Did she come in with two brothers?"

"Yes," I said. "I indicated that she was a severe suicidal risk on the commitment form. You refused to accept her for admission. I've always wanted to know why, especially since you said you would admit her when I spoke to you on the telephone."

"Because it is my judgment to avoid arguments. I always say I'll admit the patient on the phone, I decide for myself when I see the patient. My observations were different."

"Why did you refuse to admit her? On what grounds?"

"On the basis of my much longer clinical experience than the one you have. How old are you, Dr. Viscott? You're in your twenties, or something like that? Well, I'm fifty-two. And I have seen thousands of patients. I will not allow my judgment to be questioned by someone who doesn't really know what the situation is."

"Would you be interested in hearing what happened to that lady? Aren't you interested in checking out how your judgments hold up?"

"I don't need to hear anything. Now please don't bring the subject up again."

You are a phony, Dr. Frogner. I repeat, if I ever have the chance to get you, I will. At the moment, I thought about spilling something hot in his lap. Too easy . . .

Dr. Jim Sellers asked to see me. I walked into his office. The door was open. Sellers was standing with his back toward me. He was holding the football that was usually on his mantle, about to throw a pass to his wide receiver, Hank O'Donnell. It was third down and fourteen to go. His arm moved back slowly; he set his feet, waiting for O'Donnell to get in the clear; such poise, even though a defensive tackle had just broken through the line.

I coughed gently. "Hi," he said, turning around, not at all embarrassed. "We used to start scrimmaging in August." Sellers patted his gut, still flat as a board. "You've got the luck of the Irish, my boy. You're getting four little student nurses starting tomorrow."

"Fantastic!" I was putting it on, the enthusiasm. I'd been getting pretty frustrated. I'd spent several weeks reading records and interviewing patients. I was scoring brownie points discussing the patients with Gracie Obermeyer and Sue Corwin, but I also felt I was spinning my wheels. Interviewing these patients could seem an awful exercise in futility.

Mr. Daly was sixty years old. According to his record, he had been a teacher, a missionary, and an alcoholic when he was younger. When he was thirty and on New York's skid row he had a visitation from the Virgin, who told him "to seek the River of Waters and lead mankind across." He was picked up trying to walk on the Hudson River. He had been in the hospital since then. Poor Mr. Daly should have waited a few years; the Hudson is so polluted now almost anyone can walk across it. However, even if he could, Mr. Daly still wouldn't know what to do when he reached the other side.

An interesting case, you say. A pleasure for a bright young inquisitive mind to investigate, you add. Just listen to this interview. Sue Corwin is sitting in on it because she wants to see how I talk to patients.

"Mr. Daly, I'm glad you could make it," I began. What, I wondered, would Mr. Daly ever be doing that would keep him from seeing me? After all, Mr. Daly just sat all day long in his chair by the window. With Rudy pushing Mr. Daly into my office with both hands, his attendance was guaranteed.

"Tell me, Mr. Daly. How have you been doing?" Is that a stupid question or is that a stupid question?

"Hnnh," said Mr. Daly. I couldn't tell whether he was responding to me or just grunting.

"I've been reading your record. Do you remember anything about coming to the hospital?"

No response. I had the feeling Mr. Daly was staring at a spot behind his eyes.

"Do you ever have any visitors?" I asked, and then remembered that no one has visited him for ten years.

No response. Of course there was no response.

"Is there anyone you are friendly with on the ward?"

No response. This was a question I really didn't expect him to answer. It was very rare to see a patient talking to another patient on the ward. They saw the outside world as a blur. Only each one's inside world appeared clear. Mr. Daly was focusing on the inside world; I was just part of the blur. I could imagine Dr. Gelb asking in his supervisory tone of voice, "Well, how are we going to get through that blur you have so well described?" "Well, I'll tell you, doctor, I'd try a bold tactic. Maybe shout at the patient to try to make my reality break into his world." "Good, try it, Dr. Viscott," I imagined Gelb nodding. . . .

"Mr. Daly," I suddenly yelled at him.

Sue nearly fell off her chair. "Jesus, Mary, and Joseph," she said, looking at me as if I'd suddenly gone crazy.

Mr. Daly just sat there. He didn't even blink!

"Mr. Daly"—this time in a conversational tone—"I want you to come to the window with me." Mr. Daly would not move.

Sue helped me. Mr. Daly was stood up and pointed in the general direction of the window. Outside, the tops of trees were brushing against the building in the soft summer wind.

"Mr. Daly, there's a world outside." I couldn't tell whether he was listening or not. There was a huge cemetery just beyond the hospital grounds. The dead and the living dead. "Don't you want to try to do something to get out of here? You don't want to spend your life here."

No response. Apparently it didn't matter—or maybe I didn't know how to get through—maybe both.

Mr. Daly did not sit down, he was reseated. He seemed like a nonhuman object in the shape of a man. What was going on inside the man's head? I wondered if my grandfather had been like that— had his resident shouted at him? I felt badly, powerless and a little ashamed of myself for almost forgetting Mr. Daly was human. It wasn't difficult to do. . . .

There were at least forty patients like Mr. Daly on my ward. I I saw some patients, though, who did talk; they were in the minority. Joseph Kelly talked.

"What would you like, Mr. Kelly?"

"The power of the ancients. The Asunder. I want the Asunder."

"Did you ever have the power before? Was it something you lost?" If I had known a little more, I would have picked up his feeling of powerlessness and asked him about it. But the confusion of his words stifled me; the words of psychotics often are intended to push others away, away from their feelings.

"Holy, Holy, Holy, *Adonai Echod. Te deum Laudamus.*" Mr. Kelly stood up and added, "*Ex Post Christo, Ex Post Facto,* Ex Rel Post Office," and concluded, "There you have it."

Mr. Gildea, a white-haired, round man, also used words to push me away.

"My sister is coming to visit me," he began, as soon as he walked into the office.

"Really! When?" I asked.

"Why do you want to know?" said Gildea.

"I was just asking," I said.

"Why?"

"To be polite."

"Why do you want to be polite?"

"I think it's the best way to start a conversation with someone I don't know well and would like to get to know." That should do it, I thought.

"Why?" asked Gildea.

"Why, what?" I was getting lost. Gildea was winning.

"If you don't know, there's no point going any further," Mr. Gildea said, and before I could say another word he walked out.

"Well, at least patients are talking to you," said Sue, not realizing that what had just happened was nontalk, evasion, rejection.

The hours I sat with mute, staring patients who'd played the silent waiting game for years . . . their long, once distinct histories began to blur. . . . Was this the patient who lost his mother when he was ten or was it his father at five or was it only a fantasy he had and were both his patients still alive? . . . I couldn't keep it all straight, too many records, too many patients, no human contact to make it real to me. Even after seeing these patients I still felt as if I'd only read about them. Paper people.

How much longer was I going to take all of this before I started to crack up?

Not much longer!

Crack!!

I screamed as Rudy took the last patient for the day back to the day hall. I terrified Sue when I did that.

"Cut that out. The first time it might have been funny, it's not anymore."

"Sue, I'm going out of my fucking mind."

"Don't swear," said Sue. Sue was a "good" girl—that is, she never did anything in public that anyone could ever comment unfavorably upon—her definition.

"Sue, I believe I am going crazy. Your beloved ward doctor, the rider of the purple sage, is dissolving in the sunset of schizophrenia."

"You should give it more time—Mrs. Muckian," Sue called out abruptly and pointed behind me.

Mrs. Muckian was a licensed practical nurse who worked on D ward. She chatted with Sue about how her husband was coming along and how glad she was to be back with all her children on D ward. Mrs. Muckian was an overprotective, smothering woman who'd worked on D ward for twenty-five years and treated all the patients like babies. I think she actually needed the hospital more than the hospital needed her. She played a role in her job that allowed her to see herself as a warm, sensitive, and giving person. Mrs. Muckian's son had committed suicide years ago by hanging himself from a hook on the inside of her bedroom closet door and she was still doing penance. Mrs. Muckian left to pat the patients on their heads.

"There's something I forgot to tell you, Sue," I said.

Sue looked down at her feet as if she were expecting a romantic confession. If I told her I was irresistibly attracted to her, needed her, and wanted to leave my wife and kids and run away with her, she could understand even though it might embarrass her. Sue could always manage things that embarrassed her, but intellectual challenges devastated her.

"You're getting four student nurses tomorrow," I said, and watched the lovely bloom in Sue's sweet Irish face fade like a note at the end of a John McCormack recording. Sue lowered herself into a chair. I suddenly felt sorry for Sue. She was in over her head and knew it. Sue had never been much of a student. She'd taken the job at the state hospital because she didn't want night duty. Her training in psychiatry in nursing school had lasted only four months. Sue felt she really wasn't qualified to teach anyone, and told me so.

"Don't worry. I've been working on a plan," I said. (Well, at least I had a few ideas.)

When the nurses—Rita, Rosalind, Julie, and Linda—arrived on the ward I revealed my plan. "Until right now it has been impossible for anyone to make headway with the patients on this ward. No one has ever been successful treating them. We've been caretakers. I would like to try an experiment, requiring your help and cooperation. Since no one before us has ever succeeded we cannot fail."

"What do we do?" asked Rosalind, who seemed worldlier and brighter than the others.

"There are seventy patients on this ward. There are now four student nurses, two aides—Rudy and Nicholas—Miss Corwin and Mrs. Muckian, and one psychiatrist, me."

"That's nine," Rita said, counting.

"I have an alert crew this morning," I said feeling myself fitting into the role of chief.

"It's nothing, really," said Rita, who would graduate in the spring, having been voted "Miss Personality" by her class. Rita was a sparkling, interested girl, open and honest about her feelings.

"I am going to divide the patients into small groups and assign a group to each of you. They'll become your patients, your therapeutic responsibility. Each of you will be assigned some patients who talk and some who never do. I want you to work individually with the patients who talk and to work in groups with the ones who don't. I'll help you organize your day so that you have something to do all the time. I want the patients to do something besides sit. Anything we can accomplish is a victory. I'll supervise each of you personally. We will go over your patients' charts and medication and make adjustments together. It's too much work for one person and I really need your help."

Everyone was given one week to read and summarize their patients' charts. The morning schedule was reorganized. Gym period was expanded. I felt that as much movement as possible would be beneficial, if it didn't cause too much strain. After all, the men *were* older. Hell, it would be better for them than just sitting in the same crummy chair all day long.

The patients resisted, but we pushed. In order for a patient to get any privileges, he had to do ward work. That was another new rule. What had once been a dull and uninteresting ward now appeared bustling. Or were we kidding ourselves? Were we just pushing dehumanized patients around like so many pieces on a chess board and attributing human characteristics to their actions? Were we calling patients motivated merely because they complied? Were we anthropomorphizing them? If we were, and I'm sure we often were, it was to make our work more tolerable.

The student nurses were only young untrained girls. Some did not understand that a person could really give up. (Maybe I didn't either.) Sometimes the student nurses appeared like cheerleaders.

I had read somewhere that even though a stroke victim might be unable to remember certain words in speaking, he was sometimes able to remember them when singing. Maybe there was a special musical mental pathway. I decided that a daily songfest might be helpful. I got the idea at a party on one of the other wards, watching some patients join in the singing who usually reacted to nothing. Generally psychiatrists think of mental disease as a verbal entity. Defenses are verbal. Music is not, although I'm not sure my theory is correct. Anyway, some former mute patients did respond and join in the singing.

That's worth something. Tell me that's worth something, please!

The patients also began to respond to the nurses. They talked about the hospital, about the weather, rarely about themselves. I cut down on their medications and to my surprise nothing much happened—that is, the patients did not become wildmen, running around sinking their teeth into the furniture. Some became a little restless, but the student nurses found ways for them to use their energy. And I'd left the gym open all day now.

The student nurses started to get ideas of their own. One afternoon they got a football game together, involving everyone on D ward. I pulled rank and had Sue on my team. The line consisted of some of the younger schizophrenics, men in their thirties and forties. Bert saw us from his office window and immediately formed a team with patients from his ward and challenged us. Unfair, I thought, because Bert's patients were much younger than mine.

I was unanimously elected captain and quarterback—the advantages a medical degree had given me! In college I'd only played a little touch football, but the hours playing sports were lovely times. I remembered hanging around the Dartmouth College green in the fading glow of a spring afternoon, the sweet smells of New Hampshire balsam, the calls in the dewy air, "Throw it to me, throw it to me," and the sound of feet running over the soft moist ground. I was always stuck on the line then. I really couldn't throw or catch, but I still felt I should be quarterback. Thanks to my diligence in medical school, today I was a quarterback.

Jim Sellers, his sleeves rolled up, wearing tennis sneakers he'd brought with him for a squash match at his club after work, came running out to play with us. Guess who also wants to be quarterback? Because I had worked through my authority hangups with supervisors in working with Jerry Gelb, I said, "You can be an end on my team, Jim, but we already have a quarterback, me!"

"So you'll have another one," Jim Sellers protested like a hurt kid. "What difference would it make if your team has two quarterbacks? You already have a fifteen-man line."

I counted. So we did, but I convinced Jim to be inside receiver, whatever that was.

In all, Bert and I fielded forty-four men and women at the same time. Twenty on my side and twenty-four on his. Rita counted them. The game, like so many projects, was her idea.

We won the toss. I called a series of numbers. "Eleven, forty-one, vermicelli, number twenty-three—hike." Bert's line and my line faced each other in anticipation of brutal combat.

I threw the ball to—who else?—Big Jim Sellers, who actually caught it and ran all the way to glory. He really *could* move. I know his mind wasn't with us. He was back in good old BC stadium again, third down and fourteen to go.

My line did not move one inch. As a matter of fact, not one player had moved on either side. The patients just stood there motionless, looking out past each other, staring down the narrow corridor of their vision, staring through time, past life.

We played for about an hour. I know this will sound terrible, but the reason that we stopped was I was afraid to have my patients stand in one position for such a long time without moving.

"How about another game?" said Sellers. "That really did a lot for the patients."

Sellers, I'm afraid, was an asshole.

The summer was fading. The treatment program on the ward was going well. I was pleased with it. I reviewed the old laboratory studies on all the patients on my ward, ordered some new tests and discovered that Mr. Daly had leukemia. I transferred Mr. Daly to the medical building, a hospital within the hospital.

I had night duty once every two weeks. There were always two doctors on call. We were supposed to stay on the hospital grounds, although some of the doctors who lived less than a mile away took calls at home. It was a practice much frowned upon. One doctor covered the medical hospital, which had three hundred medical beds, and the entire chronic service with its eighteen hundred patients. The other was in charge of the emergency floor, the hospital admitting room, and the acute service. It was the busier of the two rotations, and rarely did the doctor on emergency call get a chance to sleep through the night. At least I never did.

My first night on call I decided to spend some time with Nicholas Karas, the aide on evening duty on D ward. He was a body-building devotee and at the same time he was shy, almost timid. He preferred D ward to the others because it was quieter and, as he said. "I don't have to worry about being knifed every time I turn around."

Nicholas was less than enthusiastic about my ward plan, but I'd done better with my other staff members. By the middle of August, every patient on D ward was spending at least an hour each day with the person specifically assigned to him. Two patients even got part-time jobs at a local car wash. Denny the manic even tried a visit home, his first in years. The social service department had been actively trying to get patients into a nursing home who didn't have a home to go to.

Nicholas said encouragingly, "It's just a new name for an old thing."

I was disgusted and walked into the gym. The door closed behind me and I picked up a cue stick and played pool. I was irritated with Nicholas and furious with Mrs. Muckian, who had gone out of her way to undermine me that afternoon. After one rack, which I played dreadfully, I decided to give up pool and make rounds in the medical hospital.

The door to the gym had locked behind me and would not open from the inside. I was locked in.

I went to a window and could see some of my patients sitting on the back porch of the ward. Mr. Hasbro, another of my schizophrenics, was pacing back and forth. I called, "Mr. Hasbro." He kept pacing.

"Mr. Hasbro. It's me, Dr. Viscott," I called, but louder this time.

Mr. Hasbro stopped, looked up and, apparently taking my voice to be just another of his hallucinations, continued pacing again. I could have predicted it because he never responded to me when he was looking right at me. How could I expect him to answer me when all he heard was a voice? He heard voices all the time. Rita's goal was to try to get him to ignore a voice unless he could see the person who belonged to it. To answer me, only a voice, would have been anti-therapeutic, I guess.

There was another patient on the porch, but I didn't know his name. He sat behind Mr. Kelly at the ward meetings. Try putting that into a request for help, "Hello there, you who sit behind Mr. Kelly at ward meeting." I doubted he even knew who Mr. Kelly was. After all, he's only been on the same ward with Mr. Kelly for the past fifteen years.

Richard appeared. My salvation! He had been walking around and apparently just found himself on the back porch in the summer air. Richard was brain damaged, beyond a doubt, but he wasn't psychotic! He would respond! And his major expression from my first abortive meeting was my name and his proved repetition of it.

"Richard," I called.

Richard stopped, turned around, and walked inside, thinking someone must be calling him to come in from the porch. I gave up. Wait, he's back on the porch.

"Richard," I shouted. "Stay where you are. It's me, Dr. Viscott."

"Dr. Viscott. Hi! Hi, Dr. Viscott! Dr. Viscott!"

"Look, tell Nicholas to come out on the porch. I'm locked in."

"Hi, Dr. Viscott."

Good God. I'm going to be locked in here forever.

"Richard," I said sternly, "tell Nicholas to come out."

"Nicholas?" said Richard, puzzled. "You're Dr. Viscott."

"Tell him I'm here."

Richard was off and shuffling. What if Nicholas didn't understand him? Worse than that, what if Nicholas understood him but thought his comment was just another part of Richard's peculiar behavior and ignored it? The shoe was on the other foot. When I wanted to penetrate through a patient's insanity to reach him, I frequently couldn't. Now that I needed a patient to break through an aide's sanity, I doubted I would succeed. There were so many defenses operating on both sides.

How many of my own patients' clues was I missing, shutting out? Was it just too disturbing for me to look at the world through my patients' eyes? Was I afraid to discover I didn't care enough? It was always easier to blame the patient's craziness than to deny your own humanity.

A key turned in the door and it opened. Nicholas was laughing his ass off. "Boy, is that a funny one. You're just lucky Richard was out there. He's the only one besides Denny I listen to on this ward, and Denny is out on a visit." Hell is a place where the people you need to believe in you the most don't believe in you at all.

I headed down the stairs toward the medical building, followed by Nicholas' laughter echoing through the halls. It was a warm night. Behind the administration building I could see the lights of a traveling carnival which had set up its equipment on the hospital grounds. Dr. Benjamin Fazio, the hospital administrator, thought it would be a good diversion for some of the patients. They rode the amusements for half price in the afternoon and full price at night. It was still quite profitable for the carnival operator.

I walked down to take a closer look at the carnival. It was a bizarre scene—waxen schizophrenics spinning around on the merry-go-round. An old lady refused to go on a ride, saying, "But it moves!" One young man gawked at the Ferris wheel as if it were a live creature about to attack him. An old man placed his bet on a number and then forgot which number he bet on. A lady in a stained coat walked about collecting empty popcorn boxes to take back to her room. Another woman lost the last of her canteen money, trying to win a doll for an eighteen-year-old granddaughter who never visited.

I walked back toward the hospital and decided to take a shortcut across the lawn. It had grown quite dark. The calliope was fading in the background. I was alone on the broad sweep of lawn with the deep shadows of evening. I suddenly became frightened. A movement in the bushes—a person about to spring at me? No, a bird. To the side, a person lying in the black grass? No, a rock.

The moon was just rising over the steamy tenements along the hospital fence. A little light now, where before it was dark. Ahead, on the grass, I could see another rock. As I got closer, the rock began to move and turned into a man sleeping on the grass.

"Which building do you belong in?" I asked.

"Go away," said the shadowy form. He was one of the drunks who lived unofficially on the state hospital grounds. I left him alone.

Mr. Daly was dying, he had gotten worse after his transfer to the medical building. He had little time left. His white count rose every day. He had an infection that was not responding to antibiotics. "You better take a look at him," said the charge nurse. "I think he's going."

"I—are there any relatives?" I couldn't remember his case very well. He had never spoken to me.

Mr. Daly looked very pale. He had a high fever and was trembling. "How are you feeling, Mr. Daly? It's Dr. Viscott. Can I get you something?"

"No," he said softly. Mr. Daly had responded! "Am I dying?" he asked.

"I'm not sure. You're very ill."

"I'm dying, aren't I?" he asked, looking right at me.

I nodded. I didn't know what else to do.

Mr. Daly smiled. "I always secretly believed I would get better, you know. I planned on retiring at sixty-five and living off social security and taking it easy. It's funny how your plans don't work out."

This man hadn't uttered a coherent word in more than a decade, and now that he was about to die he spoke as if his entire illness had been a voluntary confinement, or only a pretense.

"It must have been hard for you all these years," I said.

"You don't know the terror I've felt every day of my life since the Virgin spoke to me. I've been so afraid of saying or doing the wrong thing."

"Do you remember talking with me?"

Mr. Daly studied me and then, shaking his head, he asked, "Who are you?"

"I'm your doctor."

"No you're not! My doctor is on D ward."

I was out of place. This was not D ward and so I could not be Mr. Daly's doctor.

Mr. Daly died the next morning. In some way it was a personal loss.

I found Dr. Rutberg and told him about Mr. Daly.

"Yes, I've seen that," said Dr. Rutberg. "It is almost as if imminent death releases some patients from their psychosis. For them the ultimate punishment becomes so real that it absolves them from all their guilt. They are free if for a short while. You never forget it once you see it. You learn to respect the strength of psychotic defenses. You know how powerful the forces against you are."

My ward program was going very well indeed. Denny decided to try an extended visit home, one of the patients who worked in the car wash, Ken Mahoney, started taking weekend visits with his uncle, and four patients had been transferred to nursing homes.

"Great going," said Jim Sellers, "your game plan's working."

I wasn't so sure. There *was* more activity on the ward. There *was* more movement at least on the outside, but I didn't know what was happening inside my patients. The student nurses accepted their responsibility and worked hard. Some patients had now become extremely difficult to manage with their medications reduced and there was a lot of pressure to increase the dosages again. I resisted because the student nurses had the interest and willingness to encourage their patients to work and to take pride in it. In a sense we told the patients how proud we were of them for acting almost human.

The summer may have been exciting for me, but for Judy it was pure hell. She hadn't been able to walk since July, and spent most of the days in bed. The pain in her legs was so great that I suspected she had thrombophlebitis, but I couldn't get any of her doctors to agree with me. In August she stopped gaining weight and looked terrible. And in September Judy went downhill every day.

"Is mommy going to be all right?" asked my daughter, Elizabeth, who had just started first grade.

"Yes," I said, with my fatherly assurance voice. I wasn't sure at all.

My son Jonathan was born three weeks premature, and my exhausted, pale, edematous wife still looked terrible.

"Something's wrong!" Judy said later that day. "I don't feel at all like me."

Dr. Ryder, her internist, a dear close friend, said, "I think Judy's depressed." If I want your opinion I'll ask, I thought, stick to medicine. "She's been very demanding on the nurses, asking for pain medication," he added.

"Maybe she's having a lot of pain," I said.

"But her reaction to pain is . . . well, a little overreacting."

"People differ in pain threshold, you know that."

"The nurses feel there's something emotional going on."

"Look, let me be the judge of that. She's had a rough time. I don't think it's emotional."

"Perhaps you're too close," Ryder said.

"Look, if something is going on, it's physical. Judy looks toxic to me."

"I'll make a deal with you," said Ryder. "You stick to psychiatry and I'll stick to medicine."

I didn't like the deal!

Judy was five hours postpartum. It was noon. I left for the state hospital. At one thirty I got a call from Dr. Ryder. Judy was hallucinating and toxic. Please come down.

"I can't understand it," said her obstetrician, Dr. Sam Meckler. "She has a fever of 106 and we don't know what's causing it. Where's the infection?"

"Maybe the episiotomy," I said angrily. Meckler winced. "Maybe her legs, her uterus. I don't know, Sam. She's been very sick for the past two months. I haven't been able to convince you or Ryder of that. The first time you believed her was today. It's all been in her head, according to you two. You've given me all this crap about Judy not wanting the baby. That kind of psychological bullshit has been pounded so deep into your obstetricians' heads you can't think any other way. It may be true for some women, and it may even be partially true with Judy, but Judy's sick in your terms—physically sick."

Why didn't I try to convince Judy's doctors that she needed more attention when she was pregnant? (Maybe I could have prevented this. Perhaps it was my hope that they were right, that she wasn't so ill. They'd tried to reassure her, to get her to wish her symptoms away.)

Dr. Meckler's obstetrical associate once examined Judy briefly and told her, "There's nothing wrong with you or your legs. You should start exercising and walking a mile a day." I was ready to throttle him. I didn't though because I was intimidated by him. Doctors act most intimidating when they are most unsure of themselves and when they are unable to admit their weakness. That's when their patients have to be wrong just so they can be right.

I went into Judy's room and held her hand. Her sheets were soaking. She looked flushed and felt feverish. I started to wipe her face, and images of me helping my grandfather flooded over me. Judy was saying something, but it was garbled, I couldn't understand. I probably didn't want to hear it.

Ted Ryder had left by the time I came out of Judy's room. I couldn't find anyone I knew around. Doctors—they think they know absolutely everything. Meckler was terrified he was going to lose a young mother in puerperal sepsis—that's what they call "childbed fever" where I come from. There hadn't been a case of it in this state in years. Certainly not in a nice kosher Jewish hospital like this that catered to all the lovely Jewish princesses and their doctors who sweetly promised, "No, dear, you won't feel a thing. Just call me at the very first pain."

I knew what was going on. My wife was dying and I couldn't find anyone I could talk to. I finally reached Dr. Ryder on the phone. "Look, David, we're doing everything we can. We still don't know where the source of infection is, or what the organism is."

I spent two days practically living in the hospital. The nurses hated me because I wanted to know everything that was going on. None of the hundred cultures grew out anything. Judy was growing weaker, and her temperature was still 106 degrees in spite of high doses of Gantrisin, a sulfa drug which obviously wasn't helping. The staff felt Judy was being uncooperative by being in pain and asking for medication. Judy was also being uncooperative by being allergic to penicillin.

David Rosedale, who'd gone to medical school with me and

was on the infectious disease service of that hospital, had come by
to see Judy several times a day without even being asked. He took
several cultures himself and was scared that she wouldn't make it.
For some reason, which he could not explain, he decided to get up
in the middle of the night and look at her blood cultures again. At
two thirty in the morning he discovered alpha hemolytic streptococci
growing in the latest batch of cultures, and started a different antibiotic in massive doses intravenously. In twelve hours Judy was out
of crisis and her temperature was nearly normal. I've never been able
to thank Rosedale in any way that showed how I really felt.

During this time I found it impossible to work at the state hospital. I was not really myself for several weeks afterward. I was still
shaking from the closeness of losing Judy; I was overjoyed with having a son. I was angry at Ryder and Meckler; I felt sorry for them
for having such a problem and in some way I was grateful—all at
once. Like most people, even when I knew my doctor was wrong I
still wanted to believe in him.

When a person becomes a patient he in some sense gives up his
personal independence to his doctor. Patients should never forget
that doctors are not perfect. Each doctor lives by his own personal
standards. The extent of his wisdom is limited by his openness in
accepting his errors, and in admitting his ignorance. Doctors get into
trouble most when they try to maintain an image of perfection that
never really exists. It's then that doctors risk becoming charlatans,
and their patients risk becoming pawns to their splintering egos.
When a patient must get better for his doctor's sake, both are in
serious trouble. The idea that a doctor must know the answer to
everything simply because he is a doctor never set well with me
when I was dealing with patients. Being on the other side and seeing through the flimsy excuses for not knowing, for not admitting
that something went wrong, made me furious. Ryder and Meckler
were professors in medical schools. They *were* good. They became
bad only when they forgot that they could be wrong.

If I ever started to be that unbending, that frightened that I had
to be sure I was right in spite of the facts, I would quit medicine.
I swore it. (Or was I just angry, thinking all this out of fear and
helplessness?)

By Christmas, twelve patients had been discharged from D ward
to nursing homes. By the end of January, Denny had left the hospi-

tal, and Kenny Mahoney and another patient who worked in the car wash had both left the hospital to live with relatives. They still kept their jobs.

"The population of D ward is now fifty-four," said Rita, who really *had* counted.

There was a small farewell ward party for me the week before I left for the acute service. Mrs. Muckian walked around as usual, patting patients on the head.

"You really did a good job up here, Dr. Viscott," said Sue.

"Do you think it will last?" asked Gracie, being her usual cynical self.

"What a terrible thing to say," said Sue. "Of course it will last!" Sue poured the lukewarm lime Kool-Aid into a row of paper cups.

Painfully beautiful Sue, you grew up in a different corner of the world from the rest of us. The real world, lovely creature, is full of people who smell, who swear, who may sometimes have sexual feelings about the young priest offering mass even though they're not supposed to, and who learn to live in spite of it all. In some funny way you are as much of a dreamer as these patients walking around the day hall as if nothing real existed. Were they ever really awake? Had I been little more to them than a remembered dream? "I don't know," I said.

"I'm sure it will last," said Sue, looking as innocent, as hopeful as ever.

I hadn't *cured* anyone. I'd just rearranged some dust.

"Dr. Viscott," said Richard, the mental defective, "I know your name. I know your name." Would that fame and glory were not so fleeting.

CHAPTER EIGHTEEN

TWO PATIENTS—MIDDLE GROUND

COMPARED to the chaotic world of the Dutton Building, the hours I spent treating Roberta Goldman and Donald Johnson in therapy seemed like an oasis. I saw them each week in an office in the outpatient building, which was located right near the large iron gate. I could have seen them in a small office in Dutton Building, but I thought it might be too upsetting to both of them. Anyhow I needed a change in scenery and the half-mile walk each way was good exercise for me. Psychiatrists spend too much of their lives sitting on their arses.

Roberta made excellent progress during the past year. Progress of course depends on who is measuring it. Sometimes patients in psychotherapy appear unchanged or even worse to other people in their lives, while they may appear totally new people in their psychiatrist's office.

When a patient who has always acted dependent and compliant at home begins to get healthier and more independent, he may seem troublesome to those around him. "I don't know what that doctor is doing for you, George. You used to be such a nice guy. You'd give a guy the shirt right off your back. But now look at you. You're a bastard." Of course, no one understands that before, George was so afraid of being rejected that he felt he had to play doormat and wear a "Kick me" sign just to stay on everyone's good side. Now that he believes he's worth something simply because he's himself, he feels he can risk getting angry when someone hurts him. So he's a bastard more often now, but he's a healthier bastard when he is.

238

Roberta seemed healthier, and while it is not an inevitable consequence in every case in which a patient improves, she also happened to become a little bit more of a bastard. Ever since she first was able to get angry at me, be direct in expressing her feelings, she was better able to tolerate the threat of being rejected, abandoned. She'd kept her anger inside her and was afraid that someday if would all explode beyond her control. When Roberta learned she could get angry at me and that I would not run away, she discovered she could get angry at other people and make legitimate demands on them, especially her husband Gary. And because the anger was no longer trapped inside, she could also be more loving.

Because Roberta had not come to terms with her father abandoning her or with her anger at him for doing so, she married Gary, who re-created the situation of her father leaving by threatening to run under the slightest stress.

During the year, Roberta decided she wanted to continue in law school. Gary still didn't like the idea, wanted Roberta to play a role that he felt comfortable with, a role that suited him but had little to do with the person Roberta felt she was or wanted to be. The idea of Roberta becoming anything at all was very threatening to Gary. "What's wrong with staying just the way you are?" he would ask her. "You don't have symptoms now!"

Gary also didn't like Roberta talking back to him. "Viscott should help us get together. He's not doing that," Gary told her repeatedly. I was neither interested in getting the two of them together again, or breaking them up. I was interested in helping Roberta become Roberta, perhaps for the first time, and for Roberta to make up her own mind.

Roberta was also having an affair.

"When I'm with Roy," she said, "I feel like a different person. It's as if being with him brings out all of the good things that just never were there with Gary."

"Like what?" I asked. (Once therapy got underway, I found I didn't have to talk much with Roberta.)

"Like feeling that it's worthwhile just being me, or being a woman. You know, it's a feeling that I've never known. I find living with Gary very rough now. And trying to get him to discuss anything is almost impossible. I come out of these sessions with you with all kinds of new ideas and insights, and I want to share them with him. Forget it! He's too busy, or says he just doesn't want to hear about it. He thinks it's my personal business and that I shouldn't be dragging him into it. He thinks I'm looking for an argument, when I just want to talk."

"Are the two of you arguing a lot?"

"No, I just sort of gave up. I guess if I didn't have Roy to take the pressure off me and make me feel less desperate we'd be fighting all the time. Still, I wish we were arguing a little. At least there'd be *something* to talk about. We sit and watch television most nights after dinner. He goes into the den and reads the paper. I clean up and join him after the news around eight. If I ask him a question, he'll pretend not to hear it, or he'll give me a one-word answer. Mostly, he just shuts me out.

"When I get upset about something he does, he tells me to discuss it with you. He says that's what I'm seeing a psychiatrist for. I told him you offered to see us together."

"What did he say?"

"He said he didn't have any faith in you, that you hadn't really done anything for me, and that now all I seemed interested in was making trouble. After all I've learned about myself, who I am and what I feel, I still can't seem to use any of it in my marriage."

"What gets in the way?"

"Gary, pure and simple. I've thought out our problems and wanted to talk about them with him. I say, 'Gary, would you like to talk?' He says, 'Sure, about what?' I say, 'About the way we get along.' Then he starts screaming at me, 'We get along just fine. It's that Viscott who puts all these crazy ideas in your head.'

"Gary still accuses me of sitting and waiting for a time when we're getting along and then ruining it by bringing up something unpleasant from the past. Well, dammit. I'm not. I just want to get the air clear, and Gary won't ever let me. It's got to be his way. Everything has to be his way—and all the time.

"God, I'm sick of it. I put up with that sort of crap from my mother for years and then what did I do? I ran smack into the arms of the first creep who reminded me of my mother. Except he's even more helpless. He's not doing great in architecture. The firm he's with won't give him a raise. At one of the company cocktail parties I found out that several of the people who started with him are getting raises and their own projects. Gary is practically doing the same jobs that a draftsman could do. He just won't take any initiative. He needs to be led like a student. I really married a winner." Roberta was going full blast.

"And sex . . . well, that's become ridiculous!"

Asking questions about a patient's sex life can be a very tricky business. If a patient suspects that you're asking for your own entertainment, he may overwhelm you with sexual information just to try to please you. After such a deluge of sexual material, it becomes difficult to sort out what the patient is really talking about.

Asking about sexual feelings is a common interest of every beginning psychiatric resident. Residents are concerned about familiarizing themselves with what is normal and developing an understanding of how sexual behavior varies in different emotional states. One soon learns the sexual drive is decreased in depression, and often absent in chronic schizophrenia.

Sexual experiences are seen differently by different people, and I suppose one needs to develop his own collection of case experiences in order to make judgments. Also, patients sometimes feel that they *should* be asked questions about sex. Sometimes residents act out of curiosity when they ask questions about their patients' sexual behavior and I suppose sometimes a resident's interest in sex is prurient. "Nothing wrong with a good healthy prurient interest," Marty Di-Angelo used to say. "As long as you're aware of it and keep it under control, it won't hurt anyone." But a prurient interest on the part of the shrink is a waste of the patient's money. A neat trick—to get someone to pay for your perversion.

You could learn a great deal about a patient by the way he talked about his sexual life. Was it a symbolic act aimed at proving his worth, pleasing someone, or was it an act of sharing? Was it selfish and mechanical? Was it so ritualized and twisted that the people involved had no real identity? You learned a great deal asking about sex, providing you knew what you were looking for before you asked the question, and you were sensitive to your patient's needs and feelings about the subject and your own reasons for asking were to help the patient, not to titillate yourself. If a psychiatrist needs his patient's comments to titillate himself, he's not getting enough action in his own life and should take care of his own business before coming into the office.

It was appropriate to ask Roberta why she felt sex was ridiculous. I waited to see if she would follow her own opening, so I wouldn't have to make a direct inquiry. Why shouldn't I make a direct inquiry? Well, she's married to an unresponsive man, she's having an affair, she's looking for something better, and she has very positive feelings about me. Why should I take the chance of building up her sexual feelings about me by asking a question about sex unless I had to? They'd only get in the way.

"Ridiculous?" I said after a moment, repeating her description and avoiding a personal comment about sex. I hoped this would open the door for other responses by her and was a statement of my desire to understand. It would not be a statement of my curiosity about her sex life. If Roberta left the hour with the impression, "Wow, all that guy is interested in is my sex life," I would have framed my question improperly, and "improperly" would be the perfect word to describe it.

"Yes, ridiculous," Roberta said, "At ten thirty he says—God I'm embarrassed to say it—'You wanna pat the pillow?' Can you believe that? Two grown-ups who can't even talk to each other, directly and frankly. Do I want to 'pat the pillow'! Why can't he just say, 'Let's make love'? Even 'How about a great big juicy lay, there, honey' would be better. What's the matter with him?

"No," said Roberta, looking around the office, pressing her lips together. "That's the *wrong* question! The question is what's the matter with me for staying with a miserable, childish man who can't do anything on his own. He can't be a good architect. He can't take care of me. He can't stand me going to law school. He can't make me happy. He can't talk to me. He can't argue with me. He's a hopeless case. All he can do is sit every night in front of the television and 'pat the pillow' at ten thirty. And he's not very good at it. He always has to be on top and he comes off in thirty seconds, Speedy Gonzales. There, you have it, the confessions of a Jewish housewife. Makes great reading, doesn't it?

"God, it doesn't," Roberta went on, looking downcast. "It's an absolute bore. With Roy it's not that sex is so good. I mean, it *is* great and it's fun, but just being together is always good because we feel closer. It's more than that. Because we're open with each other I'm not interested just in sex. I can't see myself picking up a guy and running off to a motel and screwing till my back gives out. That's my idea of nothing. I could never do that. I'd feel so down and depressed and angry with myself afterward that I couldn't stand it. That's the way I feel after having sex with Gary—no feeling, just used.

"Roy likes me as a person. He likes to talk to me, to listen to me. And when we have a disagreement, we can talk about it without Roy getting hurt. He doesn't run away or pretend he's too busy to talk to me or say that I'm ruining the good times by bringing up the bad. It's just an entirely different way of living and feeling. Gary doesn't want to feel anything.

"Being in therapy isn't easy," she said. "I don't know how it is for your other patients, but I do know that it hasn't been easy for me. I've hated coming here some days and putting all my heart and soul out for you to look at, but I do it because I want to get better. Gary wants me to stay the way I am. I can't live that way."

Roberta opened her handbag and took out a cigarette. "If things were more definite with Roy, I'd consider getting a divorce, but he's not sure about his wife. His marriage is a mess. I don't know what to do."

"Roberta, I think it'd be a mistake to base your decision to get a divorce on your feelings about Roy."

"Why?"

"You have to decide whether or not you want to stay married to Gary, independent of your feelings about Roy or anyone else. It's your decision alone and one that Roy really can't help you make. If you decided to get a divorce just because you wanted Roy more than Gary, it would put a terrible burden on Roy, on you, and on the relationship. Roy might feel obligated to love you after all that you gave up for him, and he might even resent you for it. If you want to divorce Gary, you have to divorce him because you don't want to live with him, not because you want to live with someone else. To use Roy as the reason to leave Gary only avoids dealing with the problems that you and Gary have. And that just opens the door for trouble in the new relationship."

"I never thought of that.... Maybe you're right, maybe I *am* using Roy to make Gary look worse."

"It's not fair to Gary, Roy, or to you. Look, any new relationship has its newness going for it. That feeling of newness is very special. In any new relationship people often mistakenly call feelings of newness 'love.' No matter how good Gary's feelings toward you may become, they can't become brand new. So that comparison with Roy isn't fair. More than that, any new relationship is full of discovery. It's flattering to be accepted by another person and loved, and it's an enormous boost for your ego. And you don't have all the old miserable problems to talk about with the new person. You don't share the same unhappy past, just a hope for the future.

"If you get involved with Roy to avoid the problems that you and Gary have, what will you do when you and Roy start to have problems? There's no way two people can get involved in any meaningful way for more than a few months without having some problems. You have to sort out which of your problems in your marriage are caused by Gary and which are caused by you, and which are just part of the living and being human—the problems that you would have with anybody."

Roberta thought for a moment. She was very quiet. "I guess I haven't been willing to face the problem of Gary and me without keeping Roy as a safety valve. I'm just terribly afraid of being lonely and of finding myself without anyone. I've never really made it on my own. You know, my mother ran my life before I got married, and Gary took over afterward.

"I know you showed me how I really was the strong one in my marriage and how I convinced myself that Gary was the strong one because I needed to think he was caring for me. I even believe you, but that doesn't mean I'm not still afraid of being alone. The idea of being all alone is *terrifying* to me."

"Roberta," I said quietly, "I think you feel lonely already, but don't see it because you're afraid of admitting something so frightening to yourself."

"Oh, I guess you're right. I guess I *am* lonely. I'm lonely when I get up in the morning and make breakfast. I'm lonely when we eat breakfast. I'm alone after he leaves. I'm alone at law school, and when I'm studying in the apartment during the afternoon. I'm lonely when we eat together, lonely cleaning up, lonely watching television. I'm even lonely when we're making love. I guess I'm loneliest when we're making love because he's so quick about it, I can't even pretend he's someone else. I can't even have a fantasy to keep me company. Isn't that terrible?"

"You just said something interesting, you said you felt *lonely* when you were with Gary but that you felt *alone* when you were by yourself. There's a big difference between being alone and being lonely."

"That's right," said Roberta, brightening up. "I did say that. When I'm alone I at least have myself and my interests. I really like law school and my life there. It's when I get home and I'm with Gary that I feel badly. Then I realize that I'm not really being me, that I'm just someone to please Gary. When I'm with Gary I can't really be myself. Maybe the person I'm lonely for is the part of me Gary won't let come out. Maybe if I were alone, I wouldn't be so lonely. Does that make sense to you?"

It was a real insight and damned well put. I didn't want to be

a cheerleader, though, so I answered her by simply assuring her that
it did make sense and I thought I knew what she meant.

Roberta sat looking out the office window. It was a dreary De-
cember afternoon. Three thirty and the sky was already dark. I
could hear the muffled sound of traffic in the wet snowy streets, red
and orange taillights moved slowly along their way home. Lights
came on in the tenements across the way. On the sidewalk some
visitors shuffled through the snow toward a bus. Strings of colored
Christmas lights, with Santas in the middle, hung over the boulevard
and were swinging in the gray afternoon wind.

"It can get terribly lonely out there," Roberta said after a while.
"I could be alone for a long, long time. But look how long I've felt
lonely already. In my marriage I can't even have my real self to keep
me company . . . You're right," she said energetically, "I have to decide something because it's what I need, because it's what I want
to do, not because I have Roy as an alternative. If I find another person and love him, it has to be because I love him, not because I need
someone to rescue me from my marriage. Otherwise that person won't
really be himself either. He'll just be like I've been in my marriage.
I have to admit to myself what's missing in my marriage and decide
if I can get along without it. If I can't, I'll just have to leave."

"That's a very tough decision to make."

"I know, but I think that I have already made it."

"Oh?" I said, a little surprised.

"Look at those cars," said Roberta, pointing to the window. "In
a few minutes, I'll be driving in that traffic. I'll just melt into it. Who
will I be going home to? To someone who loves the real me? To
someone who brings out the best part of me and who I do the
same for? To a relationship with a future? I don't think so.

"I've gotten up in the middle of the night too many times, walked
from room to room and looked out at the city and wondered what
was going on behind each lighted window off there in the distance.
I knew somewhere out there someone was staying up being with
someone else. I knew someone out there wanted to talk to someone
else. I knew it didn't matter to them if there was work tomorrow and
they both had to be up early, because they felt that the other person
was important and wanted to talk to her. And I knew I was all alone.

"I've envied too many people that I knew just by the look on
their faces that they cared about someone and someone cared about
them. I can't stand anymore the jealousy I've had all these years
watching the other couples in restaurants who seemed so interested

in each other. I've hated with envy the couples sitting close together in their cars, or talking, or just being together—or people standing and hugging in the park. I got so upset that I even refused to see any friends who were in love because it hurt so much.

"I've sat up too many hours at night on the edge of my bed waiting for the television to go black and wondering if I'd have to spend the rest of my life with someone who I really didn't love. Why do I have to serve such a long sentence for the crime of being a coward? All I really ever did wrong in my life was to be afraid of being myself."

Roberta reached across the table and put her hand on my wrist.

"Do you understand how I feel?"

"Yes, I think so."

"I guess I really made up my mind to get divorced a long time ago." Roberta smiled, getting up to leave.

I walked Roberta out. The waiting room was empty. Magazines were piled everywhere.

"I'll see you next week," I said.

Roberta nodded and suddenly put her arms around me and hugged me. I put my arms around her for a moment and just held her. What was I doing? Come on, David, this is just what you're *not* supposed to do. What *was* I doing? Roberta squeezed my arms, smiled, and left.

My God. I must have lost my mind. You're not supposed to put your arms around a patient. Jerry Gelb had told me, "It just complicates everything. The patient will distort your intentions and you never know what will happen." Would Roberta begin to see me as a sexual object and mess up therapy by trying to make holding each other at the end of the session a regular event? Would she try to seduce me? I was really shaken.

I am ordinarily a very physical person. I enjoy hugging my friends. I'm usually spontaneous and open about my feelings. I was sure that this represented my natural response to a lonely person I cared about. It had been entirely genuine and was really a sign of friendship and understanding. If Roberta had been one of my wife's friends and we had been talking about one of her problems and she hugged me and I hugged her at the end of our conversation I wouldn't have given it a second thought. It wouldn't have meant that we were going to have an affair. This peculiar business of psychotherapy had taken a normal feeling and made its expression (probably a necessary expression) seem self-conscious and embarrassed.

Just a minute! What is all this nonsense? I was not being seduced, and I was not seducing Roberta Goldman. I was sharing a sense of closeness with her and responding to her like a human being. Goddammit! There is nothing wrong with being a human being so long as you don't let it get out of control. Just look at how contrived all this is, how torturous all these thoughts are. Isn't the purpose of therapy to help the patient become more human? Maybe I did do the wrong thing. Maybe I should have pushed Roberta away. But that would have been abandoning her again, and I just didn't have time to think. I merely reacted the way I normally reacted.

I was to learn that Roberta Goldman took it exactly the way I meant it.

How do you like that? It was possible to be a human being and a psychiatrist at the same time!

I was waiting for Donald Johnson to show. He was usually right on time. He was ten minutes late today. Odd?

Donald had called me only once during the past year. When I picked up the phone he seemed to have forgotten why he called and for almost a minute he hunted for a reason and then began to tell me how frightening it could be staring up at the skies alone at night. It didn't sound terribly convincing. I asked him if he was just checking to see if the phones worked, if he really was allowed to call me. He laughed and said, "Yes," added, "Well, I'll see you next Tuesday."

It had been a very good year for Donald. He became very involved in therapy, which means he was willing to discuss his feelings. He was more willing to endure a painful feeling and think about it instead of getting into trouble or translating his feelings into hectic action. Donald was beginning to take life more as he found it, without getting entangled in as many disturbing little "sideshows," as we called his episodes of running away and his grandstand plays for sympathy. Donald was in college, just finishing first semester, and was doing exceptionally well. He was making friends for the first time, not many to be sure and as yet no one close he could confide in, but he did have a few friends he ate with and went to the movies with. He had even been dating!

Donald knocked on my office door, which was ajar. "Anyone home?"

"Hi, Donald."

"Sorry I'm late," he said, looking at the wall clock. "Is that the right time, quarter past? Jesus! You never saw such traffic in your life! You'd think they'd know how to handle a little snow by now. I've got something important to tell you." He was grinning wide, kicked the door closed and shouted, "Guess who isn't a virgin anymore?"

This *was* an exception to the rule that a psychiatrist should not appear interested in the sexual activity of his patients. One of Donald's problems was his inability to get close enough to people to trust them. He had always been afraid of sexual contact. Both his parents were cold, superficial, and rejecting, and he'd had no friends to talk to. Donald needed the support of someone he knew was interested in him and he could share his experiences with. While I did not want to play the role of one college roommate asking the other about every little pubic detail of a first sexual encounter, I felt I should be more like a friend at this moment than a typical psychiatrist with a patient. Donald needed to feel that it was OK to be sexual.

I looked up at him with a half smile. "Let me guess," I said. "You!"

He jumped up and down like a madman. "Mr. and Mrs. Alan Johnson of 34 Brainaird Road are proud to announce that their son, Donald, is no longer cherry. Remember that girl, Rosalie, I was telling you about? She's *the one*. You wanna hear what happened?" He didn't give me a chance to answer.

"Well, I was very upset last week after coming here. I guess it was because we were talking about my cousin Rennie. I began to realize how much I missed Rennie after he died. I mean, we were very close. You know, Rennie and I were closer than you think. I mean, we used to do everything together. We even used to jerk off together." Donald turned his head away, not being sure of how I would react.

"When was that?"

"When I was about twelve, the summer just before he died."

"It's common at that age for that sort of horsing around. Most boys do."

"Yeah," said Donald, "except I got very upset about it because I wasn't sure whether or not Rennie's illness had anything to do with jerking off together. I know it's crazy, but that's what I worried about."

"You were just feeling guilty over something you didn't understand. Feeling guilty can make you imagine some very strange things and worry about things you ordinarily wouldn't give a second thought to."

"Well, I still always felt I had something to do with Rennie's

kidney disease." Donald looked down at the floor. "I also remembered something else after I left the office last week. I remembered
what happened that made me go haywire last year."

"What was that?"

"This is embarrassing as shit, but I'll tell you if you promise
not to laugh at me."

"I promise."

"Well, I used to masturbate a lot. I mean, I still do, but not as
much as before. Sometimes, I'd try to shoot right into the toilet bowl
from a couple of feet away, like target practice. When I was a little
kid I used to piss from across the bathroom and try and get it into
the bowl, or I'd float something in the bowl to aim at, but when I
got older I would beat off into the bowl. Well, one day my sister
Michelle had to use the bathroom right after me because she was
going out with her fiancé. I was just about to wipe up since I had
missed the bowl and come was all over everything, the seat, the basin,
and the floor. My mother would have died if she knew because she
was such a nut on keeping things clean. I mean, this year at college
is the first time in my life that I've ever worn the same shirt two
days in a row! Well..." Donald looked down at the floor again,
trying to see if he could think up anything else before making his
"confession."

I could almost always tell when one was coming. Patients either
spoke more slowly or asked permission to confess or tried to extort
a promise not to punish them. Sometimes they just looked away
and seemed hesitant, then resolved, then hesitant, and then finally
resolved again. And the secret would start to come out.

"Jesus," said Donald, "this is going to sound terrible. I got out
of the bathroom in a hurry. I was afraid Michelle was going to force
open the lock. She used to yell through the door at me, 'Are you playing with yourself,' and really embarrass me. Once I got so mad at
her I masturbated inside one of her fur-lined gloves, and ruined it.
Michelle didn't know what was wrong with it, but it was stuck and
stiff and she was sore. Anyhow," Donald said, gathering up his courage, "I got out of the bathroom without cleaning up and Michelle
went rushing in, pushing me out of the way. I could hear the toilet
flush so I knew Michelle used it, and I was sure there was sperm
on the toilet seat and I was sure she sat on it." Donald sighed. "Well,
anyway, I didn't know that much about the birds and the bees, and
when Michelle got married two months later I was sure it was because I got her pregnant from the toilet seat. That's when I started

to worry that what I wanted and thought about really would come true. I was scared to death, I felt I couldn't do anything to stop these awful things from happening unless I had the power of God and could rule the world and everything that happened in it. That's why I guess I was so hung up with the stars at night and talking to them. I'm really fucked up, aren't I?" Donald asked anxiously. He was seriously asking me if I thought he was crazy. I didn't think so.

"Sounds like the sort of thing I've heard from a lot of other people," I said, "people who weren't necessarily mental patients, normal people. Donald, those are very common feelings and fears, including the one that your own fantasies will inevitably come true. Most people at least had more friends than you did as a kid, and they could confide in them and know that other people had thoughts and feelings just as weird and scary as theirs. *You* thought you were the only one to think and feel like you."

"The only friend I had was Rennie, and I thought beating off together killed him. I had no one to talk to about it. I couldn't tell anyone about the way I felt about Rennie because it would be like confessing a murder. This business with my sister was another thing I kept to myself. So when my sister got pregnant months after she got married, I really thought I'd done it.

"I didn't know how long a pregnancy takes or anything. I was only about fifteen. I mean, I knew a lot about school stuff, but I didn't know much about life. What was I supposed to do, raise my hand in class and ask, 'If you beat off on a toilet seat and your sister sits on it, how long will it take for her to become pregnant.' I mean, everyone would know what I did. I mean, I couldn't ask a thing like that, and certainly not of any of the priests at St. George's.

"So like you said, I kept it all inside me and worried about it all the time. Except I didn't worry about it. I just went out and did crazy things. I wanted to get away. I may even have wanted to get caught and punished for the things I'd done—just like you said."

I'd told Donald that his stealing cars and turning in fire alarms sounded to me like a wish to be punished. Jerry Gelb had been fascinated by my reports on Donald and felt early on that Donald's turning in fire alarms was related to some sexual guilt.

"Anyhow," Donald went on, "I did a lot of thinking about all this last week, and the guilt about Rennie and Michelle came back even though I knew down deep that I'd nothing to do with Rennie's death or my sister's pregnancy. I decided to go to a graveyard. You know the way I used to wander around graveyards all the time before last year."

Donald sometimes stayed out all night then and even slept in graveyards, especially when he got upset about Rennie. Sometimes he felt so guilty about Rennie he would get very sad and wander off to the nearest graveyard and stay there, pretending he'd just lost someone. After a while he'd feel better, even though he actually didn't know who it was he'd just pretended he had lost.

"It was Rennie all the time," said Donald. "Can you imagine, I just realized that last week. I suddenly wanted to go to a grave-yard again, but this time it was one graveyard in particular. And I wanted to go to Rennie's grave but I didn't want to go alone. I mean, this felt much sadder to me than going to a stranger's grave like I used to and standing there and hoping bystanders would see me and feel sorry for me. I felt I needed someone to go with me. I was thinking of calling you, but then I decided you must be busy and instead I called Rosalie. I mean, I really like Rosalie. She's very sweet and very sympathetic. She's the only real friend I've ever had besides Rennie.

"We took her car and drove out to Rennie's cemetery.

"Christmas week is an awful time to go to a cemetery. It was cold and raining. I had to ask the caretaker where Rennie was buried. He gave me directions to, get this, the Garden of Saint Francis, chil-drens' section, row H.

"I walked right by the gravestone. Rosalie saw it. My aunt and uncle put up one of these stones with angels on each side. Rennie hated that sort of thing. I'll tell you this right now, I'm leaving direc-tions to be cremated when I go." Donald was trying to be light-hearted at the same time he was barely able to hold back his tears. "Standing there was very strange. It *was* very different from the kind of pretending I'd done before. I was standing over the grave of someone I *knew*, someone I really cared for, someone I really needed. It was finally real, not fake. I didn't want Rosalie to feel sorry for me, just to make sure I was OK and didn't do something crazy. I was afraid something would happen. I just stood there for about a half hour and cried. I don't think I ever cried like that in my entire life.

"Rosalie drove me back to her apartment. It was cold and wet out, and we were both soaked. But I somehow felt very relieved. I finally wasn't afraid of something that I didn't even know I'd been afraid of before, and that I could only admit being afraid of when I *wasn't* afraid anymore. Sounds weird, I know. . . .

"I felt very different than I'd ever felt before, very strong. Rosalie asked me to start a fire in the fireplace. Rosalie has a great apartment in an old townhouse. I guess her folks have lots of money. She said she had to take off her clothes and change them, and that I must be freezing and that I should take mine off. I was shy, but like I said, I also felt very good. Rosalie came into the living room and pulled off my sweater and unbuttoned my shirt. Before I knew it, we were both completely undressed.

"I never saw a girl undressed before. I just stared at her and she smiled at me and told me I was cute. She dried me off with a towel and then I started to dry her off. But I had this fantastic hard on and I just held her very tight. We were standing in front of the fire. I got a cramp so we lay down and start kissing and hugging and I could feel her hair against me and she was wet there. She reached down and put it in and we just lay there for a minute without moving and it felt so good and I felt so close to her. I never felt close to anyone before, and we started to pump and screw and it was incredible! It was unbelievable! She was so smooth and warm, and I just got lost in her. I spent the night there. Well, not the whole night. We were screwing so much that we forgot to eat, so we went out for a pizza at two A.M. and then came back and went to bed."

Donald was leaning back in his chair with a big smile on his face. He seemed very pleased with himself.

Donald had come of age, in so many ways.

CHAPTER NINETEEN

THE ACUTE SERVICE:
END-OF-TERM STATE HOSPITAL—
AN END TO MADNESS

IF IT was excitement that was lacking in my life I found it when I left the Dutton Building. I was assigned eleven female patients on ward Able in the reception building. None of my patients on the acute service had been in the hospital longer than three months. They were all very active. I split the ward with Bert Feinstein so I had at least one familiar face to look at. It wasn't much consolation. The six wards in the reception building were almost always full, with thirty patients each. Patients were admitted to the wards in rotation straight from the emergency floor, so they could be pretty hairy at times. Everything happened at a much faster pace than I had seen on D ward. People here even interacted with each other. Maybe they did it in crazy ways, like one patient offering prayers to another, but they did interact. Why, I never even saw a patient on D ward so much as bum a cigarette from another patient.

A young, sylphlike black woman named Honey Lomax was the RN who ran the ward. Miss Mühler, a practical nurse who had worked on the ward for years, resented Honey Lomax because Honey Lomax *was* black, beautiful, brainy, and young. Honey's rundown of our charges wasn't very encouraging but it was fast and to the point.

A Theresa and Marcia were involved in destructive behavior toward the ward personnel and themselves. They were also sexually involved and flaunted it. They upset visitors and other patients. They were both slashers and just the previous week Marcia had slashed her legs so badly she needed thirty stitches. Marcia Patton was fifteen. She had a very raunchy vocabulary and propositioned Bert the first moment she saw him on the ward. Not sexy. Not funny.

"The rest of the patients are pretty good," Honey said, "as good as you can expect patients in a state mental hospital to be. I know I've been here too long when I think these patients are 'good.' Ramona Rogers is a paranoid lady who thinks she's being murdered. She's always running off the ward, so we try to open the door carefully. Georgia is a twenty-year-old chronic patient who was out of the hospital for a while. She got upset and is back in again. She's angry and very brittle. She looks like she's going to blow any minute. Dr. Frogner, the doctor you're taking over from, didn't believe in putting patients on medication, but I'd appreciate your looking at her to see if you agree with that."

I had a meeting with Dr. William Standish, the director of the reception building. He was tall, skinny, dressed in tweeds, wore horn-rimmed glasses and hiking boots. Dr. Standish was an interested and helpful man. He told me how bad Dr. Frogner had been, that he hadn't trusted him, and that my patients were in worse shape than necessary because of him.

"If he's so bad, why is he allowed to stay in the residency program?" I asked.

"Well," Standish said, cleaning his glasses, which he did several times an hour, "if you question another doctor about his treatment plan, he can always say that what's best for a patient is a matter of opinion. Dr. Frogner refused to give medication to his patients because he said he believed that psychotherapy was better than medication."

"He did? I'm surprised Frogner would say that."

"I'm not," Standish said angrily, "because Frogner never did any psychotherapy either. It was the damndest situation. When I told him to start using tranquilizers he accused me of being antipsycho-analytic." And Standish was an analyst. "As far as I could tell, Frogner didn't do much of anything. I'm just hoping that I never see him after this year. Thank God, it's his last year of residency."

My patients needed a lot of attention. Frogner had written less than a single page of notes on each patient. He would see each patient for five minutes a week, and that was to write orders for home visits. Essentially, all he did was to let patients stay in the hospital and quiet down on their own. Frequently the only benefit to them while they were in the hospital was that the frantic, upsetting home situation that existed before had cooled off. A considerable number of admissions did result from stress and turmoil at home, so Frogner *could* argue that his method worked.

I felt a great deal of pressure to see and find out more about my patients. Georgia, the chronic schizophrenic woman, had been a patient in the hospital on and off for the past five years. When she stayed on her medication she did well. When she did not, she deteriorated. Georgia refused to visit the hospital outpatient clinic after her discharge, or follow instructions. I started her back on her old medication again. Frogner had to be a complete idiot—or maybe he was psychotic himself and was not taking the patients' symptoms seriously because he didn't take his own symptoms seriously? Who knows? It was only a theory, but there had to be a reason for Frogner's behavior. Psychiatrists tend to label behavior with big words too much. Maybe Frogner was just a sick quack.

A Mrs. Gold was also my patient. She was almost mute. When she did speak, it was all garbled. She never expressed a complete or logical thought. She had been in the hospital the year before and had received electroshock therapy for her psychotic depression and improved quickly. Since her hospitalization six weeks ago, Frogner had seen her only twice. Unlike Mr. Brodner on Bamberg 5, if ever there was a clear case for giving electroshock therapy this woman was it. She was depressed, restless, suicidal, woke up each morning at three or four, and had a history of dramatic improvement in shock therapy. She refused to sit, let alone talk, with me. I scheduled her electroshock.

By the time I had gone through these patients it was getting late. Almost without exception, Frogner had done nothing for them, and they all needed something which was clearly available. Many of these patients could benefit from medication. Many had done so before. That didn't take so many brains to figure out.

I also saw Miss Fogg, schizophrenic and alcoholic. She'd frequently been "raped" in the back booths of bars in the dock district. She continually went into bars where she would be the only woman and where she was certain to meet her previous "rapists." Miss Fogg needed more than medication, psychotherapy, or a hospital. She needed a caretaker to watch over her twenty-four hours a day.

I spoke to Maggie Shapiro, the social worker for ward Able, about Miss Fogg.

"Miss Fogg?" Maggie said in the hoarse voice of a chain smoker. "You want to do something with Miss Fogg. Why not? Everyone else does whatever they want with Miss Fogg."

Maggie Shapiro was half thirty-three-year-old Jewish grandmother, half horny schoolgirl. I don't know a better way to describe her. Maggie had gone to Goucher, spent some time as an assistant editor for a woman's magazine in New York, and then had gone into social service. Maggie was practical—very practical. She was also very much in the market for a husband.

When I walked into her office, she took off her blue plastic glasses rimmed with rhinestones and said, "I have two questions: first, are you married and second, are you Jewish? If you're married it makes a difference whether or not you're Jewish. I could cope with you being married, if you're Jewish. If you're not Jewish, you've got to be single. I can only break one taboo at a time. You want to talk about Miss Fogg?"

"Yes."

"Well, I don't know why. That girl has a sex life, let me tell you, like an alley cat. Don't waste your time trying to do something about it. You can't stop her. No one can."

"Isn't there anyone who can take care of her?" I asked.

"She has a sister, but even she threw Miss Fogg out of the house last year when Miss Fogg brought home a sailor *and* his friend."

"What about calling Miss Fogg's sister and seeing if she'll take her back?"

"It's the state's dime."

I could see Maggie Shapiro was going to become my biggest ally.

"Do you know anything about Sophia Beck?" I asked her.

"Do I know anything about Sophia Beck? Ask and I'll tell."

I could also see how Maggie could become something of a pain in the ass.

"When Sophia Beck was thirteen she was picked up by Germans invading Russia and was forced to travel with the troops as a prostitute. Only the Germans could do that, a lovely people. If we had enough beds I would commit the whole lot of them. She was branded by her people as a German sympathizer and just before the war ended she married a German private, with one leg yet. Two cripples. She got pregnant and he got killed and the war got finished."

"A real horror story," I said.

"She won't tell it to you. She told it once eight years ago to a doctor here, but she refuses to talk to anyone now. Her son refused to speak Russian at home and married a girl she didn't like and left home. Every year on his wedding anniversary, she gets angry and cries and then goes paranoid and ends up here."

It was a familiar situation. People who suffered tremendous losses during the war seemed able to endure them well because they did not take the war as a personal attack, but when a member of their own family left them they took it personally and seemed to fall apart.

"Last year," said Maggie, "I got her boss to let her go back to work as soon as possible. She'll need a little medication to do it. You believe in medication, I hope? You look like a good boy, not like Dr. Frogner. You know, even though Mrs. Beck was the only patient on the ward Dr. Frogner was interested in, he alienated her because he spoke to her in German. Now there's a sick man, if you don't mind me saying so."

I had only two more patients to see. Ina Kahn, the evening nurse, was on duty. She was a harried, wornout-looking woman of indeterminate age. She looked exhausted, drained.

"I'd like to see Elaine Jenkins," I said.

"You're probably the only one in the world who does," said Ina, holding the back of her hand to her forehead as if she were trying to tell whether she had a fever. "She really drives us crazy here. I just *hate* manic patients."

Elaine Jenkins was rummaging through the seams in the day hall furniture, looking for change. When she finished with one piece of furniture she would move it to another place, even if someone were sitting on it.

This place really is a madhouse. What the hell am I doing here? It's seven o'clock and I should be home with my family.

"Elaine," I approached her cautiously, "I'm Dr. Viscott. Can I see you in my office?"

"Why not? Cry not!" Elaine stopped pushing furniture and started to stack magazines and then followed me to my office. "If you don't try, you won't die. I used to have an office which opened and shut with regularity, you see. I am very happy to be here. Where is this?

"Are you going to open the door?" Elaine shouted when we reached the office, "or am I going to have to get someone to break through it? Are we going to have a breakthrough? It would be something new. Do you? Who?

"I grew eight or ten inches between my twelfth and thirteenth birthday," Elaine said, sitting down. "That was a good thing to say to a doctor. Do you like to say things? I say things."

I tried ignoring what she was saying. Manics say a lot of words that sound like they'd be worth looking into. You have to keep them on one point, your point. "Why are you in the hospital?"

"Don't you have all that written down? I'm here because I like to play with myself." Elaine was suddenly getting sarcastic and bitter. "They say it makes your mind go. Can we organize a search party to find where my mind went? I'd like it back. I wouldn't like to keep it locked up. You're not going to lock me up, are you?" Elaine got up and moved toward the door, suddenly terrified.

"No, I'm not!"

"They locked me up. It was in what they call seclusion. I did it in my pants. I haven't done that since I was four years old! Do you know what a grown-up feels like when he does that? I cried. I felt like I was a baby." Just like that, Elaine sounded like a reasonable person. She was talking about feeling hurt and angry in seclusion, not running all over the place associating words by rhyme, trying to avoid me.

"That sounds unbearable," I said. "I certainly have no intention of putting you in seclusion." I knew very little about Elaine Jenkins because the admission note in the chart was vague, and Frogner's notes were usually illegible and irrelevant anyway. At best he only described Elaine's ward behavior, calling her "hostile, uncooperative, and hyperactive," not why she was acting the way she did.

"It was horrible in there," said Elaine. She sounded very sad. It's important to get manics to talk about sadness because their hyper-activity is a way of avoiding it. "I was upset, but I'm not upset any-more," she said, suddenly cheerful again. "Right now I'm ready to go back to work," and added haughtily, "You can discharge me tomorrow morning right after breakfast."

"Where will you go?"

"I work in a bakery. I sell things. Would you like a roll in the hay, today? What do you say?" Elaine sounded frightened again.

"Which bakery do you work in?" I asked, trying to keep her on track.

"Gino's. It's an Italian bakery on Fields Square. Do you like pignoli? They're great. I eat a couple of dozen a day." She patted her round tummy like a pie-eating champion after winning a contest.

Elaine was short and dumpy with brown stringy hair. Although she was probably under twenty-five, she had already acquired the "state hospital" look; an expression of confusion and preoccupation, a drabness and a disarray in dress, all combined with a certain in-appropriateness in everything she did. Elaine's movements in a group stood out because she moved at continually different tempos. Some-times she rushed desperately. The next moment she seemed suddenly slowed down and hesitant, like a child afraid to approach a strange animal. There was no predictable flow to her actions at all. . . .

It became easy to pick out such people walking in a large crowd in the city. Other people usually don't notice them or don't want to notice them or take them for bums and brush them aside. They are the chronic psychotics finding their ways through two worlds at the same time, theirs and the world around them. They understand neither world well and struggle, trying to decide which world is real, whether the voice they hear calling their name is real or just a voice, whether the bus they are riding on is owned by the local transit authority or by their imagination. The place where they began feels so unbearable to them that they have changed the world to try to forget it. Their destination? They have none, except to run from their pain. . . .

"I'll bring you in some pignoli tomorrow night when I come back from work," Elaine said, calm again.

"Where's home?"

"Home? I live with my aunt and uncle."

I wondered if her parents were dead. Manic people often deny death. "How long have you lived with them?" I asked.

"Five years," said Elaine, now looking restless.

And now I had an opening. "Where did you live before?" Maybe someone died five years ago. Maybe that had made her acutely manic.

"In Albany," Elaine said anxiously.

"With whom?" I felt I was on the right track.

"My mother," she said softly. Then she started sobbing. In a moment she was kneeling on the floor, praying loudly, "Holy Mary, Mother of God. Pray for us sinners now and at the hour of our death. Pray for me Mary, Mommy . . ."

This had not really been a breakthrough to lost feelings in Elaine's past. Elaine went through similar outbursts several times a day. The point was that the feelings she had expressed did not seem to help her mourn her mother who had died five years ago. The death Elaine could not cope with was not her mother's, but the threat of her own. When manic patients fear death, they often become more active, as if to prove to themselves that they are still alive. As their fear grows, their activity increases.

"Elaine, we have a lot to talk about—"

Elaine had run out to the day hall to ransack a pile of coats. . . .

The last patient to see was Sheila Duggin. I never had seen anyone like her.

She was my age and dressed in a herringbone suit, wearing thick glasses. She looked as though she had just been kidnapped from behind a librarian's desk.

"I have been waiting for you," she said. "It is, of course, very appropriate of you to have waited until you had seen all the other patients so that we could compare notes. I have mine all here." Sheila showed me a notebook filled with pages of well-organized notes.

"I was a psychology student in college until I switched to sociology," Sheila explained. "You'll find these quite complete." Sheila had been in graduate school, but couldn't keep up with the work. She had been seen in therapy by Tanya Milhady at the state hospital OPD until she decompensated and had to be hospitalized. Sheila saw the world only in intellectual terms, expressed in jargon, a little like a certain resident you're by now familiar with. That's not really fair because Sheila, of course, was much more rigid, completely out of touch with her feelings although she could describe everyone else's beautifully, mine included. Sheila used her descriptive ability and her insight to push people away when they got too close. It was her *style* of thinking that made Sheila psychotic. Just because her defenses were more logical and well-organized than the other patients, their object was still the same, to numb reality's sting.

Her notes were fascinating.

January 2nd: New Doctors
PATTON: Disgusting verbal seductive attempt on Dr. Feinstein in A.M., obviously a reaction formation to her own homosexual strivings.
BECK: Uncommunicative and disorganized.
GOLD: Should have shock treatments. (*At least one other person agrees with me!*)
RAMONA: Needs medication. If new doctor continues Dr. Frogner's policy, call the health commissioner, 544-7820.
(*I took that as a direct threat.*)
GEORGIA: Seems worse. More hostility, less internalization.
JENKINS: Still complaining about her leg. After two months I suspect there is no pain. This woman is a hypochondriac.
(*I'll bet Sheila picked up something everyone else missed. If Jenkins had to stay in bed to take care of a leg injury, she might have been upset about being sick—afraid of dying—and could have become manic as a result.*)

"Well, this is a very interesting list."

"Thank you," said Sheila, confident her comments were good before I told her.

"But it's missing something."

"Oh, yes, I forgot the notes about the nurses and the doctors."

That was not what I meant, but I was fascinated to read what she had written.

> Dr. FEINSTEIN: Businesslike, perhaps too businesslike? Is he covering a sense of anxiety over the new ward assignment?
> (*Probably, but who isn't. I never thought of Bert as businesslike.*)
> Dr. VISCOTT: Friendly. Smiles easily. Perhaps this, too, is a cover for anxiety. I question whether or not he can be trusted.
> Miss LOMAX: Continues her sweetness as a cover for being angry at patients.
> Miss MÜHLER: Trying to make Feinstein and Viscott believe she is running the ward. Continues to be threatened by me and Miss Lomax.

"There's still something missing," I said. "There's no report on you here."

"And?" said Sheila, eyeing me carefully.

"I'd like to know about you."

"You, Dr. Viscott, are merely my ward administrator. I am Dr. Milhady's therapy patient. I'll talk to her and to no one else. My conversations with Dr. Milhady are privileged. I expect you to respect the secrecy of our doctor-patient relationship and ask no further questions. I will address you when I need something. I do not think there is anything else I need from you at the moment."

I stood up and bowed a courtly bow. "If it pleases Your Grace, there being nothing else you desire of your humble servant, might I ask a favor?"

Sheila was a little shook, but kept up her disdainful facade. "Yes, go ahead."

"When you talk to me, Sheila, you will cut the shit! I am not a servant. I am a physician, and this is not room service." I wasn't really angry at her charade but I felt she needed it played back to her, to show her how she came across to others.

"You can't talk to me like that—"

"I can talk to you any way I please. What's more, Sheila, as your ward administrator I can also do as I please. If you want anything from me, such as weekend passes or privileges of any kind, you'll have to act a little differently around here."

"I . . ." Sheila was upset. Good! I got through a little.

"I think your comments are very valuable. You do write very clear, insightful notes and you do have the skill to observe things that

other patients don't. That's useful but while it separates you from the
other patients, it doesn't really get you any closer to the staff. I'll look
at your notes with you, but only on one condition. I also want you to
write notes on Sheila Duggin each day," I said, borrowing an idea
from Fern Woods, the occupational therapist from Bamberg 5.

"Very clever," said Sheila, admiring the technique and intellectualizing her response as much as possible. "That's like role playing
in a way, isn't it? You want me to play the role of you, observing me!"

"What do you say?"

Sheila's glasses had fallen down on her nose. She pushed them
back up and stared at me. "That's suitable," said Sheila, maybe even
smiling a little.

I tried to spend between fifteen minutes and a half hour with
each of my patients nearly every day. That may not seem like much
time compared to the academic world of Bamberg 5, but it was a great
deal more than patients in the state hospial were accustomed to.
Things even started to happen after a while.

Marcia Patton calmed down when Bert told Theresa, who was a
prostitute, that he would send her back to the penitentiary if she
got involved in any more trouble. Theresa, like many psychopaths,
tried to make the trouble she started appear to be someone else's
doing. Theresa promptly leaned on Marcia and told her to behave.
Since Marcia was a follower, the slashing and window-breaking
stopped.

Georgia responded beautifully to her old medication and was
discharged in a few weeks. Miss Mühler helped her pack, she was so
glad to see her go.

Ramona, the paranoid who thought she was about to be murdered, also responded well. High doses of tranquilizers changed her
from a wild crazy lady, always knocking people over, to a more routine
crazy lady. She still had disorganized thoughts and feelings, but she
was at least willing to sit in one place and sometimes tell you what
she felt. Ramona's cousin spoke to Maggie Shapiro and said she had
never seen Ramona looking so well in her entire life and demanded
to know when Ramona would be released.

Ramona was discharged the next day. Her cousin recommended
me highly to her parish priest in case he ever needed to send someone
to a psychiatrist. I shuddered at the thought of being referred an
endless series of Ramonas.

Mrs. Gold got along even better with electroshock than I had expected. She stopped trying to escape. She talked about going home. Mrs. Gold was even knitting me a sweater, baby blue, as a matter of fact. Maggie Shapiro made a special effort to enlist the support of Mrs. Gold's relatives and the Jewish Family Service. Maggie knew all the ropes.

If you're thinking that all this is presented just to make me look the great psychiatrist, you're wrong. These are some of the patients I found on my ward who were getting better just by my following the cookbook. There was nothing really remarkable about anything I was doing. Honey Lomax summed up my magic formula: "As far as I can tell you don't do anything any different; you just spend a lot of time on the ward making sure everyone is doing what they're supposed to be doing instead of goofing off."

Whatever I did accomplish seemed to have more to do with my effort than with my personality. A psychiatrist's personality seems to play a less important role in the treatment of psychotics than it does with neurotics. Psychotics just don't allow that much from the outside world to penetrate. Although they still respond better to someone who is kind and caring than they would to someone who's nasty and critical, they don't seem very subtle about other aspects of their doctor's personality. In fact, a doctor's personality may be overlooked entirely by a psychotic patient. Psychotics tend to see a person merely as another source of stimuli from the outside world, not as a human being with feelings. The psychotic is mainly interested in knowing whether the outside stimulus will be painful to him or not.

It was easy to see how a psychiatrist who was unsure of himself as a person, who didn't want to engage other people in intense personal relationships, might prefer to treat patients like this; how he might thrive on it and how, in fact, his patients might do very well. Such a psychiatrist and his patients both depend on a sense of distance between them and a respect for the integrity of the other for their comfort. Since many psychotics have or have had intrusive, smothering parents who pushed them into a shell, this sort of therapist may be just what the doctor ordered, so to speak, even if it is a choice made more often out of necessity than intent.

Of course this was not true for all doctors at the state hospital. Many enjoyed the academic setting or the "action." You just never saw patients this sick anywhere else.

Miss Fogg's cousin was willing to give her another chance and take her in again, and she left once the arrangements were made. There was no real treating Miss Fogg. It was a holding action at best.

I could do nothing with her. My choices were either to pump her full of medication and lock her up or handcuff her to someone who would look after her. I let her go back to live with her cousin, but I expected her to be returned to the ward the first time she acted up.

One morning Sophia Beck announced in her thick German accent that she wanted to go back to work again. Just like that! No explanation at all! Whatever was going on inside her remained buried. Just as most of what went on in these patients remained hidden to me.

Elaine Jenkins stayed manic most of the time. During the first few weeks I kept increasing her medication until she showed signs of settling down. She took huge doses of tranquilizers. I was amazed she could still walk, let alone run, which she still did most of the time. She returned to work, commuting from the hospital with little difficulty, but every attempt to discharge her made her manic, and it also made her complain about pains in the legs. She couldn't take separations. I asked Maggie to see if she could get Elaine transferred to the halfway house, which was like a boardinghouse except it was run by the state hospital. There she could work out of a home setting and still feel the protection of the hospital until she was ready to make it on her own.

Sheila Duggin stayed exactly the same. Nothing I did or Tanya Milhady said seemed to work. Every day Sheila became more rigid in her thinking and more fixed in her beliefs. She did write interesting notes. Even if those she wrote about herself were distorted to make her appear the only sane one on the ward, at least she was still talking to me.

Because Sheila continued to get worse, I thought she should be on medication. I felt it was self-indulgent wishful thinking on my part to use only psychotherapy in treating her. I decided to have lunch with Tanya Milhady, her therapist.

"Look, David," said Tanya, sounding *very* Hungarian, "why don't you stop playing sweet games like taking your adversary to lunch and talk to me straight? You want to start Sheila on tranquilizers!"

"Yes, I think—"

"I can understand what you think. You think that it's ridiculous to allow the patient to regress when medication would probably help her heal over."

"Well, it's—"

"Easier to manage the patient," said Tanya.

"Not merely that, but—"

"Let me finish. Sheila might be easier to manage but there would be no real change in her. I am letting her regress in order to reach her psychotic core and to work through some of the difficult issues in her past—to *change* her." Tanya had said her piece.

"But Sheila is becoming less communicative. She's less willing to deal with the real world. Tanya, I think you're playing with fire. Are you so sure that once she regresses and understands her problems she'll act any differently? Are you so sure that once she regresses you will be able to put her back together at all?"

"No one can be sure, of course, but it's worth a try."

"You wouldn't settle for allowing her to feel a little better on medication and to get back to work?" I asked, knowing the answer would be no.

"She'll only be in for more difficulty next time," Tanya said, omnipotently, I thought.

"At least there may be a next time," I said. I went along with Tanya reluctantly. I probably shouldn't have.

A lot of patients did get better on the acute service, but it was a strange process. Sometimes I felt so far removed from the healing process that I could neither claim credit for successes nor be blamed for failures. After a certain period of time some patients suddenly seemed better and wanted to go home. I'd known a great deal about my patients on Bamberg 5 and discussed the minutest details with Jerry Gelb and the other residents and nurses, examined them under an analytical microscope. The patients on the acute ward were like icebergs—hidden, unknown and when they got better they didn't want to talk about being sick! . . .

Patients often have amnesia for the time when they are psychotic. The gnawing doubts that often plagued neurotic patients, that made them question everything they did or thought following their illness, were often absent in psychotic patients. Psychotics were blessed with a powerful abiilty to block out everything painful. When they returned to reality, or whatever it was that for them passed as reality, they seemed content because they had walled off their problems. They lived in an incomplete reality when they got better because they always denied a part of reality, usually the feeling part. That denial was the flaw that kept them from recognizing and solving the problems around them. The next time they were overwhelmed with pain they would deny all reality again.

Who knows, maybe psychotics had the right idea. When things get really bad, who wants to be aware of them or remember? In many ways psychosis is kinder to those it torments than neurosis, although psychotic patients can experience terror beyond anything neurotics can imagine.

The nights on call on the acute service were always frantic. On one night in particular I must have sewn up six people who had slashed themselves. I put in over one hundred stitches in all. And I thought I would never be a *real* doctor again! I also had nine admissions that night and felt like admitting myself to the hospital and calling it quits. I sat with the aide and admitting room nurse watching television, waiting for the clock to move from 12:30 to 1:30. If you go to bed before 1:30 you almost always get awakened. (Things hadn't changed much in that department since the early days at Bamberg 5.) So I made it a ritual to stay dressed, watch the Late Show and *then* go to bed.

I got eight calls between two and four and another early the next morning, around six thirty.

"Dr. Viscott, you're wanted in the north cafeteria," said the operator.

"That's the chronic service," I said, rubbing my eyes.

"Yes, it is, doctor," the operator said.

"I'm on call for the acute service," I said angrily. "It's bad enough to be on call for one service in this place."

"I'm sorry, I'll call the doctor on call for the chronic service."

"Good, terrific!"

"Sorry for waking you."

Since I was up, I called the emergency ward to see how one of the patients I'd admitted that night was doing and then went back to sleep.

The telephone rang again.

"Dr. Frogner?" asked the same operator.

"No, this is Dr. Viscott."

"Oh, I'm sorry. I must have made a mistake."

Another try to get more sleep. I looked at my watch. Seven. The hell with it. I got up, showered and got dressed. The phone again. The same operator again.

"Dr. Viscott, could you cover for Dr. Frogner? We can't reach him." She sounded desperate.

"What's wrong?"

"A patient collapsed in the cafeteria line and is in the hospital."

"Christ, why'd you wait so long to ask?" I said, and ran out the door.

I got to the hospital in five minutes. But it was too late, the patient died just after being admitted. Probably a heart attack.

Frogner and I were called in to see Dr. Benjamin Fazio, the hospital administrator, at ten. Dr. Fazio was known as a very tough but fair man and very big on responsibility. He had the physique of a hydrant, short and stocky. I told my story. Fazio looked at me sternly.

"Why didn't you offer to help?"

"I offered to help as soon as I knew there was a problem in getting hold of Dr. Frogner. Before then it sounded like a routine mixup and there was no indication of an emergency." Fazio looked furious.

"And you, Frogner, what's your excuse?"

"I signed out to Dr. Viscott," Frogner said, matter-of-factly. "It was his entire responsibility."

"What? What the hell are you talking about?" I shouted.

"I signed out to you," Frogner said calmly. "Are we not allowed to sign out to the resident on service with us?"

"Yes," said Dr. Fazio, looking at me oddly. "Yes, you are allowed to do that."

"Well," continued Frogner, "that's what I did. I signed out to Dr. Viscott."

"Well," I said, getting angrier, "this is the first time I've heard about it. You never asked me to cover for you. As a matter of fact, the last time I spoke to you was over a month ago!"

"You don't need to check with a doctor when you sign out for a moment," Frogner said disdainfully.

"A moment," I shouted, "is the same as a week as far as I'm concerned. Your service is your responsibility until another doctor agrees to cover it. Even so, I did what I could when I understood the situation."

"You should have been there sooner. Shows bad character," said Frogner. I wanted to throw a punch! I hadn't felt that angry in years.

"You weren't on the grounds last night," I asked, much calmer, "were you, Frogner?"

"Don't be ridiculous," he said.

I let go with both barrels. "The operator said you always take calls at home, and when you were being called your wife said you were driving to the hospital."

"Is that true?" Fazio asked, rising to his feet and standing in front of his desk.

"Yes, but I signed out to Dr. Viscott." Frogner's cool was finally slipping.

"You signed out to the operator," said Fazio, correcting him. "That doesn't relieve you of your responsibility. That doesn't relieve you of anything. The only thing that might conceivably relieve you of is your position as a resident at this hospital. You can go, Dr. Viscott."

"Tough luck, Dr. Frogner," I said.

"That will be enough, Dr. Viscott," Dr. Fazio said.

"What happened?" asked D.J., who was waiting in the hall. She had come by for moral support. I drew my finger across my throat and said, "Frogner."

D.J. kissed me and gave me a hug.

"Coffee?" I offered. It was like old times.

The year was going pretty well. Miss Fogg was returned to the hospital in April after too many bars and left again in May when Maggie got her cousin to give in once more. Maggie Shapiro apparently could talk anyone into anything, except someone into marrying her.

I had been working extremely hard these last few months, and my system of seeing patients every day, discharging them as soon as possible, seemed to be working out well. I was able to keep my patient census down to about nine.

Bert and I shared the ward meetings. That's where group process or pressure, or extortion, depending on how you look at it, really took place. The ward meetings became more manageable as we felt more comfortable. I began to wonder about that, and questioned if patients often reflected their doctors' insecurity in the way they acted. Patients still went running through the meetings yelling or hallucinating. Strange. Even though there was more activity in these meetings than there had been in my meetings on the chronic service, the amount of real feelings expressed was about the same. There's a clue to the nature of psychosis somewhere in that.

In June I received a letter from Dr. Noyes.

Dear Dr. Viscott:
It is with great pleasure that Dr. Gavin and I offer you the position of chief resident at the outpatient department next year. Would

you please contact Dr. Eugene McKee at your earliest convenience to make arrangements.

Sincerely,
M. Austin Noyes, M.D.

And I thought he hated me!

I invited Bert, D.J., and Stanley to be my lunch guests at the doctors' cafeteria. At twenty-five cents a head, I was really splurging.

"I have an announcement to make," I said.

"Speech, speech," shouted Bert, hitting his fork against the water glass and drawing attention from Drs. Fazio, Sellers, Milhady, Rutberg, Standish at the bordering tables.

"Quiet," I said.

"Tell us," said D.J.

I waited till the onlookers had turned away.

"I am going to be chief resident in the OPD next year."

"Wonderful," said D.J.

"You mean you're going to be my boss?" Bert said.

"Right."

"OK, it could be worse," he said, pointing to Stanley, pretending he was joking.

"How did you find out?" asked Stanley, looking pained.

"By mail, just today."

"What did the letter say?" Stanley asked.

"Just that I was appointed chief resident and should speak with Dr. McKee." I took out the letter. D. J. read it and passed it to Bert.

"But you're not even in psychoanalysis or planning to become an analyst," Stanley said. He really had his heart set on being chief. It was really not such a big deal. "They usually have analytic candidates. I mean, Larry Danielson was an analytic candidate." Stanley was really disappointed.

"I don't know anything about that," I said. "They probably pull the name out of a hat."

"When do I get my raise?" Bert asked.

"What do you think this free lunch was all about? This is it." Stanley looked ill.

"Is it the food?" asked Bert.

"Something you can't swallow?" asked D.J.

"Knock it off," I said, just like Larry Danielson used to.

Standish asked me into his office. "Well, you're moving on next week, and I wanted to tell you that I think you did a fine job here."

"That's very kind of you, Dr. Standish. Thank you."

"I think your being here made quite a difference with these patients. You worked hard and kept the time they were in the hospital to a minimum. I think that's important."

"Well, I don't know if it was me or not."

"This is no time to be modest."

"Look, Dr. Standish, the one thing in my life I've never been accused of is being modest. I just tried to keep up with my work and make things as easy for myself as possible. That means taking care of details. It was no big deal, really. I was more administrator than therapist. I hate administrating so I tried to keep the lid on things. And compared to Frogner, anyone looks good."

I returned to the ward to say good-bye to Honey. She told me that Ramona had just returned, that Miss Fogg had escaped again, and that my application for Sheila Duggin's transfer to the chronic service had been accepted.

A fine job.

CHAPTER TWENTY

THE OPD (OUTPATIENT DEPARTMENT), INCLUDING "THE ANALYST'S LOVE IS HIS SILENCE"

ΛRRIVING at Union Hospital was like a homecoming. I saw Jerry Gelb in the parking lot as I drove in. He didn't see me, though. I thought of chasing after him, but I had a meeting in the outpatient department. I couldn't be late, you know, now that I was one of the members of the big team. (Color me Establishment and change my name to Dr. D. Steven Viscott.)

The outpatient building was a red brick Romanesque monstrosity, complete with a pointed tower. It enjoyed a charming setting on the south side of a large brick-paved courtyard. To the side was a small lawn with two picnic tables where we would eat lunch and watch and sometimes join the medical students playing softball in spring and summer, and football in the autumn. The medical school, marble, covered with ivy, was directly across the courtyard. Walking through always gave me a warm feeling.

I met with Dr. Eugene McKee, the director of the outpatient psychiatric clinic, to discuss my duties. Like most of the people in M. Austin Noyes' psychiatric department, Dr. McKee was a psychoanalyst. He had a corner office upstairs in the outpatient building with carpets, drapes, and furniture from Design Research, and prints by Vasarely and Joseph Albers on the wall. Class.

Dr. McKee didn't even wait to say hello before he began, "I thought it would be a good idea to discuss the coming year with you. There will be two second-year residents in the OPD this year, Dr. Cushman and Dr. Yancey. Dr. Yancey may be a bit of a problem. He

271

was very erratic and headstrong last year on Bamberg 5, according to Alex Karlsson. You'll need to keep an eye on him to make sure he's staying in line. You'll also have two medical students to supervise. And you have to make sure that the residents keep the records up-to-date and that they're doing their work, whatever that is.

"The schedule is easy. There's a morning intake hour at eight when new patients are evaluated every day. At nine we have a presentation conference in which all of the new patients are discussed briefly and a disposition worked out. You discuss all the new cases with the residents briefly before that time to decide which patient will be the best one for the ten o'clock conference with a formal presentation and evaluation, together with a sparkling interview by me. Ask that patient to wait and make sure he does. It's a very important session and the major teaching conference for the OPD. So you have to pick the patients that will interview best and look for some variety. Please avoid chronic mute schizophrenics. They interview lousy."

"I know," I said, my experience showing.

"That conference is the thing I like to do best," said Dr. McKee, lighting up a cigar, "so do your part." Eugene McKee was a handsome man who dressed like the president of a successful conglomerate. He was pleasant, cheerful, and had a great sense of humor, when the joke wasn't on him. He was also very sensitive and hated to be bothered by small problems, such as secretaries quitting or residents rebelling. He preferred such conundrums as deciding whether a patient's identity crisis came from a weak father or a poorly defined sense of reality.

"You will have been a great chief resident," Dr. McKee said, "if I never see you except at the conferences or in supervision."

I heard the clue, loud and clear.

I would become fond of Dr. McKee, but I was never allowed close enough to call him "Gene." I don't think he liked me very much. I even worried about it at the beginning of the year, but decided it was probably unimportant because he didn't seem to like anyone else that much more. Which is not to say that he wasn't friendly. He was, but at a little distance. Maybe that's why he depended on wit as well as wisdom. That way he could seem to get closer to us and others than he really was. I recognized no little of myself in that.

The outpatients were different from the patients on Bamberg 5 and in the state hospital. Exposure to such overwhelmingly obvious pathology in the past two years had made our group relatively insensitive to more subtle symptoms.

"Dr. Marley," Dr. McKee asked D.J. after she'd presented a patient she had just worked up the hour before, "what do you think is the matter with this woman?"

"I'm not sure," said D.J.

"You're not sure. What the hell have you all been doing?" McKee laughed. "OK, let's ask the medical student, what's your name again?"

"Townsend," said Townsend.

"OK, Townsend, what does the patient have?"

"I don't know," said Townsend.

"How about you, Trixie?" Trixie Beyers was the psychiatric social worker attached to the clinic. She was also attached to Dr. McKee. Dr. McKee liked Trixie, but was not attached to her. Trixie was a tall, leggy blonde, bright as hell, not afraid to be as sexy as she was seductive.

"She's schizophrenic," said Trixie, tossing her hair behind her shoulder.

"Schizophrenic, I agree," McKee said. "Dr. Marley, you've been with blatantly ill people too long. Remember the people you'll see this year are all ambulatory. That means they are all more or less functional. You will wonder how in hell some of them manage, but they do and it's up to you to make a diagnosis quickly and accurately and begin a treatment program rapidly.

"The problem is that you're seeing patients essentially in remission compared to the ones you have been seeing. That also means you have to look more deeply into what they say for the subtleties they are shutting out. Think of meanings in their words beyond the obvious. This patient of yours, Dr. Marley, showed ambivalence, an inappropriateness of affect, a disturbance in thinking, and a tendency to be autistic. OK, so he didn't wear a flower in his nose and call it macaroni. But he still had several classical signs of psychosis.

"Maybe I should have the patients carry signs with their diagnoses so you people won't miss them. There are a lot of schizophrenics walking around out there on the street. Many of them are working. Some of them come to the clinic now and then. They look like just other people except, if you look for them, they tend to show these classical signs."

"You're not saying everyone is schizophrenic, are you?" asked Townsend. I thought he actually looked frightened.

Dr. McKee laughed. "There's a little schizo in each of us. It's just that there's more in some than in others."

Being the chief resident, as I told my forces at the celebratory lunch, was no big deal. I was never one to lord it over other people and I didn't have the power to if I wanted to. But I *was* obligated to keep the clinic running smoothly. I had one enormous advantage; Mary, the clinic secretary. She reviewed the charts of the patients who had been seen in the clinic each day and picked up errors and omissions. They were usually too long, too wordy, and filled with extraneous personal detail, material that would be extremely embarrassing to the patient if the record fell into the wrong hands. I'd been badly chewed out by Alex Karlsson during by first year after he read just such a report of mine. I learned my lesson.

"You'll have to do something about Dr. Yancey," Mary said. "Look at his evaluation reports. They run almost five single-spaced pages."

"And from only one interview!" I remarked, leafing through one of them. He must be making up most of this, I thought. How do I handle him? I could simply tell him that his reports were too long. I mean, you'd think a person who was becoming a shrink, for heaven's sake, could take a little constructive criticism, but Yancey was a very strange guy. He always had a big bright smile on his face and seemed anxious to contribute ideas about what he thought was going on in a case. His ideas, though, didn't seem related specifically to the case in point. Yancey seemed to be turned into a different wavelength. The rest of us were not always in touch with him, often didn't want to be. It would be one thing if he had the special insight of Dr. Rutberg or Gavin and could cut through defenses with dramatic perceptions, but he didn't and he couldn't.

Yancey's ideas were frequently a reformulation of his own personal problems projected onto the patient at hand. Of course he disguised them in vague and obscure words. However, some of Yancey's comments were quite transparent and revealed his concern about homosexuality, being crazy, being worthwhile, and being intelligent, whether relevant or irrelevant to the case at hand. Mary was going crazy trying to keep up with his endless reports.

I decided the only way to handle Yancey was to be light about it and not insult him. I asked him to schedule a free hour for me and invited him to have coffee with me in my office. I had the best office in the OPD. That was my only payoff for being chief resident. I used a W. C. Fields voice, complained my eyeballs were being afflicted, that his material was competent, well-written, but too generous in length. I told him I wanted everyone's psychiatric report reduced to less than two and a half double-spaced pages—outlines, with one specific detail here and there.

"What do you mean?"

I picked up one of Yancey's ten-page tomes I'd red-penciled and handed it to him, edited. All those days as editor-in-chief of the *Dartmouth Quarterly* might finally be paying off. Mary had typed the edited version, now a neat two pages. "You mean this is all I have to do?" Norman asked.

"That's all you have to do, Norman."

"That's easy."

"I knew it would be for *you.*"

Managing people is a pain in the ass.

Enid Rust, the psychologist, was still Enid Rust, still insisted on doing extensive psychological diagnostic tests whether or not it seemed likely they would be of any help. Psychological tests are almost useless in themselves. Without knowing what the patient is like clinically, they *are* useless. Different IQ tests vary and give different results in the same person, and the same test will vary in the same patient if given by two different psychologists. Rorschach and other projective tests are highly subjective, and even though they are enormously well-documented and carefully evaluated their results may also suggest deeper pathology than actually exists. These tests can become a jumping-off point for the clinician who tends to look for evidence to back up the test findings. In this way he may prove the diagnosis of a disease that sometimes does not exist. Used with insight and restraint, projective tests save time and may *help* point to diagnoses.

An example of the dangers of misused test results: When a group of teachers was given the correct IQ scores of their students before the school year, the students tended to be seen and to respond the way their teacher expected people of their IQ to respond. When teachers were deliberately given incorrect IQs for their students, the students tended to be seen and to respond more like people who had the incorrect IQs. All I'm saying is that expectations of behavior often drastically color performance. When a patient's tests reveal him to be very crazy, in spite of a benign clinical appearance, residents and supervisors tighten up, decrease the patient's privileges, or consider hospitalization, and the patient frequently responds by getting worse; had the tests been otherwise, the doctors might have given the patient the benefit of the doubt and he might for the same reason have improved.

Psychological tests are of immeasurable importance in evaluating brain-damaged or mentally deficient patients. They measure and point to disabilities and, more importantly, to strengths which should be kept in mind in educational or vocational training and placement. However, the psychological projective tests that are offered as a guide to the patient's psyche are often imprecise and misleading. A good clinical impression is worth a thousand tests.

Enid Rust saw herself as the keeper of the truth. The last and final judgment of a patient's sanity and of a resident's competence. D.J., Bert, Stanley, and I all felt she had it in for us from our previous group experience.

She did.

"Well," asked Dr. McKee, after Bert had presented a difficult patient for the second time, "any comments?"

"I think," I began, "that this woman is beginning to sound like someone who has dissociative reactions in which she momentarily fades out of the picture."

"Good point," said Stanley Lovett. Stanley and I were getting along better when he saw that I was only interested in letting everyone do whatever they wanted, providing they kept the paperwork done. In fact, Stanley was even beginning to look up to me. Strange what a title does. "She is a little like Eve in the *Three Faces of Eve*," Stanley said, "except she doesn't take on another face. She just goes blank. Good point, David." It wasn't that good really, and I think Stanley knew it. I also think he was trying to score a point with me. Can you believe *that*?

"Well, *I* have some *very* interesting data," said Enid Rust. Enid always called the results of her tests "data." It was more impressive and sounded more scientific than "impressions." They were the same, though. Enid never doubted she was right, either in her methods or interpretation. She had Russell Townsend, the medical student, convinced because he didn't like uncertainties. He was going into dermatology, where the diagnosis would be right there in front of him, staring him in the face. Wait, I thought, until he discovers how many psychological vagaries there are in dermatology.

"Tell us about it, Enid," said Eugene McKee, getting ready to begin his hunt for something in Enid's argument that he could refute or make a joke about. I tried not to make jokes in front of Dr. McKee. He had to be center stage. In a way it was as though he was the host of a TV talk show one hour a day. Everyone in this goddamn department had to be managed.

Enid began reading her report: "This woman has extraordinary lacunae in her superego which allow her to get entangled in inappropriate social situations without much introspection, but the intact portion of the superego is more than rigid enough to inflict great amounts of self-punitive and self-destructive behavior when they reassert their primacy, not to mention a great deal of guilt. Some of her responses to *card three* were highly atypical, showing marked degrees of repression. The attention to minutiae in the test, I felt, was abnormally high and, at times, served to provide an embarkation point for regressive fantasizing. Also there was a mixed combination of Oedipal and anal strivings which was curious. On *card four* there was a great deal of what could best be called figure and ground relationship reversal, with a resultant uncertainty about her other responses on other cards. This had retrograde as well as anterograde manifestations as she then doubted some of her previous responses to *card three* and showed some perseveration in doubting to *card five*. It was *card six* that *really* told me what was going on and what the *real* problem was!"

The day is ours! Let the band play . . . the triumphal march from *Aida* will do. Such power! Such great and singular insights! Such a unique private channel to the world below the surface. Danny Mellick, Enid's boss, the chief of the clinical psychology program, couldn't much stand Enid either. Danny would make most of his diagnoses by talking with the patients and carefully evaluating what the patients told him. He used projective tests only when he wasn't sure of a particular point, so then he was looking for specific information. "You can't treat a patient based on a projective test, boys," Danny once told us. Enid never listened to anyone.

"I can hardly wait," said Dr. McKee, "for what you found on *card six*."

"This woman's responses," Enid continued undaunted, "showed fragmentation, disorganization, and a tendency toward sexualization of sensory inputs. I would have to call her a regressed oral hysteric with depressive features."

"Wonderful," said Dr. McKee. "Now how would you recommend we treat her?"

"What do you mean?"

"This lady comes into your office off the street and says she needs help. What are you going to talk to her about?"

"Controls," Enid said. "Reestablishing controls. I think if she were able to reinstitute controls over her impulsivity she would not suffer from such severe guilt and depression when the punitive part of her superego reassumed function."

Townsend smiled. He loved it. The medical student didn't understand it, but he loved it.

"Can you give an example of how you would do that?"

Enid stared across the table and fell silent. Dr. McKee knew all about setting one person against another. He looked at Trixie with a smile and very sweetly said, "Trixie?"

Trixie smiled back at him. "I'd get her to talk about her feelings about male figures in her life—her husband, boy friends, her father. And when she talked about the loneliness and anger she associated with them, I would try to sympathize with her and help draw them out more. I think she gets angry about men leaving her and the anger makes her have these blackouts whenever something reminds her of it, of the loss that's associated with it. It *is* a dissociative reaction and I would help her reattach the anger to the people that caused it." Trixie crossed her legs and smiled.

"Trixie," said Dr. McKee, "you should have been a psychologist."

"You're right," said Trixie. Enid looked murderous.

As you can see, our happy little clinic was rapidly becoming home for the residents who worked there. What *happy* means, of course, depends upon who's defining it. Dr. McKee was happy when he was able to run his ten o'clock intake conference every morning and show off his skills, charm, and wit, and he had formidable skills! McKee was an experienced psychoanalyst with a lot of feeling for his patients. He liked to appear logical, hard, and resolute, but he really was a softie who seemed a little out of place in the Union Hospital residency program. He loved to teach and hated to administrate. He liked joking with the boys and flirting with the girls at conference and pointing out their professional faults adroitly, candidly, warmly, and humorously. You can learn a lot in a setting like that, and we did.

To give Eugene McKee his further due, he had everyone's number. "OK," he would say after presentation of a case, "we're about to hear a detailed, precise, and breathtaking evaluation of this patient from Dr. Marley," or, "Dr. Viscott will now give us a shattering insight about this patient that we all missed. Right, Dr. Viscott? Perform for your peers," or, "Dr. Feinstein will now reveal how each member of the patient's family contributed to his distress," or, "Dr. Lovett, please describe in irrelevant detail everything about this patient's drives and defenses," or "Dr. Yancey, would you like to obscure the issue by adding something?" or, "Dr. Cushman, would you like to tell us about the patient's problems with authority?" or, "Trixie, tell us something sexy about this patient, and then tell us something sexy about Trixie."

We obeyed our leader. We reported our feelings, observations, and opinions over the year and gradually expanded our points of view. We learned to consider the possibility that there might be alternate ways of seeing patients, and to recognize our own blind spots and to take them into account.

The patients in the OPD were more active, more alive than any we'd seen before. Trixie wasn't the only one on the staff who noticed sexual aberrations. While there might have been one homosexual on Bamberg 5 or one prostitute on my ward in the reception building, this place seemed to be crawling with people who had sexual problems of one sort or another. Maybe sex was still so interesting to us that even after we had come to terms with our natural, and prurient, curiosities we still often encouraged patients to display their sexual concerns. Perhaps the patients, with all their usual misconceptions about psychiatrists, felt a need to present a lot of sexual material on the first visit. Maybe outpatients were sexier than inpatients. Regardless why, almost every morning at least one sexual problem was presented at the nine o'clock intake conference right after the new patients were evaluated.

Dr. McKee was very interested in the problems of erotic transference, sexual feelings of the patient toward the doctor. He had spoken about it at grand rounds, telling how to recognize it and what to do about it. His formula was to keep the patient on strictly "Miss" or "Mr." terms and to be very structured about every session to avoid the patient's attempts to set you up and to point them out by saying things like, "Why do you wear such low-cut dresses to the sessions?" Above all, Eugene McKee's motto was, "Look but don't touch."

One morning in particular the clinic seemed overloaded with sexual deviants. My patient that day was an eighteen-year-old homosexual, Mr. Olsen, who had been sent over by the hospital chaplain at the request of the boy's father, who worked as a custodian in the hospital.

"How can I be helpful to you, Mr. Olsen?" I asked. Russell Townsend, the medical student, was sitting in on the interview. The patient had terrible acne and some scarring from badly cared for skin lesions.

"I want you to make me straight," Olsen began. "I'm sick of being a fag. It's a lousy life," he said, patting his teased hair into place. He was wearing mascara and posing for my benefit, crossing his legs and smoking, holding his cigarette with his wrist bent back, being as affected as possible. Olsen looked like someone doing an impersonation of a homosexual doing an impersonation of Bette Davis.

"What would you like me to help you with?"

"Do I have to tell you your business?" he asked, affecting a Yiddish accent. "Aren't you smart enough to know how to change a fag? Haven't you ever done this before?"

"Why do you want to change?" I asked.

"Shit!" he said, "I just told you. I don't like my life. It's a drag. So what are you going to do, already?" He started gesturing and throwing his hands in the air like he was dancing the Charleston.

"How long have you been homosexual?" I asked.

"Since I started sucking off the kids on my block when I was five."

"Five?" I repeated, disbelievingly. Townsend was really shook.

"I was the most popular kid in kindergarten. When I was ten I was tricking regularly. I used to go to the veterans' conventions in town when I was twelve. I could get twenty-five bucks a trick. Those old farts are the biggest floozies of them all. Shame on them! Old men with grandchildren paying me money to go down on my tinkle. Can you believe that? God, I think everyone in the world is queer. Look at him!" He pointed to Russell Townsend and said slowly and with feeling, "Now, *you* . . . can't tell me that *he* isn't gay. With all my experience I ought to know, sister. I can spot a prospect a mile away." Russell sat bolt upright in his chair. This is all I need, to have a medical student go into homosexual panic during an evaluation. I was waiting.

"OK," I said, "knock it off. The problem is you, Mr. Olsen, not Dr. Townsend. I'm trying to find out how badly you want to give up *the life* and how deeply entrenched you are in it."

"I think you're probably a little that way yourself. There's a little homosexual in everyone, isn't there, doc?" Townsend was squirming. "You might as well tell the facts of life to your sidekick there. Oh, I get it now. The two of you have a thing going. Yes, sir! There's a little queer in every straight."

"And vice versa."

"Bullshit," he shouted. He was angry at the insinuation he might be heterosexual. "I'm not straight. I'm pure fag."

Obviously Mr. Olsen wasn't terribly well-motivated to change his life style. Apparently he'd gotten upset over several recent rejections. Because of his worsening acne and growing older and uglier, he wasn't desirable anymore. That was what Olsen was really upset about. All of a sudden I felt I had a group therapy session going. Townsend was crossing and uncrossing his legs. Olsen kept winking at him.

Townsend was shaken and obviously couldn't keep his mind on the interview. After Olsen left I tried to reassure Townsend that it was common to feel anxious under such circumstances and that everyone had to come to terms with their feelings and learn to accept themselves. The only diagnosis medical students not interested in psychiatry felt comfortable about was conversion hysteria.

"Do you think I'm a homosexual?" he asked, blanching.

"I think you're just *worried* about being a homosexual. Now go make out an appointment slip for that guy for dermatology clinic." That made Townsend feel better. . . .

"So essentially I sent him to the skin clinic and then back where he came from," I said, concluding my presentation to Dr. McKee at the nine o'clock conference.

"Just make damn sure you send a note to the chaplain," said Dr. McKee. "He'll want a follow-up. He always does on all his referrals. He likes to feel involved. You might get a little flak from him for not treating Mr. Olsen."

"Very bad treatment case," I said. D.J. nodded agreement.

"Who else do we have this morning?" asked Dr. McKee.

"I have a young man who was found by his mother tied up, trying to hang himself while masturbating," Bert announced.

"That's a classic symptom seen in some disturbed adolescents," McKee began in his usual energetic way. It was a fascinating case. There was even an episode of fire setting and masturbating while watching the fire hoses putting the fire out. "Another classic symptom that Freud described," McKee said. A second diagnostic interview was suggested by McKee.

"D.J.?" asked McKee. I think D.J. intimidated McKee a little.

"I have a twenty-year-old man who—" D.J. smiled—"was picked up in the Public Library exposing himself and sent here for evaluation. Our workup will be given to the court. I think like most people who expose themselves, the man was looking for help. He's engaged to an overpowering woman he really can't stand and wants to get out of it. I guess this should do it."

"Who have you got, Stanley, a rapist?" asked McKee.

"No," said Stanley earnestly, "I have a man who is having relations with his daughter."

"My God," said McKee. "And now I'm sure Trixie has something uniquely lurid for us. Briefly, Trixie, who do you have?"

"A twenty-two-year-old woman who became upset after her mother's death."

"Thank God."

"And then," continued Trixie hesitantly, "she quit her job and became promiscuous and asked men to whip her after she had relations with them. I think it probably had something to do with lessening the guilt over her mother's death."

"This clinic is going to hell," said Dr. McKee. "All we have here is polymorphously perverse patients. Sex, sex, sex! Is that all you people ever think or talk about? Or see or look for? Tell me, what's going to happen when you jokers go out into private practice and a nice little old Irish lady comes in fresh from a meeting at Saint Michael's Sodality and talks about feeling anxious? What are you going to do? Are you going to ask her about the strength of her orgasms or whether she indulges in oral sex with her husband or if she has erotic fantasies about her confessor. She'll have you arrested. So would I." He said it with a straight face.

"OK, Yancey and Cushman," McKee said, staring at the two of them, "if either of you have patients with sexual problems don't bother to tell me about it. Just please to get the hell out of this conference room." Yancey and Cushman stood up as one and started for the door. We started laughing. Dr. McKee smiled. "You've got to be kidding."

"A frigid housewife," said Cushman.

"An impotent bus driver," said Yancey.

"A roomful of perverted psychiatrists," said McKee.

"Is that being redundant?" I said. The muted laughter from the others and the guidance from McKee reminded me he didn't like competition.

"I've seen worse though," Dr. McKee said reflectively, deciding to join in. "You know how much I talk about erotic transference when the patient falls in love with the doctor. Well, there's another side to that story, erotic countertransference, when the doctor falls in love with the patient. I was asked to see a patient in consultation last year sent by the colleague who had gotten into an erotic transference and erotic countertransference jam with her. He wanted me to see if I could figure a way out of their entanglement for him. You see how well-respected I am in my specialty."

We all said we did.

Dr. McKee laughed, shaking his head. "My mother would never believe this, that her son is running a clinic filled with such perverted types. Anyhow, the patient told me she was developing a relationship with the psychiatrist and while it hadn't yet turned sexual they had started to see each other after hours. She had hopes that they would soon be consummating their affections. The woman said her hopes were raised when her doctor sent her a Valentine card. She was, in fact, thrilled with it."

"Sweet," said D.J.

"Loving therapist," said Bert.

"Hmm," said Trixie dreamily.

"Be serious, you people," said McKee. "The patient said the Valentine really excited her, but the rug was pulled out."

"Ohh," everyone said together. McKee pretended to be annoyed, He loved it. He really loved it.

"Several months later her doctor sent the patient a Mothers' Day card. His relationship had deepened but it had also changed. He became dependent on the patient before they could consummate their relationship."

"The moral being, when your doctor stops sending you Valentines and begins to send you Mothers' Day cards, the honeymoon is over," said Trixie.

"Yes, and the relationship becomes perverted, just like this group of patients here today," McKee said, not to mention the doctors. "Viscott, you make sure the next sexual problem I hear is something nice and old-fashioned like a young girl who's afraid of men. You know, something simple and phobic. Masters and Johnson write a book, and everyone reads it and thinks he has to try it out. At least my generation read Kraft-Ebbing and managed to keep its pants on *some* of the time."

I don't think he smiled when he said that.

One of the chief resident's duties was to organize the monthly OPD cocktail party, which started at five on the last Friday of the month. Some years ago it was the first Friday of the month. McKee would decide which after checking the calendar and seeing which arrangement would yield the most parties each year. The tariff was a dollar a head. I was supposed to collect it from everyone attending.

Trixie handled the food. Enid, our favorite psychologist, also brought some—her homemade delicacies. One month it would be a platter or two of Greek appetizers, another an Italian antipasto plate. Enid had been married for three years in her twenties and became an excellent cook. She only cooked for herself these days, and her displays of food were almost like an advertisement.

I had three duties according to Dr. McKee: "Make sure there is plenty of ice and not the cheap crap that you get from the hospital ice machines. It's flaky and makes lousy martinis. By the way, you do know how to mix drinks, don't you, because you'll also be mixing the drinks. Do you know how to make a martini? Don't tell me. I won't believe you. You also have to buy the booze. And make sure you keep it locked up so the janitor around this place doesn't swipe it. Your final and most important duty is to make sure that under no conditions am I to have an empty glass in my hand."

I was prepared. I could have married off both my daughters with the amount of liquor I bought for the first party. It was wild. What do psychiatrists and other members of the mental health profession talk about when they are alone at a cocktail party? Each other, that's what!

"Here you are, Dr. McKee," I said, pushing through the crowd and handing him my special martini—two ounces of gin and a half teaspoon of Scotch. I never tell what's in it. The Scotch takes the edge off the gin and makes it very dry. Dr. McKee held the drink up to the light, gave it a critical examination.

"The color?" he said.

"Just try it," I urged.

"Humm," said McKee, taking a sip. "Well, Viscott, you may be a crummy chief resident, but you're the only one I've ever had who knew how to make a proper martini."

Alvin Cushman cornered me. Actually, I was already cornered. The conference room, where we held the monthly party, was very small. I really hadn't gotten the chance to know very much about Cushman. He was bright and conscientious. I knew he was considering becoming an analyst but couldn't make up his mind. He was in analysis trying to decide. I had also thought casually about the idea of becoming an analyst during the first two years of residency. I even sent for an application form to apply to the Psychoanalytic Institute, but I never even filled it out. I guess I was just nervous about deciding whether I should be analyzed and used the procedure of applying to the institute to delay my decision about a personal analysis. Many of the residents did go into analysis. D.J. had started the previous spring. Stanley, of course, had been in analysis for two years, and Bert had also gone into analysis during the first year. I didn't feel any pressing need for it, but thought it might be helpful to me in doing therapy with patients as well as for understanding myself better. I was still toying with the idea. I was, let's face it, a little afraid. (A little?)

"Dave, maybe you can give me some advice."

"Sure, it's cheap. From me—it's free." I made another pitcher of martinis and reached over Yancey's shoulder to fill up Dr. McKee's glass.

"The old man really swills the stuff down," said Alvin.

"All analysts booze," said Yancey, filling his glass up from the pitcher and walking away, muttering to himself.

"Look," said Alvin, pulling me back into an alcove, "I had an experience this morning that really shook me up. You know I'm in analysis."

"Who with?" I asked.

"I prefer not to tell you."

"Why such a big mystery?"

"I'm not sure, we talk about why I'm afraid to tell people his name. Maybe it's my reluctance to admit I've allowed another man to have so much power over me. I have a problem with authorities, I get angry and resentful at them. As a matter of fact, you're the only authority I don't get angry at." Talking with Alvin was like being with a patient after hours.

"I'm not much of an authority, Alvin," I said.

"Look, I want to discuss something with you, seriously." I relaxed on the windowsill, reaching over from time to time to mix drinks to order for people and listening to Alvin. "I saw my analyst today. I have a six thirty appointment every day during the week." (Six thirty, only robins and surgeons are up then!) "I told my analyst how I felt about a comment he made the day before. I said, 'I think you were wrong.' Usually I can tell how he reacts to something, but this morning I couldn't tell because he was silent. I mean, he's often silent, which means 'keep talking.' Right?" I nodded. I guessed so. How the hell would I know what his analyst meant? "So I'm lying there on the couch trying to figure out what he means. So I repeated my comment," Alvin continued. "Still no reply. So I said, 'Well, it's obvious that by your silence you're indicating you don't think I'm on the right track.' He still says nothing. So I started free-associating and opened up a whole new area. Still no comment. I said, 'I understand you're trying to see how much stress I can take!' Still no comment. I'm starting to feel paranoid, maybe even angry at him. It scares me to do that. I tell him. He still says nothing. So I get anxious. I said, 'I'm afraid something's happened to you.' Then I get this brilliant insight and I say, 'It's this way with all authorities and me. I get afraid of my own anger at them and knuckle under. I'm afraid of my own anger. How about that?' I'm saying to myself this guy is really a brilliant analyst! What brilliant technique, superb self-control, being quiet like that and not saying a word, letting me go through all this anxiety, knowing just how much I can take, knowing I'm safe because he won't let me go too far. So I told him how much I appreciated his ability to stay silent. I really did, and for the first time I understood what they mean when they say the analyst's love *is* his silence. I suddenly understood something about my anger, about my feelings. And it was the result of his brilliant technique. He's the first *authority* who has helped me."

It sounded pretty impressive, listening to Alvin carry on.

"I actually started to cry," Alvin continued, "and when I stopped, I asked my analyst what he thought. He was still silent. I could hear him breathing heavily in the background. Maybe something had happened, maybe he's had a heart attack, I thought, after all, he *is* over sixty-five. Maybe he's still testing me, I didn't know.

"I asked him to comment again but he was still silent. So I said, 'I'm going to turn around and see if you're OK.' I was afraid because here I am lying on the couch, never have done anything in almost a year but lie on my back and talk. The idea of sitting up and confronting my shrink seemed so strange, bizarre almost. But I had to. I said, 'I'm going to give you a chance to talk'—still no comment. So I turned around, and there he was, *sound asleep.*" (Oh my God, the old joke comes true, I thought.) "I started coughing to wake him up. I had an awful time explaining my feelings because the hour was almost over. He merely said I had a great deal of ambivalence and guilt about my feelings toward him and that we would continue to discuss them."

"You've got to be kidding," I said.

"No, no. It actually happened. What should I do?"

"You mean you just got up politely and left."

"Yes," said Alvin, nursing another drink.

"Wow," I said, "I would have gotten up and walked out without even waking him—let *him* try and figure out what happened."

"What should I do?"

"Tell him how angry you are with him and that you're not going to pay for the hour. Look, Alvin, if you want an analysis as good as that you can come over to my house at six thirty every morning and lie down at the foot of my bed and free-associate. If I don't have to wake up or get dressed or listen to you, I'll even give you a professional discount and throw in breakfast."

Dr. McKee's drink was running low again. "Excuse me, Alvin." I walked over to the chief. Trixie was all over him. She didn't have a great figure, but she did move it around well and it seemed to improve with each drink.

I was feeling the unmistakable symptoms of a rising serum ethanol level (increasing sense of drunkenness), as Stanley Lovett would have put it. I wandered over to Dr. McKee. What does Dr. McKee talk about when Dr. McKee gets drunk? At this moment, at least, he talks about his mother.

"Trixie," Eugene McKee said, putting his arm around her, "what's going on with people today?"

"Gene," said Trixie—Gene!—"young people are more open about their feelings. They're more willing to give, to take and share. I think it's a beautiful thing. Don't you like the closeness of other people?" she asked, practically crawling into his shirt.

Gene glowed but said, "I don't know, there seems to be a lot of flat-out screwing, without any real relationship between people."

"Gene," said Trixie, brushing back a lock of graying hair off his forehead, "didn't you ever screw anyone you didn't have a relationship with?" Trixie was maybe twenty-five, -six, -seven at the most and was making an obvious play for Gene, who was pretty upset over the fact that he was turning fifty in two months (normal reaction, even for a psychoanalyst).

Fifty or not, I could hear him thinking, you can still make it with anyone, anytime . . . Enid Rust was glowering in the corner, swallowing her homemade chopped liver, nearly a handful at a time. I could hear her thinking, primitive, narcissistic, hysterical bitch, while she stared at Trixie.

"Look, Trixie," said Gene, "my mother (his *mother*, my chief) brought me up differently than you kids were. She taught me—yes, damn it, *taught* me—values and she taught me to know people, even if only slightly, before I jumped into bed with them."

I quickly refilled Trixie's and Gene's drinks, figuring he, at least, needed all the help he could get. He looked at me.

"Right, Viscott?"

"She's your mother, chief," I said. "I'll take your word for it."

"My mother," he said, "had more damn common sense in her little finger, more psychotherapeutic skill, than all of you in this room put together." Just then M. Austin Noyes turned around and smiled his great toothy smile. Noyes's mouth at that moment looked to me like the grill of a 1950 Buick Roadmaster.

"Hi, Dr. McKee, nice party," said Dr. M. Austin Noyes. "Fabulous martinis." Rumor had it that Dr. Noyes wasn't even on a first-name basis with his own wife.

"It's Viscott's secret!" said Gene, straightening out his psyche a bit for the head of the department.

"I see we made the right choice this year for chief resident then?" said Dr. M. Austin Noyes in the forced style bosses can't seem to overcome when they try to make jokes with their subordinates.

"Thank you, sir," I said, and poured the hostile sonofabitch four ounces of my very finest. I could hear the old Dartmouth Drinking Song in my head and the chant to chug-a-lug it in one huge swallow. . . .

"I once had a patient," said Bert, chomping on some food, and getting into the act, "when I was on gynecology after I had just completed a pelvic exam, a nice lady in her fifties who asked, 'Does your mother know what you do for a living?' " I pulled Bert away.

Dr. Gavin was carrying on a conversation with Dr. Yancey and Dr. Lovett, who were both trying to score points. Gavin wanted to talk about his plans to go skiing. August was just coming up and Gavin had just bought skis for a ski trip to Chile. "It's winter down there," Gavin said. "I turned fifty two years ago [his reluctant way of admitting he was fifty-two] and I started skiing. It's a good thing to begin something new at fifty, makes you feel good about yourself. Keeps you young." Psychiatrists tend to talk about living more than they actually do it.

Terry O'Conner had just walked in. Stanley immediately sat down with her. They looked very serious together. Stanley recently had been trying to talk Terry into going into analysis. She didn't want to. She couldn't afford it. Stanley wanted her to change from a hysterical character. His analyst was giving him a lot of grief about her. Stanley really seemed to care about Terry. She was about the nicest part of him. Terry still looked great.

Everyone was pretty loaded with well over an hour of very hard drinking. Alvin was trying to score points with Dr. M. Austin Noyes.

Trixie was still trying to get Dr. Eugene McKee to stop at her place on his way home to his suburban wife in his suburban powder blue Plymouth Fury hardtop. I imagined he really wanted a Thunderbird but his wife wouldn't let him get one. Enid was getting pissed and pointing out people's defenses, without benefit of diagnostic tests, right to their face. She would have made a play for Bert because he was so interested in her food, but she hated whiskers. D.J. was shaking off one of the first-year residents who was trying to put the make on her. Russell Townsend was just practically shaking. I poured him another. (I *am* supposed to take care of the medical students, aren't I?)

With all the crazy carrying-on in that room, it could have been a party on my chronic ward at Dutton. I was expecting Richard to walk in and say, "I know your name. I know your name."

"Why the fixed smile, David?" asked Jerry Gelb, coming up. "Has the OPD got you going schiz?"

"Where've you been, you bastard? I've kept the best Scotch hidden for my master."

"And he thanks you. By the way, you going on vacation?" Jerry asked.

"Yes, I'm taking off August to fix up my back yard. It's a big hill. I plan to cut it down and terrace it. Vacation starts tomorrow. Are you taking off August?"

"David," began Jerry, "I'm a psychoanalyst. We *always* take off in August. I'm going to the Cape. I have a place in Wellfleet. You'll be glad you took August off. You'll need the rest for September. It gets busy in the OPD."

A tall, gorgeous black woman with an Afro walked across toward us. She gave Jerry a big hug and kiss and straightened his tie. Jerry introduced me to her, his fabled wife, Mara. I was—for once—speechless. No dumb cracks. Just dumb admiration.

Gene and Trixie were still reminiscing about *his* childhood. She'd heard about it so many times by now she must have felt as though she were a part of it. In a way she was, his second childhood. Trixie was hunting for her car keys. After all, *someone* had to drive Gene home.

CHAPTER TWENTY-ONE

OTHER PLACES, OTHER VIEWS
(INCLUDING DELINQUENT KIDS,
DOCTORS, PARENTS, JUDGES)

"YOU'RE really not planning to do this hill all by yourself?" said Judy.

"Why not? It's not that big a hill and besides I have all the right equipment," I said, walking around to the trunk of my car to show her the tools I just bought.

"Because you'll throw your back out. That's one good reason. Another good reason is that you'll probably get tired of working right in the middle and then we'll have nothing but a hole for a yard."

"Look at these tools, a pick, shovels, a hodder, and the—"

"You didn't need to buy all these," said Judy. "You're not building a pyramid." Wives never really have faith in their husbands' true capabilities.

Undaunted, I loaded up my new wheelbarrow and started up the hill in my back yard. I had blueprints on a sheet of yellow paper in my pocket. All I needed to do was cut the hill five feet down, one hundred twenty feet across, and make two retaining walls, one at the top, one at the bottom. Then I'd have a beautiful terrace, increase the value of my property, and have the satisfaction of seeing something I did with my own two hands. I was out of breath just from climbing to the top.

After swinging away on my pick for ten minutes I realized I was completely out of shape and sat down. I had worked on heavy construction a couple of summers, but this was ridiculous.

"You look ridiculous," said Marty DiAngelo, startling me. Marty and I kept in touch. He was in private practice, working like a dog.

"What are you doing here?" I asked.

"Just came over to talk. Maybe to let you in on a good thing. Have you decided about next year? It's going to be here before you know it. And you're never going to make a living with a pick and shovel."

"I don't have any plans at the moment. What do you have in mind?" I swung away with my pick.

"You know I'm working part-time with Dr. Max Handleman?" asked Marty.

"Handleman? Isn't he one of those guys who give electroshock for everything?" I stopped and wiped my face.

"Pretty much. Don't get me wrong, I don't do any electroshock. I just treat all his psychotherapy cases and run around doing psychiatric consultations in all of his hospitals. He sure knows a lot of internists. He has to take it easy because of his health. He has a huge practice, with more than enough therapy cases he doesn't have time to treat to keep two psychiatrists busy just on the overflow. I've been working in his office but I'm going to quit after the summer and I'd like to let you in on the same deal."

"It sounds interesting," I said.

"And lucrative," added Marty. "You charge patients twenty-five dollars a visit. You use Handleman's office, his secretray, and his answering service. You pay him what amounts to about five dollars per session just to cover his overhead. You'd cover him on nights and weekends and keep office hours one night a week and Saturday morning."

"That's not fee splitting?" I asked. (Fee splitting is actually a kickback for referring a patient.)

"No, Handleman figures he actually loses money. He just about meets his expenses."

"Then why does he do it?"

"To keep his office open at night and maintain good service to his referral sources. He wants to reduce his workload but still keep up his EST practice. You'd cover his entire practice for the summer if you decide to take it. He takes off for the mountains."

"I'd like to meet him and decide," I said, leaning on my pick.

"You'll like it. I've already mentioned your name to him. You'll do whatever you want. You'll be given staff privileges at his hospitals. He'll do all the EST, though. That's thirty-five dollars a buzz, and he wants that work because it's easy. Except you'll do his EST next summer."

"Sounds OK." I was ambivalent about EST.

"OK? You dumb bastard, it's a godsend and you don't even know it. And that's not all I'm handing you. I have a consult job at the youth center, evaluating juvenile delinquents that the court thinks have a psychiatric illness. It pays twenty-five bucks for two hours' work, but you can make your own hours and it's really interesting. I'll put your name in to the commissioner. I'm quitting that job too."

"I think that sounds fascinating." I had my wind back and was attacking the hill again.

"I have a couple of other goodies to throw your way. I have another job working twice a week at Brookfield State Hospital, the prison for the criminally insane. I'm giving that up too. It pays well and you get a chance to see some unusual psychopathology, stuff you never see anywhere else. And you get a chance to work with Dr. Leo Albee, the forensic psychiatrist."

"You really move around, don't you?" I said, swinging the pick.

"I'm a pusher. Without me, kid, you'd probably die. You have lousy pick technique, by the way." Marty was right. I wasn't much interested in running myself ragged making connections and working up referrals. Marty loved getting out there and making contacts. But I did think my technique was good. "I know that you're a good friend of Jerry Gelb, but if he sends you more than two private patients next year I'll be surprised. Remember, he's an analyst and analysts generally send patients to each other, not to us lowly guys. Do you want the job?"

"It sounds great," I said. "I'll have to talk to Dr. Albee first. By the way, why are you giving up all these jobs?"

"I've been working at the university student health clinic for the past three years and I've been trying to set up a separate psychiatric clinic. Well, it looks like I'll be getting some money from Dr. Noyes to set one up any day now. It'll be a small beginning, but in about a year I'll need several part-time people. When I do get set up I'd like you to be on my staff. Right now I'm still putting it together."

"I'd like that," I said, exhausted, putting down the pick. Suddenly I had three part-time jobs and the promise of a fourth.

"Now," said Marty, rolling up his sleeves, "let me show you what's wrong with your pick technique." Marty went at the hill for a bit. He really could swing a pick.

"Where'd you learn to do that?" I asked admiringly.

"With a name like DiAngelo you can't figure it out? The man who is swinging this pick is a direct descendent of the Romans who built the great amphitheatres." He swung. "The beautiful temples." He swung again. "The fabulous aqueducts." He did have a lovely natural rhythm to his swing.

My daughters, Elizabeth and Penny, had come up the hill and sat down next to me to watch Marty. "Mommy said you were crazy to try it alone," said Elizabeth. "Is he working for you, Daddy?"

"At twenty-five dollars an hour?" I said.

The rhythm of Marty's swing was broken by his laughter.

I used my month's vacation to become familiar with my new situations. Dr. Handleman practiced psychiatry the way some general practitioners practice psychiatry, with pills and reassurance, except he also added a large amount of electricity. Max was board-certified in psychiatry and neurology and routinely performed physical examinations on his own psychiatric patients. I suppose it used up some time so he wouldn't have to talk or listen too much. He had a fully equipped examining room just off his office. I watched him perform the morning I dropped by to meet him. He was running through an abbreviated neurological examination with a patient. He prescribed a tranquilizer for anxiety, an antispasmodic for gas pains, and sent the patient on her way.

"This will be your office," he said, leading me into a pine-paneled office directly across a common waiting room decorated in Colonial style. "The furniture is from my den at home. I had it brought in and now I can take the price as a deduction. Take my advice"—Max said that a lot—"get yourself a good tax accountant. Be straight with Uncle Sam when you report your earnings but take every nickel you can. You know how much I get to keep of every dollar I make? Eighty-five cents! That's because I have a good accountant. Otherwise I'd probably have to pay fifty or sixty cents on the dollar! You like the office?"

"Yes, very much." It was a nice office to sit around and sew a quilt in.

"You just tell Flora, my secretary, the hours you'll be working and she'll start making appointments. Marty will be finishing up in October so you'll be getting patients in a hurry."

That summer Marty continued to manage Handleman's hospital consultations and do the electroshock. I was being sent patients by Flora. In two weeks I had seen eighteen private patients, most of them interesting and relatively easy. It was an entirely new experience. I was the boss. The patients who came to Handleman were not at all sophisticated about psychiatry. They expected me to treat them as their family doctor would. They were open about their feelings, in some ways more open than the patients I was seeing in the OPD who were skilled at manipulating psychiatrists. Handleman's patients were ordinary people who wanted help and were paying for it. Somehow that seemed to make them more motivated. Maybe they valued what I said because they paid for their sessions. I was actually very happy with the arrangement. It was fairly easy just doing therapy with none of my other residency pressures.

I also began working at the Youth Center in August. It was a dreary place and looked shabby in spite of being less than ten years old. Sad children stared at me wherever I looked in the yard. Most of these children had been accused of committing a crime and were awaiting trial.

The observation section of the Youth Center where I interviewed kids was on the second floor. The first time I visited, it was a hot, steamy day outside but in the dark corridors, the stench of a decade of never completely washed away urine still prominent, it was oppressively damp, almost chilly. A young boy, no older than eight, apparently being punished, pressed against the steel bars over the window at the end of the hall. He stared down at the other children playing ball outside. His eyes were dry. After a while, tears don't come anymore.

I walked into the office on the second floor and met the Center's social worker and psychologist.

Mr. Grayson was the social worker and a former career navy man who had four tattoos to prove it. He spent his time griping about the inequities of the civil service system, the supervisor of the Center, and his co-workers. He also complained about the parents of the kids and believed that the problem of delinquency was the result of lax moral standards in the home. Whenever he made a home visit, which was as infrequently as he could, he would return to the Center raging at what he'd seen.

My job was to evaluate two kids a week and to write brief psychiatric reports in which I would make a recommendation to the court. Grayson would read my report, adjust his findings to fit, and submit it to the district attorney in charge of each case.

Each boy was usually given some form of psychological testing by Orson ("Just call me 'Happy,' everyone else does") Farrington.

Happy looked like a blown-up version of one of the seven dwarfs. He was always squinting, red-faced, had a giggly laugh, and dressed in a tweed jacket, chinos, and sneakers. He had a master's degree in psychology. He administered the same IQ test to kids over and over, using it not only as an instrument to measure their ability but also as a projective test. Apparently it was the only test Happy felt comfortable with. He wrote extensive, elaborate reports describing each kid's psychological makeup based largely on his attitude during the IQ test. He was a sort of male Enid Rust. Happy had a talent for imaginative writing, but not much clinical experience. When I disagreed with him he pouted and sometimes slammed doors.

When I disagreed with Grayson, he got almost paranoid and went overboard changing his report so he wouldn't later be shown up by a young punk. That's what Happy said Grayson used to call me when I wasn't there. Grayson said Happy used to call me a jerk when I wasn't there. To my face they both called me Doctor.

On the surface at least they were very cooperative. Each week they found two youngsters for me to see. Almost 85 percent of the children I saw in the two years I kept the job did not, I felt, belong there. They'd been detained on what was called a Stubborn Child Warrant. Any parent who so desired could go down to his local police station and make up a story to the officer in charge that his kid is "*stubborn.*" The mother's or father's word would automatically be taken over the child's and before the dust settled the child would be sent to the Youth Center and detained. The children could do nothing about such false arrests. They were powerless.

Such children generally had no legal counsel unless their parents provided it, which under the circumstances was unlikely since the parents were the complainants. However, when a child was truly delinquent and had allegedly committed a crime that threatened the well-being or rights of others, his parents frequently provided him with a lawyer. Sometimes this was done by the parent out of a sense of guilt or to save face in the community so people wouldn't think that the parents had anything to do with their child turning bad.

Frequently the children who were treated the worst were the innocent. Often their only crime was to run away from home, to be a problem in school, or to be emotionally upset. Children were also frequently used as scapegoats by an angry family who sometimes did not know what they were angry about. Such children were treated as things by their parents, not as people. They were the boys for whom no lawyer was available, no adult willing to go to bat, and no parent able or caring enough to come in and talk. For these, the stay at the Youth Center was filled with confusion and rumor and the hope that their case might be brought up before a judge who could still remember his own prankish boyhood and that boys will be boys. Some judges had forgotten that they were once children.

The children put up with the inequities of the law, with the tyranny of their parents and the threats of the bullies, the best they could. Some of the boys I saw tried to shut out their home problems from their minds and hoped without any reasonable justification that everything would somehow be better when they got home, which was wishful—if understandable—thinking.

I have listened to children, who were guilty only of being born to an unstable mother or a vindictive father, while they earnestly promised me that they would be good if I let them go home again. I would tell them that I felt they were good already, and I would explain the situation the way I saw it, simply as possible, trying not to hide anything. I figured that if I couldn't change a kid's parents, I could at least tell him what was going on so that he would know when to duck. I could side with him when it was possible and allow him to remember that some adult once believed in him, if only briefly.

Grayson thought I would infuriate some judges with my outraged letters to the court, so I toned down my letters some and tried to manipulate the judges to my way of thinking. No expert witness to any court is ever impartial, I soon discovered. I was no different. I believed in my opinions. I wrote my reports with the specific intent of influencing the judge. I was biased. I admit it.

The boys also had to put up with the personnel at the youth center. The security staff—uniforms were chino pants, blue sneakers, and sweatshirts—looked like a bunch of off-season gym teachers. They made the kids line up for everything—straight lines, very straight lines. They made the kids call them "sir" and would chew them out when they did not. In fact, they were called "the Sirs." Staff members sometimes hit kids when they were troublesome, according to Happy. I never saw any of the staff hit a boy when I was around. I was a threat because I was an outside authority, the kind most feared by the staff because I could register complaints outside their normal chain of command. The thought of being reported terrified members of the staff, many of whom were still themselves children emotionally.

Any time a boy showed a typically adolescent attitude of rebelliousness the staff was quick to be down on him and hand out punitive details like cleaning the toilets or sweeping floors. A boy who was confined to this unit after a dispute with his parents would soon feel undermined. He would also sense that his own parents felt too weak to control him. When he returned home he often feared losing control again and the nightmare repeating. If his original "crime" had been only his parents' inability to tolerate the sort of horseplay in which most boys often get involved, the boy might not be able "to control himself" at home and, in fact, he might even *want* to do the same things again—to run away, to talk back, to have a beer with his friends or come home late at night—and his wanting to do these rather innocent things might even be healthy. He knew plenty of friends who committed the same "crimes" and went unpunished. As a result of all these double standards a boy lost faith in the fairness of his parents' authority and eventually the fairness of all justice. After all, the courts backed his parents up, not him. Since he remembered with feelings of helplessness his experience with the law, he often decided that, for him at least, there was no chance through the law, that the cards would always be stacked against him. His time with the security staff at the Center would only confirm and even strengthen those feelings. The innocent would become the guilty soon enough.

The staff punished boys on the basis of hearsay evidence gotten from one of the Sirs' favorites, the boys the Sirs called "good boys." These good boys usually turned out to be disturbed psychopathic kids who set up the other boys. The Sirs continued the process of eroding the boys' confidence, of hardening their belief that all adults were punitive, cold, and unfeeling. Their despair, and anger, grew.

The stronger children bullied and tormented the weaker ones. Children do that, especially when they feel picked on by adults. They were led by the worst among them, the physically strong, the psychopathic, or those who had a compulsive need to control other people. Homosexual activity was rampant. Children varying widely in age were clustered together without even superficial considerations for differences in their emotional needs or development.

The children were treated as though they were small adults. They were bawled out for a lack of responsibility, criticized when they acted like children. They were ridiculed for being afraid, slapped for being ambivalent, screamed at for being sad, and called "uncooperative" when their hopelessness made them give up.

I did the best I could for them. I wrote the most convincing letters to the court that I was capable of and I tried to reassure them. I contacted the public defenders for help. I tried to manipulate Happy and Grayson into doing what I believed was best for the children, but it was tough because they were trying to get ahead in the system that made the injustices and were afraid to make waves. There was backbiting and undermining among all staff members. The director of the Youth Center was a politician who spent almost no time with the children personally. He knew only what the reports on his desk told him—that is, if he ever bothered to read them.

The Youth Center saddened, infuriated, and frustrated me. But at least through my reports I had a pipeline of sorts to the judge, the man who held the key. I tried, damn it. The little boy somewhere inside me refused to let his friends down.

CHAPTER TWENTY-TWO

THERAPY IN THE OPD

I HAD finished terracing the hill in my back yard by the end of what turned out to be the rainiest August on record, and I was pleased to get back to the clinic. September was delightful, a real Indian summer in the New England fields and woodlands. September was a nightmare in the OPD.

Patients appeared as if out of nowhere. Every morning there were eight people sitting in the waiting room asking to be evaluated. The nine o'clock intake conferences were so crowded that if a resident went longer than five minutes presenting a case he would be cutting into someone else's time.

Dr. Eugene McKee had a genuine gift for uncovering the event in a patient's life that precipitated his present crisis. "If you can identify a patient's precipitating event and understand what made it so special to him, you know everything you need to treat him," he said. Almost all precipitating events involve a loss of some kind. Mr. Brodner, for example, became upset at his son's birthday party. The party was a precipitating event for Mr. Brodner because it symbolized to him his feelings about not being given to as a child the way he wanted to be, the way he felt his son was. All of the old unresolved feelings from his past surfaced and overwhelmed him. He felt anger at his son and worthless about himself.

"It's also important to understand what's happening in the patient's life well enough so you can isolate the precipitating event," McKee said. Mr. Brodner suffered other hurts about the same time that *could* have done the trick. During the week of the birthday party he took some losses in the stock market and had also been fighting with a neighbor over the neighbor's children. But neither of these had the symbolic punch of his son's party. A precipitating event in a psychiatric illness is something like the dramatic resolution in a tragic play. You have to identify it by understanding its source and development before you can change the ending.

McKee could also trace the threads he had uncovered through the broader fabric of the patient's life. He made the precipitating event meaningful for both the present and the past. He could tie the patient's symptoms and history together in a way that made the patient and his illness seem logical, clear, and easy to remember, if not always predictable. Maybe the packages he wrapped patients in were sometimes too neat and too simplified, but they were still very useful. It probably didn't matter what system a therapist used. The significant thing was to have some system to give order and help you understand a patient who might otherwise seem chaotic and confounding, providing, that is, you didn't expect the patient to perform according to your theoretical expectations. It made you more able to sit with a patient and to listen, knowing that most everything he told you would fit together somehow, that in time you'd recognize his problems as something familiar, almost as old friends—or enemies. Knowing that, you also stopped being afraid.

Determining the precipitating event quickly was especially important in the OPD because of the limited time to spend with the patients. The major form of treatment in the OPD was short-term psychotherapy. Patients were seen for twelve visits or less. In that time you would focus on one specific issue—to understand the circumstances surrounding the precipitating event and to help the patient come to grips with them. It was a short affair and, unlike long-term therapy, usually dealt with only one issue. But as McKee used to say, "A short affair is better than no affair at all."

You learned a great deal doing outpatient psychotherapy. You learned that the difference between normal and abnormal was not always easy to define. Most of the patients looked and acted no differently from anyone you would meet at a cocktail party, especially one of ours. They would pass unnoticed in a crowd on the street because they were the crowd on the street.

Much of what we did in psychotherapy—short and long-haul—had to do with helping patients learn to cope with a painful reality. The first step was to establish a sense of trust between the therapist and the patient. The next was to understand what the patient's symptoms meant, where they came from, and how they related to the present. The therapist and the patient joined forces to try to make the patient more real, more in touch with what he felt, more responsive to the outside world as it really is, less hateful of the world because it's not what he imagined it to be.

The second stage of therapy is called "working through." "Everyone," said Dr. McKee, "talks about beginning therapy and ending therapy, but it's in the goddamn middle of therapy that all the work happens. And nobody says *anything* about that. You evaluate a patient and spend a few months resolving the urgent problems and then four years later you start to terminate with the patient. I don't know about you, kids, but I think those three and a half years between are pretty important. We charge enough for them, so they must be."

In the working-through stage the therapist and patient reexamined the world using a new pair of eyeglasses to correct for the patient's emotional blind spots. In the beginning of treatment, the therapist decided how much error there was in the patient's vision. Working through was the adjustment period in which the patient got used to his new perceptions and saw some things for the first time and got his bearings in a new reality. It could also be a very rough time. Patients often saw themselves in an unfavorable light for the first time. Old accepted "truths" tended to have holes in them. People once loved were often seen differently. As the patient's vision cleared he had more energy available to work and to enjoy life, because less was being wasted in blind rushes into dead ends. He had a chance to develop realistic goals, to accept what he could and couldn't expect to change. Sometimes this seemed to take forever in long-term therapy, but in short-term therapy it had to be completed in three months. Dr. McKee's orders . . .

Mrs. Norton had a phobic reaction. She was afraid to travel in automobiles, airplanes, over bridges, on elevators, up stairs, practically anywhere and on anything. She seemed a charming woman and was quite bright. Mrs. Norton's daughter, Sybil, from her first marriage was definitely not the sort of girl Dr. McKee's mother would allow in *her* house. Sybil became what her mother called a tramp when her father ran away. Mrs. Norton was overcome by the prospect of taking care of Sybil, and remarried in the hope of finding someone who could cope with her, control her.

The second marriage became a failure, and Mrs. Norton couldn't face it. She wanted to leave, but felt if she did Sybil would go wild (which, of course, she'd already gone). She looked to the time when

Sybil would be grown up and she'd be free to divorce her husband and begin life on her own. But when Sybil *did* leave the house she married the minister who saved her! Mrs. Norton became afraid of leaving the house. Mrs. Norton had married her second husband more to take care of herself than Sybil. She felt weak and helpless when her first husband left and had buried those feelings beneath the facade of a self-sacrificing mother. After Sybil left and there was no obligation on her own terms for Mrs. Norton to stay married, she panicked and developed symptoms. Her fear of traveling both obscured and expressed her intense desire to be cared for, a desire she couldn't admit and so couldn't fulfill. Since her phobia kept her from leaving, her husband would have to take care of her. There was also another side of her that *did* want to run.

"Where would you go if you could?" I asked.

"I never thought of it. That's a difficult question," Mrs. Norton said, and conveniently found a picture on my wall to look at. "That's unusual, that picture."

"Where would you go?"

"*With my daughter . . .*"

With those three words Mrs. Norton summarized much of her life. She secretly admired her daughter's sexual exploits because she always felt sexually inhibited herself. In fact, in some ways she silently encouraged Sybil to act promiscuously and to experience what Mrs. Norton believed she'd missed in life.

In the twelve sessions I tried to help Mrs. Norton accept her desires to be cared for. She began to see that many of the qualities that she thought made her husband a good father for Sybil also made him a good husband for herself. As she began to accept her desire and need to be cared for, she also complained less about her fears of traveling. After a while, she hardly mentioned them at all. She was on the way. . . .

In the Union Hospital OPD there was just about enough time to determine what the patient's problem was, how it developed, what to do about it, and to say good-bye. Please don't look down your nose at the idea of seeing someone for only twelve hours. A great deal could be and was accomplished. True, you didn't have the time to go into every detail, but at least what you did discuss was relevant to the problem, hopefully.

Termination is the last phase of therapy. In terminating, you helped the patient accept the idea he wouldn't be seeing you anymore.

It's often painful for a patient to say good-bye; rarely if ever before has anyone been so interested in what he thought or felt as his therapist is. Because his doctor has tried hard and has cared, a patient feels loss and the sadness that goes with it when he leaves therapy. These feelings had to be anticipated and discussed.

Because the therapeutic process uncovers so many old forgotten feelings, and since many of these feelings become attributed to the doctor during therapy, terminating without resolving them may cause problems in the future. For example, instead of worrying about a hated father, a patient who has abruptly terminated may spend years worrying not only about a hated father but about a therapist as well on whom he's projected that hatred. If the patient's feelings about the therapist are settled realistically, this problem can be minimized, although patients commonly think about their therapists for years after therapy is over.

Features of a patient's personality that originally made a particular loss so important to him are still in force when he terminates, and make the loss of the therapist seem equally important to him. By then the therapist has taken on many symbolic meanings to the patient. It's common for symptoms that were prominent in the first hour of therapy to appear again in the last hour of therapy as those same forces that were originally at work show themselves at another loss. It's almost as if the patient is saying that leaving his therapist is as important a loss as was the one that precipitated his illness. In fact it is, but in reverse. Because the patient has learned new ways to deal with his feelings and because the loss of the therapist has been resolved before it actually happens, the terminating event pulls the patient together rather than apart.

The reappearance of symptoms in the last therapeutic hour is almost a plea, "You can't let me go. I'm not ready yet." You can't keep patients forever. In time, they've got to be allowed to assume their independence. To postpone termination when a patient is ready may undermine the patient and risk making him dependent on his therapist. It's especially important that adolescents be encouraged to take over again as soon as possible.

In short-term therapy we didn't see much regression to less emotionally mature ways of coping with problems, because short-term therapy was directed to specific and relatively narrow goals. In long-term therapy more attention was given to understanding a patient's distortions of the doctor as part of helping the patient discover how

his particular network of defenses operated. The goal was broader—
to change the patient's style of interacting. Sometimes the goal was
reached, sometimes it wasn't. Sometimes patients underwent a sea
change in short psychotherapy, sometimes they stayed stuck even
after many years of intensive treatment.

I remember a young woman, Karen Wells, who changed drastically after three weeks. Before therapy she was barely existing in a
cold-water flat while her rich, widowed mother was living it up
around the world. Dr. McKee, who sometimes supervised me, said
after I discussed the initial hour, "Viscott, you go back and tell that
girl to cut the crap. Tell her to get on the phone and call her mother
and ask for some money to help her out. She thinks she has to be in
mourning for her father forever. The mother is probably worried about
the girl and upset because she can't get her to take any money. This
girl is just overdoing her grief reaction for her father. She thinks if
she stops grieving that her father's memory will disappear."

"I'll tell her that father left something more for her than a
memory."

"You just do that, Viscott," said McKee. "I'd belt her with the
facts."

I did. Karen called her mother the same day and they got
together between Karen's second and third visits. They went shopping
together and her mother helped furnish Karen's apartment. At the
third visit Karen was no longer depressed, no longer felt that her
father had left her nothing, and she could believe that her mother
had also loved her father and also remembered him. It was an
incredible change.

"What did I tell you?" said McKee, trying to sound unimpressed
with my report of the progress. He was so unimpressed with his own
suggestion that he discussed the case at the next grand rounds as a
dramatic example of the results of short-term therapy.

McKee stressed the value in having an organized treatment plan.
"I don't mean you should have a written script telling you what to
do every minute you spend with a patient, but you should know generally where you want to go, what your goals are. You should know
which issues are important and try to keep the patient focused on
those issues. Remember, a patient doesn't go to a psychiatrist just
because he likes the chairs in his office. He goes because he doesn't
like what's going on in his life and he wants to change it. That requires plain old hard work and the psychiatrist's resolve not to be

seduced by the patient's flights of fancy into areas that have nothing to do with the problem."

Of course the psychiatrist can only stay this sharply focused when he's sure he understands the problem. And it's also important to know when to allow a patient to describe his fantasy life because that's where the clues to forgotten or hidden ideas are found. But to allow a patient to run his own therapy by jabbering on aimlessly about anything all the time seems to have limited value. The process of psychotherapy is too long and expensive as it is now, and there usually isn't enough time to discuss all the real problems. The theory that work expands to fill the time available for it is especially true in psychotherapy. If the process of psychotherapy is needlessly extended a patient can lose a great deal. He may find himself less spontaneous, feeling that he needs to analyze absolutely every aspect of every problem before he makes any decision. All aspects of an idea are analyzable only if it's possible to know everything about that idea. Only people who feel omniscient believe this, like some therapists and, unfortunately, some of their patients. What good is an analytic answer, no matter how brilliantly expressed, if the question or the issue are irrelevant. It's been said—especially by some analysts—that the unanalyzed life is not worth living, but it is equally true that the unlived life is not worth analyzing. Needlessly protracted psychotherapy is just mutual mental masturbation. It's time that the psychiatrist and the patient both grew up and found appropriate objects for their fantasies and did something to connect them instead of just talking all the time.

Stanley Lovett passed me a note during a conference. "Can I see you as soon as possible?" It sounded urgent and I couldn't recall Stanley ever asking me for anything. We met right after the conference.

"David, I'm all mixed up, I just don't know what to do, I think Terry's pregnant."

"Have you discussed it with your analyst?" (If this exchange sounds almost humorously familiar, just as though it might have happened between two ordinary mortals, it's because that's exactly what we were—psychiatrists-in-the-making notwithstanding. Also, on my part, I was a little reluctant to get involved.)

"Yes, Dr. Fletcher feels that Terry represents a reaction-formation (translation: adoption of behavior opposite to often disowned impulses)," intoned Stanley, pedantic even in his time of genuine crisis and anguish. "Instead of marrying a castrating, controlling, obsessive bitch like my mother, the woman he says I secretly really love as well as hate, I'm seeking out the exact opposite, a sensuous, soft, accepting hysteric. Fletcher says I've picked Terry to avoid talking about my mother. He refuses to talk about Terry in terms that relate to my present feelings. He's only interested in my past anger at my mother. I try to get him to talk about Terry and how really good I feel with her." Stanley sounded desperate.

"What did he say about the *pregnancy?*"

"He said it was my unconscious attempt to get him to focus on Terry. He still only wants to hear about my mother and doesn't comment when I talk about Terry." I thought that was a crappy thing for Dr. Fletcher to do to Stanley even if what Fletcher said was true. I wasn't so sure it was true. All I knew was that I liked Stanley best when he was with Terry.

"You want to marry her?" I asked.

"I don't know. She's so much that I want . . . still, when I look at her I see neurotic traits that stick out all over the place and feel embarrassed and ashamed that she isn't perfect. I know that's stupid but—"

"Stanley, you can go around intellectualizing about Terry for the next ten years and it won't do you any good. That girl has a lot of great qualities. She's warm, she's charming, she's cheerful and very kind to you. She's a good person. OK, she's a flaming hysteric, but what's so goddamn bad about that? I mean, everyone's got to be something. Just because you can make a psychiatric diagnosis on someone doesn't mean he has a disease. Look, you miserable bastard, you're not exactly what I would call the picture of mental health yourself. I mean, you're an obsessive-compulsive from way back. And, Stanley, if I'm not mistaken, hysterics are higher up on the scale of emotional maturity than obsessive-compulsives."

"You're pretty funny, David."

Like a crutch, Stanley, like a crutch.

"Another thing," continued David-the-therapist, "Terry accepts you, and just for yourself." I thought a minute and remembered how I used loneliness with obsessive-compulsives. "And, Stanley, I think you're the kind of guy who feels lonely a lot of time. I'll bet you don't when you're with Terry."

And that *did* ring a bell! I suddenly was doing psychotherapy with a shaking twenty-eight-year-old psychiatric resident. "It's true. I *am* so damn lonely all the time," Stanley said, "except when I'm with Terry. I know I'm an obsessive-compulsive and that sometimes I don't feel as much as other people. Maybe that's why I'm attracted to a hysteric like Terry, because she feels so much and *shows* her feelings. I just don't want to make a mistake and marry someone for neurotic reasons." (He'd have known the answer to that one with a patient. But at the moment *he* was the patient and I was the doctor. So I made like a doctor.)

"Most reasons for getting married are probably neurotic, Stanley," I said cheerfully. "Some, in fact and as you know, are psychotic. I think you're *thinking* this out too much and not *feeling* enough about it. How do you feel when you're with Terry? How do you feel when you're not? What does Terry mean to you? What would it be like without her? You have to be sure about Terry before you can make a decision about the baby. How far along is Terry?"

"Six weeks."

"You'll have to decide pretty soon."

"Can I talk with you again later on in the week?"

"Sure." I actually felt warmly toward Stanley. In fact, I hurt inside for him.

"Thanks, David. You're about the only one I can talk to."

(My God, what's that guy been doing all this time with his *real* analyst?)

"I'm happy to, Stanley, anytime. By the way, am I overstepping by asking why you don't feel you can talk to Dr. Fletcher more openly?"

Stanley was silent for a moment and said, "Well, I don't want to appear too upset or disturbed in analysis or they'll throw me out of the Institute. I was only given a conditional acceptance to the Institute and they postponed their decision whether I can begin the seminars or not until the end of this year, depending on how my personal analysis goes."

"Stanley," I said, "you can talk to Fletcher. You can tell him how you feel. That's not going to kill *or* disqualify you. Stop worrying about being crazy so damn much. Being crazy didn't stop some of the analysts around this place from making it. A lot of psychiatrists are crazy. There are probably more nuts in our profession than in any other. Honestly, you know them as well as I do. The important thing for us is to be aware of our craziness and not be rigid about it. Tell him! He already knows that you're upset, for Christsake! If you can't be yourself and be an analyst at the same time, why would you want it?"

"Because being a psychoanalyst is the best I can be," said Stanley resolutely, quoting from somewhere in his adolescence.

"I used to feel that way," I said, "that being a psychoanalyst must be the furthest you could go in human understanding, but you have to do what suits you best. You can't spend your life wanting to be something if it's not you."

"I like being in control and knowing what's going on in people," said Stanley, pulling himself together.

"And you do, Stanley. From what I can tell you seem to know the name of every process going on in your patients, but I don't think you're as in touch with their feelings as you should be, and that's because—forgive me—you're not as in touch with your own feelings as you should be. Keeping how you feel from your analyst so you won't be rejected at the Institute is just silly. You're only cheating yourself. You have to face up to being yourself, the way you are, not the way you think you ought to appear to become an analyst. Otherwise, you'll sure as hell never make it. You'll just be a figment of your imagination and in the end you'll hate yourself for it."

Stanley seemed to be taking it in.

"I just haven't thought enough about these things."

"Maybe I have no right bringing them up."

"No, I'm glad you did."

I saw Stanley three times during the month. He finally decided to level with his analyst and they were able to clear up several problems that had been holding them down. All was not roses, though. Terry, like a lot of girls before her in her situation, decided she couldn't wait—not even for Stanley's analysis—and had an abortion. They broke up, and Stanley was understandably depressed all winter.

And I guess that, as they say, is life.

I was also treating Russell Townsend, the fourth-year medical student, who started to have anxiety attacks from his fear of being homosexual. Russell approached me in October. He had acne and it had gotten worse because he couldn't leave his face alone when he got an unacceptable sexual thought. His continual picking was also his way of fending off his fears, just like Mr. Harold Parker's magically touching me. At times Russell appeared psychotic and I put him on fairly stiff doses of tranquilizers. His grades improved along with his diminished anxiety. In a few months his face was almost clear.

October had gone from scarlet to umber. In spite of the heavy pressure of work, the evaluations to review, the medical students to supervise, the residents to manage, and my various moonlighting jobs, I still found I could budget my time, get a great deal done, and have some time left over. I did give up lunch, but that wasn't going to hurt me. I was feeling comfortable, very happy in my work.

It was good to be able to say that and mean it.

CHAPTER TWENTY-THREE

BROOKFIELD—HOSPITAL FOR THE CRIMINALLY INSANE

$\mathbb{B}$ROOKFIELD State Hospital was called a hospital. At best it was a prison, and by prison standards it was a slum. It was designed to confine, not treat the so-called criminally insane. There were no psychiatrists on the Brookfield staff. Just a handful of medical doctors whose experience in psychiatry was so limited it hardly mattered. The Brookfield medical director, Dr. Raymond Cortina, an old GP, once told me, "I got my psychiatric credentials the hard way, the only way that really counts, by *being around* emotionally disturbed patients." Without supervision, without the desire to read, and without any special insight, Dr. Cortina seemed little more qualified than the patients' relatives, who also had spent their lives *being around* a disturbed person. As for Brookfield's prison facilities—it had only walls, locks, cells, and officers who, for the most part, understood little about emotional illness and less about managing patient-prisoners. There was no way for the patient to get better or for the criminal to be rehabilitated.

The Forensic Medicine Institute was associated with the medical school and had established tentative ties with Brookfield Hospital several years before. Institute members and affiliates served in an advisory capacity to the staff. Dr. Leopold Albee was a professor of legal psychiatry. He wrote a great number of papers on the subject. He was always working on a study, not so often on an original idea. Albee was interested in studying patients at Brookfield and had a federal grant providing the funds to run one small ward which, for reasons I still do not understand at all, was called the rehabilitation ward.

"You'll be in charge of 'rehab,' " Dr. Albee said as we drove down to the hospital together for what would be my first visit.

Dr. Albee was a tall man, maybe six-foot-five. He was only forty but his hair was already thinning and gray. He was rather pompous and addicted to the details of the official protocol. I suppose it was partly because he was concerned about his grant and didn't want any trouble. "We've made inroads into this system here but we're here on sufferance. You should regard yourself as a privileged guest. DiAngelo was only the fifth in a short line of psychiatrists from the Institute who have been associated with Brookfield these past five years. Everyone has kept their noses clean and been helpful as possible to the Brookfield staff.

"You are going to see a lot of abuses at Brookfield that are going to make your hair stand on end. Just remember, any change in the system must come from within, from people who are regarded as friends, not as critics trying to get publicity and make the headlines. You are part of the system and you must accept it."

"What sort of things are going to make my hair stand on end?" I asked. "—Do you have to smoke that pipe?"

Leo Albee smoked one of the most obnoxious pipe tobaccos I ever smelled. After I had given up smoking, my tolerance for other people's smoking decreased. When I complained about Jerry Gelb's pipe, Jerry told me I was expressing my hostility toward him. Why do psychiatrists look for *hidden* meaning in everything? He was right. I was hostile about it because I didn't like it. Right out in the open, no mystery about that one as far as I could tell.

Albee apparently didn't hear me. He filled my car with smoke while he thought up juicy, hair-raising details to frighten me. Albee seemed to like to intimidate people, especially people who already felt intimidated.

"Well," he said, "you'll see incompetence and violence. You'll work with murderers. You'll see brutality and homosexual attacks by officers. Don't call them 'guards.' The officer in charge of the rehab ward is a bigot, he hates Negroes and Puerto Ricans more than anyone I know."

"Why is he still there?"

"Well," said Albee, adjusting the rear-view mirror to comb his hair, "he has seniority and can choose his own ward."

"Oh," I said, readjusting the mirror.

"This is an excellent opportunity for us to learn how the system works. I think those of us at the Forensic Medicine Institute have a special opportunity to observe and eventually make recommendations to the governor's commission to improve the place. You'll be treating patients and helping them become competent to stand trial. You'll evaluate the men and attend the staff conference, where they're interviewed and a decision is made whether to return them to court for trial or hold them for more observation. May I ask you a direct question, Dr. Viscott?"

"Sure."

"Why are you driving almost one hundred miles an hour?"

"Because I'm anxious?"

Dr. Albee looked surprised. I slowed down. We took a side road through the countryside.

The meadows all about Brookfield were dotted with tiny farms. Rows of tall corn stretched out toward the salt marshes that bordered on the sea. "Some of the patients work here," said Albee, pointing to one of the farms. "That's the Center for Incorrigible Delinquents," he added, pointing to a yellow-walled complex blistering bright in the late summer sun. "When kids committed to the youth center get worse or continue to commit crimes, they sometimes get sent down here. It's quite a hellhole. The officers in the delinquent division are, I'm afraid, the most psychopathic officers anywhere in the state. They have a windowless room with a dirt floor with a hatch through which they lower boys into solitary. It's just a dark hole. You just can't believe it."

I followed Albee's directions to a dilapidated red brick building. The air smelled like the country. Bees buzzed erratically around. There were huge flowerbeds everywhere, all along the turreted walls and walkways.

Brookfield State Hospital's physical structure seemed to reflect its ambivalent philosophy about the insane criminal. Its walls were not high enough to prevent some from escaping, and its facilities were not adequate to help those unfortunate enough to remain behind to get better.

We walked through the main entrance. Bob Linnehan, the chief deputy, met us. He was a big warm strapping man with a brogue so thick he seemed to taste the words he spoke.

"Mr. Linnehan, this is Dr. Viscott. He's replacing Dr. DiAngelo."

"An' it's a pleasure to be havin' another of your boys. Dr. DiAngelo is a darlin' man. We'll sure be missin 'im. Darlin' funny man. I don't know if he's kissed the Blarney Stone but for sure he's kissed something. You two gentlemen going to staff this mornin'? They'll be presenting Albert Carrol shortly now. Right after Mr. Dunphy."

"I know," said Dr. Albee, walking through the hall toward a large iron door. It slid open and we walked in. "This is the trap." The door closed with a clank behind us. An officer in the control booth waved to Albee. "Morning, Dr. Albee," he said.

"This is Dr. Viscott, Dr. DiAngelo's replacement," Albee announced to the officer. "I hope you don't mind being referred to as some-one's replacement, but it's the fastest way of making people under-stand who you are. It also makes clear your right to succeed Marty as well as inherit, I might add, not a little goodwill, as you can see from Bob Linnehan's reaction. By the way, Linnehan is your strong-est ally here. He's been very helpful. You'll learn a lot from him." (I did.)

Another iron door slid open. Albee and I walked down a long corridor. I could see a locked door at the other end. Dr. Albee stopped; he wanted to talk to me before entering the conference room. "Let me give you the criteria for determining competency"— Albee was getting stuffier by the minute. "Does the man know the crime of which he is accused, and understand what could happen to him if he were convicted? Is he able to cooperate with his lawyer in his defense? This means that he has to understand what a court proceeding is. He can't be tried if he thinks the judge is a Martian or the court is a dining room at Harvard Business School." Dr. Albee chuckled at his drollness.

Dr. Albee was very academic, slow to make his decisions and implement them. People like Dr. Albee sometimes acted this way not only out of a sense of care and informed deliberation; they also were worried about some lack of competence that might be shown up if they made a mistake. His reputation, I thought, was pretty good. Dr. Albee, a stickler for following procedure and respecting the chain of command, was leery about some of the relatively unconventional tac-tics I had used at the state hospital. "Remember you're a guest," he told me before we walked into the conference.

Dr. Albee was a pipe-smoking old lady. He felt protected by the confounding intricacies of the very system he said he hoped some day to reform. No matter how much anybody, including myself, pushed him to move, he'd find a procedure to cut through first. Sometimes he stalled to reassert his control or to demonstrate his power. At other times he wanted to slow a person down not neces-sarily because he was wrong but because he *might* be wrong. It was fine for him to take forever with a decision. He wasn't the pa-

tient sitting behind bars picking little green worms out of his breakfast cereal and sleeping on a mattress in a bare room with leaky
pipes that dripped on him at night.

The staff room was crowded. The hospital staff was interviewing
Mr. Dunphy, with Mr. Albert Carrol in the wings. Mr. Dunphy
was sent to Brookfield because he had become disoriented and was
crying when he was arrested. Mr. Dunphy was accused of breaking
and entering.

"Now let me get this straight, Mr. Dunphy," said Mr. Shea, a lean,
white-haired parole officer who'd been a former detective. "On the
night in question you were drinking."

"Yes, sir," said Dunphy, a huge, sad-looking man.

"What?" shouted Shea, apparently startling Dunphy.

"Yes, sir!" said Dunphy, shifting his position in his chair.

"You broke into the store," Shea said.

"No, sir!" said Dunphy.

"Are you trying to tell me that all these people are liars?" Mr.
Shea held up copies of the written reports of witnesses.

"No, sir."

"Then are they telling the truth?"

"Well, it's complicated."

"Yes or no, is all that I want to hear from you," Shea said.

"I can't answer that."

"Well, you'd better."

"My lawyer said I shouldn't."

"He did, did he?" said Mr. Shea. "Your lawyer doesn't decide
anything for us. That's all I have to say."

What a prick!

"Anyone else want to ask any questions?" asked Dr. Cortina, the
medical director running the show, angular, slow, deliberate, almost
alive.

"I have a few," said Dr. Bleak, the psychologist. His interviewing
technique was a burlesque. "You were thought to be emotionally
disturbed at the time of the crime," he began. "What was wrong?"

"I was fired from my job," said Dunphy.

"Why?" asked Bleak.

"I was on the booze."

"Why?"

"I don't know why."

"How come you don't know why?"

"I don't understand."

"How come you don't understand?"

Dunphy shrugged.

"Why were you so upset in my office?"

"Who wouldn't be?" shouted Dunphy, causing Bleak to sit farther away in his chair. "With people accusing me of breaking into a store I didn't break into. I don't want to serve two to five for something I didn't do. That's a stupid question."

"That's enough," interrupted Cortina. Cortina got tired easily.

Dunphy left with two officers. Dr. Bleak offered his considered opinion. "I think the patient is suffering from a borderline or schizo-affective process and that he uses alcohol to manage his anxiety and mask his depression. There are features reminiscent of a fugue state in the repressive and regressive quality of his memory lapses. I think he will be a difficult one in court and potentially dangerous."

"I think he'll be a mess in court," said Dr. Lear definitively. Lear was one to talk. Lear was a chronic alcoholic himself! His mind wandered and he often forgot the question he was about to ask. Lear used to sneak around stealing Thorazine samples from the other doctors' desks. He took almost a thousand milligrams of Thorazine a day. He was usually sweating, flushed, and eating sweets, and weighed almost three hundred pounds.

"I think he'll be uncooperative," said Shea, the parole officer. "He wouldn't cooperate with me in here." Neither, I thought, would any-one with half a brain. After all, the Fifth Amendment of the Con-stitution guaranteed people the right not to testify against themselves. It's an interesting document, Mr. Shea, you ought to read it sometime.

"What do you think, Dr. Albee?" asked Cortina, barely holding up his head.

"Well," began Leopold Albee, forensic psychiatric expert, pulling out his pipe and beginning the reamer-and-tamper pipe routine, "this young man obviously has some severe problems in controls."

The psychologist Dr. Bleak nodded, "Yes, yes!" I guessed I must have missed something.

"The impulsiveness of his actions, the denial," continued Dr. Albee. "It could be a problem in court."

There was a long silence. "Probably not competent?" said Cortina, half-asking, half-stating.

"But," I blurted out, "Dunphy knew he was accused of breaking and entering and could get up to five years for it, and Mr. Dunphy did seem to be following his lawyer's advice. Is that cooperating in his own defense? He doesn't have to convict himself to be competent, does he?"

Leopold Albee turned and gave me a look while the others stared at me. So I'm a loudmouth. So execute me or something. The room was silent. Albee's pipe was out. He lit it again and said slowly, "Perhaps he *is* ready to go back to court, but that is not our decision. It is Dr. Cortina's. . . . Remember you're a guest here," Albee whispered, "it's their prerogative."

"Well," said Cortina, feeling compelled to take a stand, "I think we'd be safer keeping him here and getting another look at him in a month. The impulsiveness and the denial and the question of schizophrenia which Dr. Bleak brought up have to be considered."

"Albert Carrol is next," Cortina sighed.

Albert Carrol was a man in his forties. A shy, quiet man, beginning to gray at the temples. He was polite and obsequious and obviously well liked—he didn't make trouble. He was the sole survivor of his army unit at Anzio and was found in a pile of his friends' corpses. He went wild and was brought home in irons. After two years in a veterans hospital he came to live with a sister. While he was babysitting for his sister, his nephew choked on some food and suffocated. Carrol's old guilt of surviving at Anzio returned and he pleaded guilty to a murder he never committed. Because he was so disorganized, Carrol was sent to Brookfield over two decades ago, longer than any sentence he could have been given had he been tried and found guilty. But Carrol never went to trial. For one reason or another it always seemed to fall through.

"How are you, Albert?" asked Cortina, much more relaxed. Cortina obviously knew Carrol. Everyone did.

"Good," said Carrol.

"Everything going well?"

"Yes," Carrol replied. "Hi, Dr. Albee."

Dr. Albee nodded. Carrol was Albee's patient, his one case here just to stay in touch.

"Any questions?" Cortina looked around. Everyone just smiled. "We're processing papers right now, hoping to get you back to court one of these days soon now." Albert nodded and smiled. You could tell he didn't believe Cortina. Albert left. In a while, so did we.

Besides Carrol there were five others on the rehabilitation ward. David Czernowicz was a butcher who thought he owned the world, invented tomato juice, talked to God, and had the power to wish anything in or out of existence at will. He was caught stealing women's underwear from a fashionable woman's boutique and resisted arrest with a toy gun.

Chester Allen was accused of knifing a man, claimed it was self-defense but became deluded during his hearing and thought the judge was really his brother. He didn't, as you might suspect, give a good account of himself.

Sonny Corena walked into a bank to make a deposit, suddenly panicked and yelled, "Stick 'em up." He reported that he had always been bothered by an urge to yell out at concerts or in church. When he was in the bank he just couldn't stand the pressure he felt and shouted. A guard fired a shot. Another guard thought it was Sonny shooting and captured him. He was unarmed. The fifty dollars he brought to deposit mysteriously disappeared.

Leslie Smith was a trustee who was accused of running his boss down with a tractor, killing him. His mind kept going blank in court.

My routine was uncomplicated, if somewhat dreary. I would meet with the men and discuss their cases to help them understand the realities involved, and I evaluated other patients. After a few months I managed to get Corena and Allen back to court. There were always new admissions. Some went right back, some stayed on, but Albert Carrol remained most difficult to move.

Carrol was Albee's patient in name only. I was the one who talked with him and handled details. Each month I would send another letter to the district attorney in the county where Albert lived. Each month I got no reply. Finally, I called the district attorney on the phone.

"Look," said the D.A. "I have my hands full. I can't do anything for this guy. I've been telling you people for years. He's a two-time murderer. We can't let a guy like that go out on the street."

"Two-time murderer?" I said. "He's accused only of murdering his nephew and nobody believes he did that."

"What about this wife he killed?" asked the D.A. "I have correspondence which indicates he also murdered his wife. Several years' worth in fact."

"But he never was married," I said, totally confused.

You may not believe this because it is so bizarre. I went over every piece of correspondence and discovered that Gordon Young, Mr. Carrol's social worker, had invented a story. Apparently Mr.

Young had been having terrible fights with his wife almost daily for years. Young was usually upset when he came to work.

"Sometimes Young was manic, sometimes he was depressed, but he was *always* crazy," Bleak told me.

His own sense of reality was foggy and sometimes he didn't know where he left off and a patient began. Young had invented a wife for Albert Carrol years ago, after an especially wild argument with his own wife, and had written into the Carrol record a detailed history of her murder. Young eventually forgot about the entry, but each time Carrol's case was brought up, so was the record of the murder. Somehow it was not picked up at Brookfield. I found the original note and showed it to Gordon Young. "Your note is the first mention of this murder. Where did you get that information?"

"What are you trying to prove?"

"I just want to know if Carrol was ever married?"

"Well, go find out. He's a *murderer*. You want to let murderers out on the street. You don't care who you hurt, do you?" The man is nuts!

Cortina overheard us talking. The idea of such an injustice made Cortina anxious for his job and he slowed down my correspondence to the D.A. In fact, he held my letters for two months. Albee also wanted me to slow down, to avoid the chance of embarrassing anyone at Brookfield. Young did quit. Albert Carrol waited. More about him later. . . .

We'd had one prisoner who'd been a schoolteacher before he killed his fiancée. He wrote quite well and together we put together a thirty-six-page orientation manual for new patients that listed the rules of the hospital, some hints from insiders on how to manage and how to adjust. There even was a section that explained all about competency, and another that described what would happen to patients during their hospital stay so new patients would know what to expect. I also tried to outline the rights of patient-prisoners and included directions on how to write a sealed letter and how to get a lawyer at state expense.

"You're going to stir up every jailhouse lawyer in this place," Cortina said wearily. "What are you trying to do? You Institute guys are trying to take over."

Some patients did indeed fulfill Cortina's prophecy. One man walked into the staff conference and announced, "I am being accused of second-degree murder. If I'm found guilty I can get twenty years in jail. I know what court is all about and I get along well with my lawyer, and he feels I can and will follow his advice. He thinks I'm competent and I refuse to answer any other questions." That guy knew more about competency than most of the psychiatrists in the state. He was allowed to go to court. Cortina loved me not. . . .

Leslie Smith, the trustee, asked to see me one evening. He had been having severe diarrhea and he felt the medical doctor on call, a Cuban refugee, Dr. Hernando Velez–Agricola, was not helping him. "The medicine he gave me made me worse. And I'm not the only one who's got it. There are several people on the geriatric ward with it."

Diarrhea in a closed institution is always a serious problem. It can rapidly became an epidemic. In a geriatric ward where many patients have heart disease and are taking digitalis it can be life-threatening because potassium is lost in diarrhea and digitalis toxicity may develop. Dr. Agricola did not take stool cultures, did not see the patients individually, but prescribed medication for the entire population afflicted, thirty-two people in all. One man on the geriatric service had died suddenly. He was taking digitalis and had severe diarrhea.

I went over to see Dr. Agricola.

"Oh, yes," he said, "we see this thing all the time. Not unusual. I've been taking care of it."

"How?" I asked.

"I give these." He held up a large bottle of Kaopectate. That might stop the diarrhea if he prescribed enough.

"How much?" I asked.

"One tablespoon in the mornings." That was so little it was useless. "You know," Agricola continued, "that these can be very constipating. So I make sure that patients don't get constipated."

I was afraid to ask. "What do you do to make sure of that?"

"I give each of them two ounces of mineral oil at night."

I couldn't help myself. I lost my temper. "You stupid asshole, you're going to kill those goddamn patients. You didn't do cultures. You don't know what's going on. You're prescribing medication that could kill them, and I think you already killed one patient. Mineral oil with diarrhea! Afraid of constipating them! I don't care if these patients don't shit for a month. They're weak and trembling. Other patients are contracting whatever they have. You have an epidemic on your hands, and you're too fucking stupid to know it."

"You cannot talk to me like that."

"I can talk to you any way I goddamn please."

"I am a member of the medical profession."

"You're a quack!"

Dr. Agricola complained immediately to Dr. Cortina, who returned to the hospital and asked me to visit. I was prepared to be fired on the spot. Dr. Cortina went over some of the charts and the order book. "Kaopectate and mineral oil," he said. He read another patient's orders, "Kaopectate and mineral oil." Cortina looked at me, "When did you find out about this?"

"An hour ago," I said.

"Agricola, go home and get some rest," Cortina said.

Agricola left.

"Well, doctor, you and I have about thirty stool cultures to take. If you still remember how." Cortina did not like me any better. He was just glad I'd caught a problem in time to save his skin. That's how he judged people. Friends help you, enemies screw you. When you're running scared, a simple philosophy works the best.

When I reported the story to Dr. Albee, Albee blew up. "You are going to ruin a relationship that took years to build. I don't care if you were right about the facts, you were still wrong and insulting. Also, you should have let me see the final version of that booklet you published. I knew it was in progress. Maybe you didn't think I had the right to see it? I'm hearing about that from everyone down there." Albee just shook his head. I knew, though, that if I had shown him the booklet he would have suppressed it.

"The superintendent even wrote the cover letter, which I published on the first page." Actually, I wrote the letter and had him sign it. The superintendent wanted to write his own letter but I gave him some crap about the letter I wrote being psychologically supportive and casting him in a fatherly role. Maybe it did, I don't know. I just wanted to keep it under one hundred words and have it sound positive.

While my relationship with Albee deteriorated, it improved with others at the state hospital. One day Linnehan took me aside. "You won't believe this," he began. "Last night there was a fire in the geriatric section. I ordered all of the cell doors unlocked and told the patients to get out of their cells because it was unsafe. This is the truth now. Most of the poor devils couldn't push the doors open because they were so old and weak. Who would have thought it? The officers had to take the men out and even carry some of them.

Now, you tell me, what sense could it possibly make keeping the cell doors closed?"

"Maybe you ought to leave the cell doors open on the geriatric ward."

"I've already ordered it," said Linnehan. The inmates at Brookfield were condemned to live out their lives behind two walls. They could never escape the infirmities of age, the confusion of their disease even when their cell doors were open. Many inmates saw their keepers as friends. They depended upon them for care and sustenance.

Because the laws which governed the insane offender were so vague, and the facilities to treat him so inadequate, many insane offenders were kept years longer than they would have been kept had they returned to court, been found guilty, and served their full sentence. A suspected criminal who was found incompetent to stand trial was held at Brookfield until he was. Unfortunately, that time never came for many of the men. Some were, of course, guilty; but others were innocent. Both received the cruelest of all punishments. They received no treatment.

As the years passed the men gradually forgot the circumstances surrounding their crime, and eventually the crime itself. For some, the criminal act was part of a psychotic process and was blotted out with amnesia. In time, all inmates became less and less able to help defend themselves.

There were few visitors because Brookfield was far away from most big cities and there was minimal public transportation. Inmates had few friends among the other prisoners. They were all loners, each in a world of his own. As the years passed, their wives found new solutions to the problem of their own loneliness and some inmates received letters from the court confirming a divorce they could not remember agreeing to. Some could not remember the person who was divorcing them.

The men found themselves trapped between the pages of an archaic law that neither provided for their needs as human beings nor took into account the real nature of the disease that afflicted them. A crime may call for a brief punishment, but schizophrenia is forever. The law that committed contained no provisions for treatment. The inmates were prisoners in a world where time was the only jury, where death was the only sentence ever pronounced, even for trivial offenses.

The seventeenth century dies hard.

A psychiatrist who has the authority to declare a criminal mentally ill holds the power of life or death over him. I found that many psychiatrists did not realize this and made their pronouncements as if doing so were just another routine step in helping the insane criminal receive care. More than likely they were unknowingly condemning him. Calling a patient mentally ill often removed him from the legal system which guaranteed his rights. Once a patient was found to be mentally ill and was committed, it was very difficult to reinstate those rights. The law says that the patient has a right to appeal, but if his doctors say he is not yet competent to stand trial, he is prevented from doing so. In time, hospitalization can make all patients incompetent to stand trial.

Much of our law regarding the insane criminal is based on the belief that once the patient is committed he will be treated by people who are skilled, who will view him professionally, and will help him return to trial as soon as possible. This is a myth, a fantasy, generated out of the sense of helplessness of the people who wrote the law in the hope that psychiatrists would know what to do with these difficult patients. They often don't. The patient needs protection from the doctors *and* the law.

Many psychiatrists do not know much about psychotic criminals and less about the law invoked to confine them. You would think that those who write the reports to the court must know, and so must the lawyers who represent these patients. Unfortunately, most of the doctors at Brookfield and even many of the patients' lawyers, did not understand the simple requirements that a patient had to meet to be considered competent for trial.

I don't think any government has the right to make laws that limit the freedom of a citizen by restricting his access to treatment or to the legal process. If the state doesn't have the facilities to treat a patient, it doesn't have the right to commit him to a mental hospital. To commit a patient in such circumstances is to violate his humanity and to pronounce a cruel, although not particularly unusual, punishment on him. It's far better for the insane criminal to be found guilty and sent to prison and serve his time than to languish in a counterfeit mental hospital for an eternity, pinning his hopes for returning to society on a doctor who incompletely understands the law, is afraid to let him go to court, and has neither the time nor skill to treat him.

"I can't let this patient go to court," Dr. Cortina once told me.

"If he's released, he'll go out and kill someone. With all the publicity that would bring, I just don't need it."

Dr. Cortina had become the judge and the jury, confessor and hangman.

It seems to me if the law doesn't protect us from the criminals' behavior, we should change the law, not our sense of justice, the way Cortina did. But any law that confines a criminal unusually because he is declared mentally ill is based on the belief that being mentally ill is in some way a crime itself. If that's true, then everyone has reason to fear.

The end of the year was coming for me at Brookfield State Hospital. I had convinced Alvin Cushman to replace me. Bob Linnehan and I had become good friends. He frequently asked my advice and, with a little encouragement, he instituted some reforms against rather stiff opposition. He found a retired florist who was willing to teach the prisoners the trade, and in a brief time the greenhouse became the center for some of the most effective psychotherapy in the entire hospital.

Dr. Albee still thought me difficult to manage and wished he had never accepted me in the program. But he always said he admired my energy and respected my opinion. If you believe he sincerely meant that, I know a good psychiatrist you should see.

Albert Carrol remained. Albee was finally convinced that Gordon Young had been crazy; Cortina was no longer afraid of Albert committing a third "murder"; and the D.A. was willing to have all charges dropped and to let Albert be sent first to a state hospital to help him make an adjustment to living outside the walls and then in a few months go to a Salvation Army home. All we had to do was bring him to court and the judge would let him off.

The day Carrol was to go to court he dressed in a suit and was handcuffed while he waited for the sheriff. Dr. Lear, the obese alcoholic, tried to remember where he'd put the court order that was needed to take Carrol to court. Dr. Lear couldn't remember where he put it. The sheriff returned to court without Carrol. Carrol took it much better than anyone else because for the first time he believed he was finally going to get out after twenty-five years of unjustified imprisonment.

I told Carrol he would have to wait until the next session of the court, which would be immediately after the summer.

"I can do two months standing on my head," Carrol said, smiling broadly. He had a nice smile. He patted my hand as if he was re-assuring me.

He was.

"You know I'll be leaving," I said, "but Dr. Cushman knows your case and will make sure you get to court and out."

Carrol nodded.

I left Brookfield feeling I'd at least been able to do something for the men, maybe not a great deal, but *something*. Probably the most lasting changes would be those Linnehan put in because he was still there to see that they were followed up. Linnehan was *within* the system. I was still outside. I found work with criminals fascinating, but the system seemed too restricting. Marty DiAngelo urged me to apply for a fellowship at the Forensic Medicine Institute, to gain some experience in the court clinics and to attend their seminar program part time for the coming year. I applied and was accepted. They must have decided on a day Dr. Albee was out of town.

I got a call from Alvin Cushman just after he began working at Brookfield.

"I have some bad news for you. Albert Carrol, the fellow you were seeing, had a massive heart attack yesterday and died in the prison yard. I thought you'd want to know. That's a tough one."

CHAPTER TWENTY-FOUR

MAC AND CHARLIE—
ME AND MY KID PATIENT

MY SCHEDULE as a third-year resident also called for spending two afternoons a week in child psychiatry to learn something about diagnosing and treating children. The program contained the usual seminars, treatment, and supervisory hours, but in almost every respect the experience was like starting psychiatry all over again.

I never was much of a pediatrician. As I've said earlier, I hated seeing sick kids and I found trying to diagnose and treat them terribly frustrating. I remember feeling that pediatricians shared a problem with veterinarians because they weren't able to get a history from many of their patients and had to take the parent's/owner's word for the way the patient felt. The only experience I'd had with disturbed children was while I was on a neurology rotation in medical school, when I observed hyperactive children running around like perpetual motion machines, squealing and knocking furniture about. It was all very disorganized. I couldn't relate to it; meaning, I really hated it.

The child psychiatry division of Union Hospital was very well-organized but everything seemed to move at half speed. Each resident received the chart of the kid he was to evaluate. Standard procedure was: First, I was to meet with my social worker, Geraldine Millis, to discuss the meeting she'd had with the kid's parents. Then I was to make an appointment with the parents. Next, Geraldine and I were to meet with one of the supervisors, a child analyst, Dr. Kibbe, to discuss how I should approach the kid. Finally I would see the kid three or four times while the social worker met with the parents again. After each meeting Geraldine, Kibbe, and I would discuss our progress and try to decide what was going on. An evaluation took about two months and obviously involved the entire family. The way I figured it, they didn't want us adult psych residents making mistakes, so we went slow! *Very* slow.

When a kid was in trouble, chances were the family was also in trouble. Very often the family's diagnostic workup alone was enough to straighten out many problems. Treatment sometimes went no further. Much effort was made to help the parents understand their child and their fears about him. I saw many children in evaluation only because their parents were concerned about something unsavory in their own past, something they'd hidden which was now coming out in the behavior of their child: like stealing, lying, cheating, or acting in an unmanageable way. Sound familiar? Parents sometimes saw their own forbidden wishes in their kids. They feared a display of traits they couldn't admit in themselves.

I evaluated an eleven-year-old black kid, Duke Evans, who was having a difficult time in school, low grades, erratic behavior, and he did not get along with his peers. Duke also had trouble with his parents, who frequently put him "on punishment," making him come home right after school and stay in his room. It was like a sentence and sometimes lasted weeks. Duke's parents really believed in punishment. The trouble was that Duke never remembered what he did wrong. He was on punishment so much that he often forgot the crime entirely.

Duke was a neat kid. He was a lot smaller than I imagined he would be, judging from all the hell-raising his parents said he did. He was perhaps ten pounds underweight and not even five feet tall. You want to see great child psychiatric technique? Our first meeting:

"Hi, Duke, I'm Doctor Viscott."

"Hi." *(Duke is looking down at his shoes.)*

"How are you today?"

"OK" *(still looking at his shoes).*

"Did your folks tell you anything about coming down to the clinic?"

"Uh, uh."

"Do you know what kind of a place this is?"

"Hospital" *(looking at my shoes).*

"Do you know what part of the hospital you're in?" *(a stupid question).*

"Clinic!" (*Duke looking at his shoes again*).

"Do you have any idea why you're here?"

"No" (*looking at my desk*).

"Well, I understand you've been having some problems at home and school, and I'd like to help you."

"Who told you I had problems? I don't have no problems."

"Oh!" (*Look, kid, I just want to talk with you. Don't blow up at me. Okay?*)

"How long am I gonna have to come here?" (*meaning, this stinks*).

"I don't know." I didn't.

Duke was staring around the office. "What are all those toys for?" The offices were all loaded with children's toys. Dr. Kibbe hadn't said very much about the toys, but I figured that playing with toys was one way to relate to a kid.

"To play with," I said. What incredible deductive reasoning!

"You got any checkers?" said Duke, getting up and walking around. That kid didn't like me. I know when a kid likes me, and that kid didn't like me.

"Somewhere, I guess." What the hell, I couldn't get a complete history from this kid if I tried. I'd just tell Dr. Kibbe that the kid was uncooperative and didn't want to talk. Why bother struggling? I'll just play checkers with him. No one will know. There was time for only one game. I played to lose, naturally. I knew *that* much (I'd forgotten the lesson of an earlier Ping-Pong match). Duke looked very intently at me during the game. Duke obviously had played before. He just kept whipping my men off the board.

"You sure you've played this before?" he asked.

(*Fresh little bastard. You're talking to a psychiatrist you just frustrated trying to get a history from you. Be polite, at least, if you won't talk.*) "Yes, I've played before."

"Well, you sure play lousy." (*Oh, yeh, kid? We'll see.*) I started to play for blood, but what were my four men against his eight kings? I was slaughtered. "You weren't moving them too bad at the end," Duke said patronizingly.

"Well, I don't get much practice," I said sheepishly.

"You gotta play a lot," said Duke, looking sure of himself.

"You play a lot?" I asked. I wasn't really thinking about therapy at the time.

"Yes, with my father," said Duke. He was looking down at his feet again. Aha!

"He any good?" I asked, and thought, was that the right question? . . . the kid just looked miserable when he told me about his father.

"Yeh," Duke said dejectedly. "I never beat him."

"Why not?"

"I dunno."

A brilliant diagnostic hour, doctor! Wait till Dr. Kibbe hears about it. "Duke was obviously afraid of beating his father at checkers," I said to Dr. Kibbe. "That's about all I got out of that meeting with him."

I sat patiently, waiting for Dr. Kibbe to jump on me. Actually, I really didn't think he would. No one in this department ever seemed to raise their voice, nice, understanding people. Dr. Kibbe was not yet forty. He was a very sweet guy, affable and kind. He didn't say anything particularly special. He just seemed to approve very much of everything you did and smiled when you did it. Maybe that's characteristic of child psychiatrists. Anyhow I liked him. I felt very comfortable with him. I felt absolutely no sense of competition with him. But I just knew he'd nail me for not getting any facts out of the kid. And if he asks me why not, what do I tell him? That we were playing checkers! Try that one on Eugene McKee sometime.

"That's a very strong first hour," said Dr. Kibbe.

"Strong?" I said, surprised. Kibbe is soft!

"I think so. You uncovered one of his interests and used it to help him express some of his concerns about his father."

"I did?" I said, starting to believe I planned it this way.

"Yes, it's a good way to deal with him. He'll open up," said Kibbe. "What about the family, Geraldine?"

Geraldine Millis was a round, gentle person. She was one of those girls who always looked as if someone had just painted her cheeks with rouge. She had the rosiest complexion I'd ever seen. She looked like an 1890s ad for a baby's health tonic.

"Mother is a very passive, helpless woman looking for direction," Geraldine began. "I think she'd like to spend more time with Duke but she has four younger children and they keep her pretty busy. She admits she loses her temper fairly easily with him and that sending him to bed or putting him 'on punishment' is the easiest way for her to handle him. She thinks Duke is probably a nice boy but doesn't mind her. By that, she means he balks when she sends him to bed with his eight-year-old brother."

"I'd mind too," I said.

"The father," continued Geraldine, "is only five-foot-two. He's three inches shorter than mother and very self-conscious about it. Father has to be right about everything. I think he resents Duke, for two reasons. Because Duke is much lighter than father, and because he's going to be taller."

"How do you know?" asked Dr. Kibbe.

"Because Duke's real father was over six feet tall," Geraldine said.

"Good luck, kiddo," I said.

"What do you mean?" asked Dr. Kibbe, smiling his smile.

"I can just see Duke's father trying to control him and getting stricter with him as Duke gets bigger, trying to show him who's boss all the time. Boy, that would make any kid feel like cutting up. You know, I'm surprised he doesn't cut up more."

"Exactly," said Dr. Kibbe, as if I'd said something insightful. "Why do you think he's holding back?"

"I guess he really doesn't feel loved enough to risk letting out his anger at his father and is afraid he'll be even worse off if he does. . . . You know, Dr. Kibbe, this whole case feels very odd."

"Why?" asked Kibbe pleasantly.

"I'm not really clear about it, but talking with Duke I felt as though I could picture him at twenty-five remembering talking to me. I dunno, I'm not sure exactly what I'm saying." What the hell did I know?

Dr. Kibbe smiled. . . .

I kept on making these simple-minded statements all year long. I felt like an idiot doing so. In one seminar in which all of the esoteric details in diagnosing children's disease were being discussed, Dr. Katrina Higgenbottom, a brilliant child analyst, asked us what we thought was the most significant concept to remember in the diagnosis and treatment of children.

Bert, who was really into child psych and spending extra hours over in the clinic, gave a beautiful statement. I couldn't get over how well organized and thought out it was. D.J. quoted several people in the literature. Stanley talked about the psychodynamics of the treatment situation. I felt really out of place. Dr. Higgenbottom turned to me.

"Well," I began, "I'm not sure. I have three kids at home, a one-year-old, a four-year-old and a six-year-old. Oral, anal, and Oedipal." At least I got a big laugh instead of a smile with that one. "And none of the kids are complete persons yet. They lack a lot of stuff"—How do you like that for a scientific word?—"that they haven't acquired yet, developmentally, I mean. I think the main point I'd make is that

children aren't little adults, they're incomplete personalities. And, and
. . ." I ran out of words.

Big silence. Dr. Higgenbottom looked at me very thoughtfully, and
said, "Nicely put. I think that's pretty close to the basic point of this
seminar and the basic philosophy of treating children. If this isn't
understood, then all of the other ideas can't be effectively applied."

I wasn't sure if Higgenbottom was putting me on. This is so obvious. I mean, it's common sense. How many times did I hear my
grandfather say, "Leave him alone, he's only a child," when I did
something stupid. It's common sense, isn't it? Apparently it was more
than common sense, but I really didn't understand it.

Duke was giving me checker lessons. He was terrific. Some hours
all Duke and I did was play checkers. He'd walk in and I'd say "Hi"
and he'd say "Hi." He'd correct my mistakes. He had all these varia-
tions. You could jump backward and forward if you wanted. And
you could have "flying kings." That means a king could move as if it
were a bishop in chess. I was getting better. One day after really
trying my hardest to beat Duke, I still lost, and badly. I pounded the
desk once with my fist and said, "Shit!" I really had tried very hard
to beat him. Let's face it, I was out of my league.

Duke looked at me very sympathetically and in the next game
started to make stupid mistakes. Now what should I do? Should I beat
him and let him hand it to me? It might make him feel good. Maybe
I should have, but I couldn't. "Look, Duke," I said. "Maybe I'm not as
good as the people you usually play but, man, I've still got a sense
of pride and no one is going to hand me a game out of charity. If I
beat you, Duke, it's going to be because I really beat you."

Duke looked at me. "I know just how you feel. Sometimes I want
to beat my father and I can't. Except he don't ever throw no game. He
just wins 'em all. He's good."

"Look," I said. "I don't believe anyone is so good that he can beat
you consistently. Get off it! If you really wanted to, you could beat
him."

"Maybe," said Duke, "someday . . . I'm just not ready to beat
him yet."

"Do you ever play with anyone else, besides me, I mean?"

"No," said Duke, "just my father."

"Why not?"

"He's got the only checker set in the house. He won't let me use it!"

I got Duke a checker set for Christmas. He really loved it. We
played four games on it. Duke won all four, naturally.

"A delightful present. I'm pleased that therapy is going so well," said Dr. Kibbe.

What's going on in this department? I'm sure you're supposed to do more in therapy than this. I wondered how Dr. Kibbe would feel if I walked into supervision with a checker set and insisted on playing with him instead of being supervised. No, I didn't wonder at all. He'd play with me. I was sure of that. He'd probably even let me beat him. I bet I could beat him, though, fair and square. Duke was a good teacher.

I don't want you to think I was casually giving Duke the short end of the deal. I taught him stuff too. One of my favorite toys was a labyrinth game which consisted of a board with sixty holes in it. The purpose of the game was to tilt the board and guide a steel ball through the maze of holes to the sixtieth and back. I could do that better than any other resident in child psychiatry, including the *real* full-time child psych residents, because I'd had one as a kid. I could go to sixty and back several times. Bert couldn't believe it. Stanley and D.J. both marveled at it. I had a gift, let's face it.

I decided to pass my great talent on to Duke. He lit up when he saw me do it. "Wow, man, you really make that thing move. You gonna let me try that?"

"Go ahead." Duke plopped into the first hole. I got him up to twelve the first day. And that is really moving! The twelfth hole is a toughie, it's a double zigzag. You try it sometime.

Sometimes we played with the labyrinth game, sometimes we played checkers. Sometimes I'd wait till it was ten past the hour when I knew his mother—his father stopped coming—was safe with Geraldine and then we would sneak across the street for ice cream. We'd laugh and talk about his friends. He had a cast of characters that would fill a book. Duke was a hilarious kid. Then we'd sneak back early so no one would know.

"You wanna see my report card?" Duke asked one time when we were at Buzzie's Spa gulping down ice cream.

"Sure." I thought that was unusual for Duke.

It was the end of second term. Duke had one C and four Ds first term, which I already knew about from a report his teacher had sent me. I spoke with his teacher only when she had a problem. She was so busy and under such stress that she was really unable to be helpful. Duke was in a class of forty kids, and in a ghetto school you got to make it on your own. Hey! Duke had five Cs and a B this term.

"Hey, Charlie, that's a big improvement," I said. I felt like Duke was one of my kids. "I'm proud of you, Duke."

"We're gonna ketch it if we don't move," he said, noticing the clock.

We were late getting back to the clinic. Mrs. Evans met us at the top of the stairs. "Where have you two been?" asked Geraldine, bringing up the rear. "We didn't know where you were."

"A walk," I said, out of breath. "It was a nice day for a walk."

"On a drizzly February afternoon?" Geraldine asked, thinking I had gone loony.

"You gonna ketch hell," Duke whispered to me. "She your boss?"

"Why do you think that?" I asked, as I walked him down to the office following behind Geraldine and Mrs. Evans.

"Well, I figure you're with me. She's with my mother. My mother's my boss, so that lady's got to be your boss."

You know, it figured!

Duke was doing great. Any kid who can learn to get that little steel ball to forty in just six sessions has got to be one helluva kid! No two ways about it! I told him so. My checker game was improving. A game of checkers could take us almost a half hour. We *really* went at it.

It happened one afternoon in early March. I made three very good moves in a row. I led Duke into a double jump that he just didn't see and let him lead me into one that I did see and knew that as a result I'd get the first king.

I controlled that board. I was mean! I was tough! I was hanging in there and I wouldn't budge my men unless he forced me to jump, which he did. No doubt about it, I *was* good. But I got careless, and he used his one king to chop my loose men to bits. Duke looked worried.

"I have you worried about your men, Charlie." I called Duke "Charlie" when I was kidding. He called me "Mac."

"You ain't got enough stuff to get *me* worried. I'm gonna take your men like they was puppies."

"Heh, heh, heh," I said, the devil in Gounod's *Faust*.

Duke really began to dig in. The hour was over. We played on. At quarter past the hour I jumped his last king.

I won! I beat him! I triumphed! Me, David the great! I finally beat the little sniveling grimy kid. I won. He lost. In that instant I had asserted my full superiority over him. My Dartmouth Ivy League education; my medical school education; countless years and hours of residency; the advantages of being brought up in a wealthy suburb by college-educated parents yet, of having my own convertible at sixteen, of being almost twenty years older and now, at this instant, so much wiser and more worldly than this eleven-year-old ghetto black!

Duke stood up, all smiles, and threw his arms around me and gave me a hug. "I knew you could do it," he said.

Duke's grades pulled up again to an *A*, two *Bs*, and a *C!* I guessed something really must be going on in therapy. I could even spell it out to Dr. Kibbe. "He seemed to be identifying with me in my struggle to beat him at checkers," I said. "Maybe that's a form of role reversal. In some way he becomes his father and I become him."

"I wouldn't be surprised if he feels strong enough to beat his father," said Dr. Kibbe. "Wouldn't that be a breakthrough?"

Maybe I should go into child psychiatry? Bert decided to take another two years of specialty training after this year in child psychiatry. I thought about it seriously. It would be fun, but I could just imagine myself lying back on my deathbed staring at the ceiling watching everything go dim. I would recount my past life and the work I had done and I would see the record unfold in front of me. "*Checkers:* won, 6,344 games; lost 1,866; ties, 275. *Parcheesi:* won, 540; lost, 5,000. (I'm a terrible Parcheesi player.) *Dominoes* (Another game Duke introduced me to. He beat me continuously. I'm a zero talent Domino man.): won, 2; lost, 5,200. *Labyrinth:* let the record show that Dr. Viscott once cured an entire class of autistic preschoolers by letting them watch him roll the ball from one to sixty and back twenty-three consecutive times, a new intradisciplinary record!" I supposed it would be eclipsed some day by the Russians or East Germans, who were coming up fast.

It was fascinating, but although I dearly love kids, I liked words too much to go into child psychiatry. Who's kidding who? I really don't think I ever grew up. I would feel too guilty kissing my wife good-bye in the morning and going in to work and playing games most of the day. I could hear Judy ask, "Did you have a good day, honey?" when I came home.

"Naw, it was a rough one. I couldn't get the ball past twenty-three, and I lost three games of Fish in a row."

Duke was making remarkable progress in school. According to Dr. Kibbe he also made excellent progress in therapy. He had finally beaten his father in a game of checkers, and, to his surprise, he didn't worry about it afterward. He seemed to have a great deal of confidence.

"You should be discussing termination with Duke now," Dr. Kibbe said. That struck me in a funny way. Such a formal descriptive term for such an informal nondescript process. With kids I was rarely sure of what I was doing. Instead of "working through" problems we had been "playing through."

"How do you terminate play therapy?" I asked.

"You tell him that you'll be ending," said Dr. Kibbe, smiling. The logic of this discipline sometimes left me breathless.

Duke was very sad when I announced I was leaving in May. As the days grew longer and the time left grew shorter, Duke grew sadder. He was managing though. He was doing well in everything and he liked doing well. His father, in a moment of rare warmth, actually bought him a bicycle and rearranged the bedroom so he would be sharing a room with only one brother the next year.

The therapeutic process in child psychiatry was finally a little clearer to me. My job was to help the kid feel better about himself. The social worker's job was to help the parents accept the changes that took place in the kid and to understand their own feelings that might have interfered before. As for insights that Duke might have gotten, I would have a difficult time putting them into words. He just learned to feel better about himself.

Actually that's not bad. Not bad at all.

CHAPTER TWENTY-FIVE

TWO PATIENTS—END GAME

THE winter had come and gone and the spring seemed to slip by me unnoticed this year. Perhaps it was all the work in the OPD—including my good times with Duke in my child psychiatry hours—perhaps I was so interested in what I was doing that I forgot to look outside and just didn't see the gray turn green. This spring was not only a season of new beginnings but one of endings. In just a few months I would be completing my residency and would be saying good-bye to this place. That seemed difficult to believe. I had grown fond of the hospital and the OPD. I saw them as warm and comfortable, even though to a passing stranger the buildings probably looked dirty, old, and forbidding. Hospitals often seem forbidding. But feelings are in the heart of the beholder, and to me the place was home, it was somewhere I was simply accepted, where I fitted in. I could remember few times in my life when I'd felt as content, as useful, or as appreciated as I had these past three years. I was not the only one who felt sad about leaving.

Roberta Goldman was in the OPD waiting room. She was twenty minutes early and looked uncomfortable, restless. There was no sense making her wait since I had free time.

We walked down the hall toward my office. What could have happened to upset her? Her divorce was settled months ago. She had broken up her affair with Roy a few months ago because she decided they were both using each other to escape from their marriages. But the divorce had been an anxious struggle for her. Many times she thought she'd made a mistake and wanted to go back to Gary. When she'd moved out the previous year, he had called several times a day and made her feel guilty and worthless until, finally sure of what she wanted, she put a stop to his calls. Law school, though, had been a breeze for her and she had received an offer with an excellent law firm in town. She had even learned to cope with her mother by being firm and saying no when her mother infringed on her rights. She had also been dating, but at the moment wasn't seeing anyone in particular. Why did Roberta look so terrible?

"I think I'm going crazy," Roberta said, near tears, collapsing in her chair. "Yesterday was the worst day of my life. Everything seemed unreal. Floors seemed to be rising and falling, and the perspective of rooms kept changing. I felt I was losing my mind. I thought I heard special meanings in the things people were saying."

"How do you mean?"

"I overheard one girl mentioning she was breaking up with her boy friend and I just felt it had a special meaning for me, too, in some way."

Roberta was anxious about not seeing me anymore.

"Did you think what she said was directed at you?"

"No. I just felt I could relate to it very strongly. I panicked in my car. I opened the windows and couldn't get enough air. It all got worse as the day went on. I felt like I was going to drift away from reality. I couldn't stand being with people, and yet I wanted someone to help me."

"Why didn't you call me?"

"I did, but the phone was busy and I couldn't wait. I went to the emergency room of Center Hospital. But when I got there I was afraid to tell my story to the doctor because I thought he might think I was crazy and commit me. And then I wouldn't be able to see you. I was so upset. I just ran around looking for someone or something to hold onto. I felt like I was just breaking into pieces."

"When did all this start, Roberta?"

"I'm not sure. I think I woke up with it."

"Did you have a dream that night?" I asked, playing a hunch.

"Oh God, yes, a horrible dream." Roberta had never been especially interested in her dreams and usually claimed she didn't dream or couldn't remember them when she did. "I dreamt I went back to Gary. Oh, yes, there was a bizarre religious ceremony! My mother was standing at one end of a synagogue with long branches growing out of her body. Spanish moss was hanging down from the branches like a veil and Gary was standing under them. I was naked and had to crawl down the aisle on my hands and knees begging forgiveness from all the relatives for leaving him. I wanted to turn around and run, but I couldn't. I just went on crawling toward the two of them. Then Gary jumped on top of me and started having sex. It was awful. I had a baby in front of everyone. Gary handed the baby to my mother. That's when I woke up. . . . Please, tell me what's *happening!*"

"I think, Roberta, that you reacted to your dream as if it were real, even though you couldn't remember it. The feelings you had during the day were mostly fear. The feeling in the dream was the fear of being caught again in the trap of your marriage. I think they were both the same fear but you didn't know it."

Roberta suddenly seemed more relaxed. "That feels very true," she said.

"I had a similar thing happen to me once," I said. "I had a dream I couldn't remember. I had a horrible day. The way I felt was the way I would have felt if the events in my dream had actually happened."

"You had the same thing happen to you and you didn't crack up?"

"And neither did you. The feelings you had were real, but the event that caused them, your dream, was only a dream."

"It's really strange," said Roberta, "the things that happened in the dream were like losing everything I've worked so hard for in here. I mean my independence, my ability to stand on my own two feet."

"Sometimes," I said, "a dream reveals a part of yourself that you find very hard to face."

"You mean, I want to go back to Gary and be dependent on my mother again?" Roberta was shaking her head. "*Not a chance.*"

"Maybe it's only a very small part of you that wants that, Roberta, but it is possible that you might still have some doubts about being on your own, even if they're small doubts."

Roberta was very quiet thinking about that. She looked as if she was going to say something, but stayed quiet.

Finally she said, "I guess I'm still afraid of being alone, and I guess I'm afraid of being better. If I'm better, it means I don't have you anymore and I'm *really* on my own. I know I can make it but I guess there always are some doubts. . . . God, you don't know how much better I feel all of a sudden. I was so afraid in that hospital waiting room last night. I was so sure I was going to be locked up. There were several patients sitting there. I just knew I was the worst of them."

I could well imagine some resident hospitalizing Roberta. Sometimes when psychiatrists hospitalize a patient, they really hospitalize the part of *themselves* that they see in the patient, the part they secretly fear and want to keep down.

It suddenly struck me how so many of my patients, like Roberta, spent their lives reacting to a feeling from a forgotten event, a feeling whose source was obscure but would be felt whether they wanted to feel it or not. And unless they found out where the disconnected feeling came from and measured it, it would make them distort the world around and inside themselves and they would begin to lose their sense of what was real. . . . I was in a reverie, trying to figure all of this out. . . . If a nonswimmer fell overboard into water he believed was over his head he'd panic whether it really was or not. If he stood in the same place but knew it was a safe depth for him he wouldn't. He'd know fear in both instances, but in one it would be terror and the other a little anxiety. The intensity of his fear would depend more on his perception of reality than reality itself. So Roberta felt terrified when she woke up because she knew she'd experienced something horrible but couldn't rmember what it was or whether it was real or not. Just like the man who thinks he's over his head believes he's going to drown, Roberta expected the worst and she lost control of her feelings until she remembered they were based on a dream, until she remembered that the water was shallow all along. Roberta had remembered what she was really afraid of—her fear of being alone.

I pulled my thoughts together. "In a way, Roberta, you were like a person swimming in shallow water without knowing it's shallow who suddenly is afraid she's about to drown. You were struggling without even trying to touch bottom."

"You know, you're really right," Roberta said, realizing something very important for the first time. "I've been pretty safe all the time. I've always thought I needed another person to make me be myself. No one can do that. I have to do it all by myself. Maybe the truth is that I've always been myself but I've been afraid to test it out. At least now I don't need to spend my life always being afraid I'm going to lose someone—for whatever it's worth I know I can't ever lose myself."

"The water has always been shallow," I said. "You were just too afraid to look."

"I guess," she said, "I should talk about saying good-bye and all that business about terminating next week. I thought I was going to be a patient of yours for another year."

"I think you were talking about termination today," I said.

"You know," Roberta said, "as alone as I sometimes feel living by myself, I never get as lonely as I was when I lived with Gary. I just don't have that nagging emptiness anymore. I could never go back. I've been looking back at the past few years. I've really done all right for myself! I've never been that bad, I don't know why I couldn't see that before. I just couldn't accept myself. I wanted to be something different."

"That's because you didn't know yourself."

"I'm really going to miss you, Dr. Viscott."

"I'll miss you, too, Roberta."

Donald Johnson had also changed remarkably over the past year and a half. Apparently his guilt over his cousin Rennie's death was the cause of many of his other difficulties. Before, he needed to be in total control, to be neat and tidy, to appear like a good boy, not like someone who would hurt another person. His car stealing and wild midnight drives were his call for help—he wanted the police to capture him and help him control the feelings that he couldn't handle and that frightened him.

That all seemed like a long time ago. Donald Johnson was finishing his sophomore year in college and doing beautifully. He was active in campus politics and part of his generation. He had let his hair grow, once even had a beard. He also now had friends and a new steady girl, Dottie.

"Better late than never," said Donald, bursting into my office and throwing his army jacket on the floor. "I overslept." He reached forward and turned the clock on my desk around. "Hey, I'm sorry, I didn't know it was that late. I didn't even have a chance to shower or eat."

"It's eleven thirty," I said. "How late do you usually sleep in the morning?"

"I dunno." Donald picked up his army jacket and went through the pockets looking for something. He pulled out a piece of paper and then, as if changing his mind, he put it back again. The sweet mysteries of life.

"Donald, why do you think you were late?"

"Donald, why do you think you were late?" he taunted. "That is such a psychiatrist question. OK. You want me to tell you what really made me want to stay in bed because you're going to tell me that my not showing up on time had something to do with my feelings about therapy. Well, I really didn't oversleep. So you can't tell me that I didn't want to come here."

"You know you've been upset about ending therapy with me," I said. "We talked about how leaving reminds you of losing Rennie and how painful that feels, even though it's necessary."

"OK, just cool it for a minute. I've got something to show you." Donald reached into his pocket again and pulled out the mysterious piece of paper. He sat back in his chair and held it in his hand. "I got up an hour early this morning just to make *sure* I would get here on time today. I didn't believe your big-deal theory that the reason I've been late recently is because I can't face leaving you and therapy. So I decided to prove to you that you were wrong and also that saying good-bye to you had nothing to do with my feelings about Rennie. I decided to take the turnpike into town because it was faster. I wanted to sit in the waiting room and watch the surprised look on your face when you went into that conference I always see you just coming out of. I had it all planned. I imagined you sitting in there with all the other doctors saying to yourself, 'I really figured him wrong, Donald's here early.' I had it all planned."

"What happened?"

"I'll tell you. Try to be patient, doctor. I got on the turnpike. I don't use the turnpike very much because it's too expensive, so I wasn't very familiar with it. Anyhow, when I started off I was sore at you for insinuating I really didn't want to come and because you were dragging me through all these heavy feelings. Lately when I come here I've been getting angrier and angrier, the closer I get to the clinic, I mean. I run through conversations in my head between you and me. You say, 'How do you feel about leaving?' I say, 'I've told you over and over,' and then we fight just like we do here, except in my head I can always put you down. In my head I also take you to lunch to make up for being such a bastard, but I eat ice cream because I know you're on a diet.

"Anyhow, this morning I was still angry when I started to drive in. After a while I didn't feel so angry, I was thinking about you and Rennie and wondering, maybe there *was* something to your idea that your leaving was like Rennie's death in some way. I wasn't sure. I started to feel pretty good after a while. I decided you weren't such a bad guy and that I was being too tough on you. After all, you really have helped me straighten my head out. OK, I said, Viscott's leaving, going into private practice to do the big money thing. It's his right. And, anyhow, I said to myself, I don't need him anymore. OK, maybe I'm angry at him for leaving, but I can face it. Look at me, I said to myself, I can talk to him about how I feel, I can tell him I'll miss him. My angry feelings are easy to control. Simple. I'm no longer the kid that used to run away from his anger because I was afraid it would make me hurt people. That Viscott has really helped me—that's what I was thinking on the way in." Donald smiled.

"I—something's missing?" I said. "This doesn't sound complete."

"It isn't. Just be quiet and listen, you'll learn something. Remember, I don't believe in this Freudian crap and I'm only telling you this because I really do like you. I'm starting to get very happy in the car. As a matter of fact, I feel like I'm high. I feel terrific. I feel very good about you. I want to be with you and see you. I realize that I do care about you very much. I'm going to tell you everything, I say to myself. Suddenly I hear a siren. I can see a state trooper's car in the rear-view mirror, lights flashing all over the place. I look at the speedometer and I'm doing over ninety. I slow down and look for a place to pull over. As I look around I realize I'm nowhere near the city, if you must know the truth. I'm on the *outbound* lane of the turnpike heading in the opposite direction, toward Albany. I'm almost forty miles from town. The farther away from you I got, the better I felt! The trooper walks over very slowly. I start thinking, maybe I should tell him that somebody in the family died. I haven't felt like saying something like that for a long time. Well, I told him I was late for an appointment and had taken the wrong ramp. He gave me a ticket and told me to slow down. That's what this paper is, twenty bucks! That's not the important part, though."

"What is?"

"I turned around at the next exit and headed back. Do you know what is right off that road? You can practically see it from the highway. The cemetery where Rennie is buried. I never realized it. The last time I was there I also used the turnpike. Jesus! You know, I must have passed that cemetery a dozen times when I was stealing cars and not realized it. Maybe I really wanted to visit Rennie all that time. Christ, I was always drifting west on that road. I was drawn out there like it was a magnet. I guess when I went out there and talked to the stars I wanted to get caught *there* for my crimes."

"I think you're right." I said. "You must have really missed
Rennie but felt too guilty to go to his grave so instead you talked
to Orion, your friend in heaven, almost the same thing as talking
to Rennie. And I think what you did today shows how hard it is for
you to say good-bye to close friends."

"Yes, it really is," Donald said, "but I don't think saying good-bye
to you will be the same as Rennie dying. After Rennie died I felt
empty and frozen. Saying good-bye to you, it isn't easy and I feel
sad about it, but I don't feel I've lost something. I feel I've sort of
gotten back a part of me. Even if that part is something that saddens
me, at least it's real and something I never had before. It's a relief
to let it in and know what the hell it is. . . ."

In becoming a psychotherapist I learned that no two men ever
died for the same country. In a real sense, each of us lives in a
world of his own, and while we may allow other people to enter
and even live in our private world from time to time, a part here,
a corner there, the total reality, the inner world of our feelings, remains
largely inaccessible to others. If we are not islands unto ourselves,
we are at best peninsulas.

In psychotherapy I saw my goal as helping patients to understand *their* own inner worlds better by giving them a new sense of
perspective. I found out that when one's perspective of his world
changes, his world changes with it, because the world *is* one's perspective of it.

How do I know that what I feel and perceive is real? How does
my sense of reality affect what my patients see? No single person
can ever be completely objective. Each of us usually can make out
only a part of the truth, the part that's similar to what we can accept
in ourselves. When the truth we see exceeds our ability to accept,
we often feel pain. Sometimes the only reality my patients were
sure of was their pain, because pain is always real even though it
makes us all distort the truth.

As a patient learned to accept himself more, his world tended
to grow and his pain subsided. I tried to help patients become more
flexible, to make adjustments for the way the world outside seemed
to be, to question whether their perceptions were false and to try
to change them when they found they were.

I believed that if something worked well for a patient, even
though it seemed crazy, I would not tamper with it. I don't think
a psychiatrist should ever tamper with something that works unless

he's absolutely sure he can replace it with something that works better and that the patient also believes works better. The patient has a right to his values.

The insane person believes in the world he perceives without questioning if it is real. He depends mostly on his inner world to support his beliefs. Every insane belief has its origins in some reality, and even the craziest idea was once a response to the outside world more truly perceived. The situation may change in time, but the psychotic will not reexamine the world again. His painful experience has convinced him he was right and he rigidly defends himself against it. His fears in turn make him misperceive the world even more and only admit evidence that supports his original belief. The problem with the psychotic is that having once burned himself with hot water, he believes all water is hot.

I learned to befriend and love the healthy side of my patients, and struggled to help my patients learn to love what was healthy in themselves. I learned that the most important question to ask myself when I wasn't sure of my direction with a patient is: "Will what I am doing help the patient?"

It hardly ever let me down.

Eugene McKee looked very unhappy during our last week in residency. I guessed he really would miss us, even though he never said so. Trixie was especially nice to him all week long. The ten o'clock conferences were getting quieter and sadder. D.J. pointed this out to us and even broke into tears at one point. Bert instinctively handed her a doughnut. Stanley Lovett noticed Bert's gesture and whispered, "Symbolization." You can see we hadn't changed so much.

Dr. McKee asked to see me. I took a long savoring look at his office, knowing that I would probably never see it again. Dr. McKee sat down and handed me a note. It was from Dr. Ryder. It was next year's OPD schedule. It looked pretty much the same as this year's schedule except in place of the nine o'clock conference there was another patient evaluation scheduled for each resident, and the ten o'clock conference had been eliminated altogether!

"That's impossible," I said. "That means that there would be twice as many patients being seen in evaluation as now. We're already filled to capacity. Where will we get the time to treat the patients?" I was still saying "we" as if I would be there next year. Saying good-bye is difficult for everyone. "And that's not even the major point, Gene"—I called Dr. McKee "Gene" for the first time—

"what about your teaching conferences? That's really what the OPD is about."

Dr. McKee nodded. "Well," he said, "it seems Dr. Noyes and the governor of this good state have decided to bring the OPD into the world of community psychiatry."

Dr. McKee didn't think community psychiatry was a bad idea in itself, but in the process of joining the OPD to the larger statewide community mental health program, he would lose the stage he'd been performing on so effectively for so many years teaching residents and social workers. It was an important part of his life.

"I'm really disgusted with this place," I overheard him say later. "I've been thinking of quitting. I've been running this clinic for almost fifteen years and it appears that Noyes doesn't feel I have any rights. You know, I do have a very nice private practice and people are always referring patients to me. I don't need the twenty-five thousand a year this place pays me and I sure as hell don't need the headaches. I'm not going to starve. It might be the best thing that ever happened to me. I've always wanted to go full-time in private practice anyhow."

It was pretty depressing. Here was a fifty-year-old psycho-analyst with all the right credentials and the right background reassuring himself by asserting how good he was just because some figure in authority had knocked him down. He'd quit! Some protest!

Noyes had given Dr. McKee two token teaching hours a week, but it was nothing compared to the twelve and a half hours he now had. The entire atmosphere of the clinic would change. It would become a service-oriented rather than a teaching clinic. You have to have service-oriented clinics to diagnose and treat patients, but you need to staff them with doctors who've learned their skills somewhere, usually in a teaching clinic. The teaching clinic must be a more leisurely and inefficient operation if only because it takes time to find and correct mistakes. If Dr. McKee was going to quit, why did he bother to tell me all of this? I was his chief resident, sure, but I wasn't his confidant or his therapist and, believe me, I wasn't his favorite. Suddenly I knew why. He wanted me to do something about it, to help him.

And I did.

I called a meeting and presented the problem to the staff. I suggested that we all compose a petition to Dr. Noyes, which I eventually wrote. Mary, the clinic secretary, typed it. It was a plea for the preservation of academic freedom, the traditions of the university, not to mention the goodwill of the staff. It had a noble ring to it. To go against it would be antiintellectual, antipsychiatry, antihumanitarian, antimotherhood, as well as against the American flag and the AMA. The petition was also tainted, ever so slightly, with sentimentality, just a touch. In other words, it was a political document.

I presented it to Dr. Noyes that afternoon. I said, "I have a prepared statement to read on behalf of the resident community in the teaching program." I read it.

Noyes said, "Hmm . . . well . . . I see . . . I didn't know you people felt so strongly about this issue."

And do you know what he did? He actually backed down! The OPD would stay exactly the same next year. Dr. McKee would stay on.

It seemed that people in authority—including even psychiatrists—became confused and stymied when they were directly and openly confronted. Few people confront them, though. Dr. McKee, a good man, was going to quit "in protest," which meant he was going to let Noyes have his way. Noyes was ready to step on him as he would a bug. Authorities only notice bugs when they bite.

Of course, I had nothing to lose because I wasn't interested in staying in the academic world. It was precisely these feelings of inhibition, backbiting, and unproductive competition that I wanted to avoid. If you do something that's not in the usual or accepted way, people stare at you and try to put you down. The academic world is filled with frightened people who undermine you because they're afraid of being shown up and being thrown on their own. Most of all they fear somebody who exists independently of their system. They call him difficult, eccentric, and they try to wipe him out in a nice academic way. He's feared because he has no allegiance to maintaining the lies of the system and because he knows the emperor has no clothes on.

There comes a time when you just have to go your own way, and do what you believe is right.

CHAPTER TWENTY-SIX

QUACKS, OR NOBODY'S PERFECT BUT . . .

IT WAS a standing joke in medical school that it didn't matter whether or not a psychiatrist was a quack because psychiatrists did so little it was unlikely that they could do any harm. It wasn't until you were out practicing psychiatry for a while that you really knew how bad psychiatrists could get. You discovered that some didn't follow *any* scientific theory or method. They were out there just hanging on, making up their own philosophy of life and the mind as they went, talking to their patients the way they talked to their kids or to their wives, and charging a fortune for the privilege of listening to their homespun advice.

The only difference between these incompetent psychiatrists and laymen was that the psychiatrists had patients who believed in them and who thought they knew what they were talking about, simply because they were doctors and they had qualifications. That meant they knew what they were doing, didn't it? Of course it did!

Many of the incompetents I have known had a long list of qualifications, often including degrees from fine universities, training experience at good hospitals, and impressive clinical affiliations. Many of these inept psychiatrists were also board-certified. The board-certification examination did not always weed out the inept psychiatrist. It measured something about his understanding of theory, history, and might even test his diagnostic ability, but it told practically nothing about his ability to relate to other people or to treat them and make them whole again. It overlooked many of the most impor-

tant qualities which make a good therapist, such as his interest, his
honesty, his curiosity, his openness, his humanness, and his willingness to help. Most of them were things they didn't teach in school.
You could have all of the qualifications on paper and still be a
quack. Academic qualifications were some psychiatrists' only assets.
Better than nothing? Maybe.

I spent the first week after I left my residency trying to get
Dr. Handleman's practice in Kingswell under control. Marty had
left. Handleman was hanging around for a few days before he left
for the summer to make sure I knew the ropes. It was busy. I had
twenty therapy hours, five evaluations in the office, and three consultations in hospitals scheduled the first week. In addition, I was
also scheduled to continue giving shock treatments to some of Dr.
Handleman's hospitalized patients. I also had my job at the youth
center and eight hours of private therapy in town. I had sublet an
office, part-time. I studied my appointment book during my first
free hour and figured out that if I just followed my schedule I
would net over eleven hundred dollars after all expenses! That was
just my first week! The court clinic job wouldn't start for another
month. Amazing how well doctors get paid.

"If you want you can go down to the hospital and take a look
at one of Dr. Anson's patients in 1018 while you have a break, a
hysteric probably," said Handleman just before lunch. "You don't
have anything scheduled this afternoon. No need to see the patients
you're going to shock tomorrow. I already saw them today. No problems, just press the button when the anesthetist tells you."

I drove toward Kingswell Hospital and noticed a small municipal
zoo on the way. I made a mental note to stop there. I'm a nut for
zoos. The zoo was the best thing about St. Louis. Every time I go to
a new city I go to the zoo.

The first person I met at Kingswell Hospital was Dr. Anson.
He was a tall, robust doctor who looked so much like a doctor he
could have gotten the part of one in a television drama. He had
a manner that even intimidated me. "I'm Dr. Anson." We shook
on that. Anson wasn't interested in social niceties. He was busy.
"This little gal in 1018 I want you to see has been on my service
for about a week. Now we've been pretty tolerant of her problem
and tried to manage it medically, but I think it's time one of *you
boys* came in and laid the law down to her."

The very model of clear, scientific thinking!

"What's she been doing?"

"Well, you know! The kind of action that is annoying to the nurses, a lot of demands, a lot of silly behavior. The girl was supposed to get married soon, but I guess it was too much for her. She got engaged last year but on and off since she's been having these moods. It's clearly emotional. I've tried some Librium but it doesn't touch her."

"How much?" I asked.

"Oh, pushing twenty milligrams a day."

I couldn't tell anything from Anson's comments except that he didn't know a great deal about Librium. "I'll see her and we'll chat," I said. "Chat" was a word I used when I was doing consultations for physicians who knew little about psychiatry. If a psychiatrist speaks clearly and simply to an internist, the internist regards him as a sage simply because what he says makes sense. If you had read as many psychiatrists' notes as I, you'd understand how unusual that often is. If you try to be a smartass and show an internist how much psychiatry you know, he'll turn you right off with "I have a patient to see in 308 now. Thanks for your consult," and he'll never read it.

I discovered that the "little gal in 1018" had a name. It was Libby. Libby also had some other interesting findings. Anson had indicated in the chart that she had episodes of blindness which came and went. Anson thought this was "conversion hysteria!" (exclamation mark, his). Medical students who are uncomfortable with any other psychiatric diagnosis but conversion hysteria grow up to become internists who are uncomfortable with any other diagnosis but conversion hysteria. Libby was reaching for a glass of water on her bedstand when I walked in.

"Hi," I said. "Let me get that for you." I noticed Libby had a tremor in her hand as she stretched. I handed her the glass.

"Oh, yes, I am, ever I am," said this pretty little freckled redhead. The room smelled of urine. "I just love it here so very much," she blurted out, slurring some words. She had a funny smile, resembling at times the odd little smile that some schizophrenic patients have, but Libby's was much softer and seemed more natural even though her mood state was peculiar. She had hazel eyes that jerked rhythmically when she looked to the side. That's called "nystagmus on lateral gaze" where I come from.

Libby got up to go to the bathroom. "I have to go," she said. Her nightgown was soaked. She had apparently lost control.

"Do you lose control like this often?" I asked.

"Just recently. The nurses have been getting angry with me for it." She started to cry and then broke into a big smile, just like that! "Everything's going to be wonderful," she pronounced.

I felt sick. Libby had many of the symptoms of multiple sclerosis. They were pretty obvious; they practically jumped out at you. I borrowed a doctor's bag to do a neurological examination. Libby had areas of sensory diminution which didn't seem confined to the usual distribution of sensory nerves. A multiple sclerosis patient's eye viewed through an ophthalmoscope often has pale optic discs. Libby's optic discs were also pale.

I completed my examination. I was afraid I knew what I needed to know. Suddenly I remembered that Libby was a person. Odd, in the ten-minute period examining her I was so engrossed in her physical signs that I had forgotten. It's so easy to do.

I wrote the briefest note possible in the chart. "The patient shows lateral gaze nystagmus, pallor of optic discs, an intention tremor, staccato speech, sensory losses, questionable related urinary incontinence, and euphoric inappropriate affect. . . . Suggest complete neurological workup for possible MS. Psychiatric problems, if any, can wait for now. Thank you for letting me see this most interesting patient." A well-written medical note by a noninternist would be a put-down, I wasn't into that. I wanted Anson to help Libby, not resent her, for his missing the diagnosis. I guess you have to manage people everywhere.

The next morning I was up at six thirty and driving like Stirling Moss trying to get to Kingswell Hospital early. Handleman told me the earlier I got there, the earlier I would get out. The electroshock room was downstairs in the hospital basement. There were about twenty patients scheduled for EST that morning. There were four other psychiatrists taking their turns shocking their patients. I was last on the list.

"Hi, there," said a familiar-looking doctor. He had once had a patient on Bamberg 5 who was one of D.J.'s patients. Mrs. Bottone, I think. She had been depressed, and he had shocked the woman into oblivion.

"Hi, I'm Dr. Viscott," I said. Nice company I'm keeping, I thought.

"Dr. Lauria," said Dr. Lauria, a thin, pale-faced man. He was wearing a light blue seersucker suit. "You taking over for Max Handleman?" he asked.

"Yes."

"Good for Dr. Max," said Lauria. "That's the life, isn't it, Sy?

Max gets this young blood in for the summer and goes off to New Hampshire for two months."

"Not to mention a six-week vacation in the winter," said Sy Talcott. "So you're the new boy in town."

"How old are you, kid?" asked a balding, fiftyish man. "Doesn't look dry behind the ears yet. I'm Bill Groper."

Nice bunch of regular guys, could be anyone. "You're up," said Lauria to Sy.

Sy walked over to a patient on a litter who had just been put to sleep by the anesthesiologist. Sy pressed the button on the shock machine and walked away, not waiting to observe his patient grimace with the electrical current.

"Did you have Litton Industries?" asked Lauria.

"I had it and sold it at the wrong time. Who gave you that tip?" asked Groper. "One of your patients?" Groper said this loud enough so that any of a dozen patients still waiting could have heard it. The others didn't notice.

"I made fifteen points on it," Lauria said.

"Who tells you when to get in and out?" asked Sy Talcott.

"My brother-in-law's an electrical engineer. He has all the inside information. You can't make money in the stock market unless you have inside information," said Lauria, walking over to one of his patients who had just been put to sleep. "I had a great tip on Burroughs." Lauria hit the button. "It was a fantastic ride." Lauria's patient grimaced with the shock. Not a routine ride either! "Keep the electrodes on her. Yes, again," Lauria called to the aide. "I want to give her a second shock. It helps them out faster." Lauria directed that last comment to me. He was being a teacher. "I made almost twenty-two percent on Burroughs—OK, hold her." Lauria hit the button again. The patient grimaced again, but there was no indication of a seizure. "Put them on again." Lauria hit the button once again. This time the patient jerked considerably because the muscle relaxant was wearing off. Lauria had just earned another thirty-five dollars on that one (a bargain, he might contend—and with justification—if you tote up the years of schooling, experience, and qualification behind that finger on the button). . . . "I got that from my brother-in-law also. You play the market, Dr. Viscott?"

"I used to," I said, "but I found it took too much time. To do it right you have to do it full-time." Doctors are notorious for losing money in the stock market. They have a great deal of ready cash.

Doctors think that because they're able to get through med school they are very bright about everything and take no one's advice. They act on their own "clinical experience" in the market, which is even less valuable than their clinical experience in the profession sometimes is. That is, it is biased and based on too small a number of cases. Naturally, they lose their shirts in the long run. They also lie to each other about it—not really lie, exaggerate like crazy.

"Where did you train?" asked Lauria.

"Union and the state hospital," I said.

"Oho, with all the analysts," said Groper, nodding his head knowingly.

Lauria hit the button. Another patient grimaced with the electric current.

"Sorry about that," I said.

I walked over to a desk and got the chart that had come down with my patient. I could overhear Groper shouting, "That's not right, Lauria, you've taken three in a row. You've got to let us get through." What a loud voice!

Mrs. Bellmon was in her sixties. Since her husband died she'd been depressed, according to her chart. Handleman wrote a fairly concise note, but he didn't vary his reports much from one patient to another. They all sounded the same. There was a social service note which indicated that Mrs. Bellmon's daughter felt her mother was confused for a year *before* her father died and had slowly been getting worse. Mrs. Bellmon had a very high blood pressure, 210 systolic over 100 diastolic. That pointed to severe arteriosclerosis. I just wondered. Her symptoms could be better explained by a diagnosis of arteriosclerotic brain disease than by depression. I looked at Handleman's progress notes. She was getting no better on shock treatments. She'd had eight to date. She was on no medication at all. I was about to decide to send her back to her room with the aide without shocking her when the anesthesiologist called me over. She was ready. I pressed the button and shocked Mrs. Bellmon. I felt very ambivalent, but figured Max knew what he was doing. If when I saw her later I was still convinced of the diagnosis of arteriosclerotic brain disease I could start her on tranquilizers and discontinue the shock treatments. Or should I have waited? . . .

I also gave shock to Mrs. Maxwell. She had been having recurrent psychotic depressions for years and usually got better with shock. I must have given a dozen treatments to her that summer, but she did not get better at all. I was surprised because her symptoms reminded me of Mrs. Gold, who had gotten better in the state hospital during my second year of residency. . . .

Groper had finished with his patients and left. It was quieter at least. Lauria was still shocking away. I could hear the cash register ringing at the Blue Cross computer terminal. Finding that the patient has insurance seemed like the most common indication for giving electroshock; the second is depression.

I soon learned that most medical insurance plans were generous in paying for EST treatments and rather stingy in paying for psychotherapy. Unless you have a very expensive insurance plan, the chances are you will have to pay for most of your visits to a psychotherapist, but even the most basic insurance plans generally pay for EST and often for outpatient EST as well. This never made much sense to me. Certainly the most common psychological problems are not the ones for which the treatment of choice is shock therapy. In making their payment policies for psychiatric treatment, the insurance companies are influenced by the psychiatrists they consult, and many of these psychiatrists tend to be the sort who used EST considerably. Many of my colleagues believed that if EST were not covered in insurance, its use would greatly diminish.

Not only did insurance pay $35 for each EST treatment, it also paid $15 for each hospital visit the psychiatrist made to the patient on the days between treatments. These visits rarely took more than a few minutes. Dr. Lauria, bragging about how well organized his schedule was, told me, "The secret is to make a timetable and stick to it. Don't waste time talking with the patients if you don't have to. I see the patients the day after EST just to say hello and ask them how they are feeling. You can't talk about anything with them anyhow because they're so confused. Just put in an appearance and write a note in the chart."

One of Dr. Lauria's typical progress notes read: "Mrs. X is still confused—a little brighter today. Treatment #10 tomorrow." To visit his eight patients hospitalized for EST and write eight such notes would take Lauria less than forty-five minutes, providing he didn't get involved in a conversation with another doctor or a patient's relative. In forty-five minutes Lauria could make eight times fifteen—$120.

If Lauria's progress note was brief and uninformative you would think it would be justified by the incisive psychiatric history that a psychiatrist with his breadth and reputation surely must have written on the occasion of the patient's admission to the hospital. You would think that, and you would be wrong. Lauria's usual admission note:

> Mary X is a 35-year-old mother of two. She has been chronically depressed for the past three years. There is a bad family situation. She has no insight into her problems. Her husband is uncooperative. Physical exam reveals no contraindication to EST. Admit to semiprivate.

The note did not indicate basic information such as what had happened three years ago when Mrs. X became depressed or what her family situation was really like or why her husband was uncooperative. Someone who didn't know any better might think that the doctor hadn't asked or didn't know enough to ask. The solutions to Mrs. X's problems come from answers to these and similar questions.

I read many psychiatric admission notes at Kingswell and at other hospitals over the years where I have seen patients that differed only slightly from Dr. Lauria's. Groper's notes were similar, except Groper couldn't spell. Handleman's notes were a little better. Talcott's notes were illegible.

Of course there were other psychiatrists who primarily used shock and other somatic treatments who wrote longer notes with more clearly outlined dynamics, but even these notes often sounded like long-winded rationalizations for using EST. No matter where you started reading they tended to point to the inevitability of giving EST. . . .

During those first months, reading other doctors' charts, I discovered other patients who were being treated with shock therapy who probably shouldn't have received it, and not just at Kingswell. . . .

A Mrs. Forman had looked shaky when I observed her lying on the litter. She was scheduled for her third shock treatment. She also seemed very bright and coherent and not at all depressed. Her admission note indicated that she had been complaining of severe weakness and fatigue for the past several months which did not respond to the usual treatments. Her doctor concluded in his consultation report that this was the way she manifested her depression. There was a discharge note from another hospital where she had been hospitalized in the winter for treatment of a heart problem caused by hypertension. She had been given a potent diuretic, Renese, 4 mg. a day, for the past several months. There wasn't a serum potassium level reported in either chart! Unbelievable!

Renese not only removes excess water from the body, but with it a great deal of potassium which must be replaced. Any patient taking this drug must be closely followed and his serum concentration of potassium frequently determined. With very low levels of potassium, one sees profound muscle weakness, emotional changes, and cardiac arrhythmias. Mrs. Forman probably was suffering from a low serum potassium. I pointed it out to her doctor, who then ordered a stat (which means immediate) serum potassium determination. He stopped the diuretic and started replenishing Mrs. Forman's potassium.

At another hospital I discovered a Mr. Ford who was waiting to be shocked. I scanned the chart. At last a patient who really looked like he needed treatments. Except he had already improved drastically and was supposed to be discharged that day. *His doctor had simply lost count.*

On another occasion I noticed a Mrs. Porter lying on a litter, trembling and awaiting treatment. She looked odd. I took her right hand and as I did her hand closed on mine very suddenly. I removed my hand and her grip tightened as I did. I repeated the procedure by moving my finger and then a key across her palm, and each time her fingers and thumb jerked closed on my finger. She had a positive grasp reflex! (A grasp reflex is a pathological reflex. It is positive when a moving object across the palm causes the patient to grasp the object involuntarily. It usually means that there's disease in the frontal lobe of the patient's brain on the side opposite the one where positive reflex is found.) She also had a very slow pulse, a sign of increased intra-cranial pressure. . . .

When the internist, Dr. Anson, next saw me at Kingswell, he thanked me for my diagnosis of Libby. "Very subtle, very strange how multiple sclerosis masquerades as other diseases. I appreciate your note." At least Anson didn't feel put down!

Subtle? Why, with one foot in a homosexual panic and the other in a psychotic state, Russell Townsend could have made that diagnosis of MS. What the hell was going on. This *is* a hospital. These *are* doctors, well *aren't* they? Didn't these doctors have medical school degrees on their walls? Weren't they board-certified? Why didn't they pick up the problems with their patients? Why didn't Anson pick up the MS?

You may or may not think that it was very clever of me to make these diagnoses. I assure you they are not rarities. They are boringly routine. Tragic, perhaps, but they are still commonplace diseases, and the possibility of their presence should occur to any physician as a matter of course if he does his minimal routine work.

Mrs. Bellmon was suffering from diffuse hardening of the arteries, I finally decided (and hardly to my credit), after giving her more treatments without any appreciable signs of improvement and after reading her chart more closely. She eventually improved on tranquilizers and on medication for her physical problems, and she was able to return home. For my own deficiencies in this case, I can perhaps plead inexperience—but not too loud—but how did these experienced psychiatrists miss these diagnoses? Were they perhaps too interested in eliciting the indications for giving electroshock? I can hear them: "depressed, recent loss, behavior slowed down, EST!" Hike!

Mrs. Forman's low potassium was a straightforward problem. A druggist knowing that she was taking Renese and no potassium supplements would have made the diagnosis. Why? Because there are two pages of warnings in the prescribing literature about the drug, and the first warning is to make sure you watch out for a low serum potassium. In four days of a high potassium diet with supplemental potassium she was markedly improved.

Mrs. Porter was a little more subtle for me to make a diagnosis based on the grasp reflex and the slow heart rate. OK. I'll take a little credit for that! But not that much! After I examined her record I almost flipped. Her pulse rate was consistently below sixty, and that was charted on a graph. Mrs. Porter also complained of severe headaches and mentioned waking up at night to vomit; very suspicious symptoms. I hoped if they transferred her to neurosurgery and opened her skull they would do it on the correct side.

I also saw patients who were given shock to treat depression when they were in fact depressed because they were taking Reserpine, a drug used to reduce high blood pressure and which may cause severe depression as one of its side effects. Patients may even commit suicide while taking the drug, and the depression can last for months after the drug is stopped. But the only proper treatment—perhaps self-evident—is to discontinue the drug, not continue the shocks.

Still other patients received shock for treatment of menopausal depression without receiving hormone replacement and remained depressed after many treatments.

One afternoon I became extremely upset thinking about all of this. I went down to my car and not knowing what else to do I drove to the zoo. At least this zoo wasn't disguised as a hospital. I bought two bags of peanuts, one for the elephant and one for me. I spent an hour feeding the peanuts one by one to the elephant. I like feeding elephants. Their trunks feel like vacuum cleaners. So I have a fetish! Elephants are lovely. They're big and they move with grace. Elephants are charming. . . . I was in a sweat and it had nothing to do with it being hot.

It's not that I don't believe in electroshock. I do, but I think its use is limited. I simply had no idea EST was being abused this much. And, dammit, Marty DiAngelo considered Handleman one of the better doctors in this area. Better than what? . . .

I've always felt quite free to question anyone's authority about anything. Dr. Leo Albee once even suggested that I go into analysis specifically to straighten out that problem. . . . Why was I shaking so? Obviously, I wasn't sure about myself. . . . This *must* be wrong. These doctors just couldn't be that bad. I must have seen them at their very worst. Is this what I wanted to be associated with? . . .

I was upset because I realized how easy it is for any doctor, me included, to fall into the rut that these doctors had. It is so easy. The money is fantastic. Several made over a hundred thousand a year. And practicing out here is low pressure. The doctors all feel secure. They stand behind each other; they back each other up. They have to, they have no choice. To question what another is doing would mean that they would have to question themselves and their own methods, and they certainly didn't want to do that.

Shouldn't I do or say something about what I saw? What do you think, elephant? Stupid elephant! I did not go to medical school to become my colleagues' keeper. To begin with, I just didn't know that much myself. When errors as flagrant as these were committed, pointing them out was a sure way to upset people, not to mention to sound like an impudent upstart. Doctors hate to admit that they are wrong. Often the only time doctors will admit that they are wrong is when a world-famous specialist, whom they have recommended, is called in and spends several hours with the patient, orders several rare diagnostic tests which have to be done in the specialist's hospital at great expense, finally makes a diagnosis so rare that the patient is only the eighth known case, and then compliments the family for choosing such a bright family doctor. The specialist calls the family doctor "bright" only because he knew he was in over his head, but the family doesn't know that.

I could understand why many bright doctors stayed in the academic community and put up with the backbiting. If this first peek at medical practice in the suburbs was any indication, the frustrations to anyone who had an open mind and any diagnostic skill were enormous.

My opinion changed little over these past months, even though I met some excellent physicians in the suburbs, first-rate. I found many competent surgeons, probably because surgeons are the most closely watched. They always have a pathologist on their neck, but some still do too much unnecessary operating. There were many capable internists in the suburbs, but then there were some awful ones. Psychiatry in the local suburbs was generally the worst of the group. Lauria would argue that at least he and the others were doing something while I just talked to patients.

I discovered that the doctors in Kingswell who were good were often very good, but the doctors who were not as good were often terrible. When their competence ran out, it really ran out. Strangely enough, these doctors' reputations had almost no relationship to their competence. What gave a doctor a good reputation was not his performance—the patients usually don't know how to judge that anyhow—but his availability, his bedside manner, and his reasonableness in demanding payment. Apparently that's especially important to people in the suburbs.

Doctors in private practice were exceptionally forgiving of each other's mistakes. The best would cover up for the worst, because the best depended on referrals from the worst, and rather than put a bad doctor out of business, the competent practitioner would accept what he called the interesting, challenging patients from the incompetent doctor whenever the incompetent doctor got into trouble. These were the same cases the incompetent doctor called "rare" or "unusual." In time these doctors would refer away their more difficult patients to other doctors, leaving them with a practice that was slightly more intricate than the practice of a nurse in an exclusive overnight girls' camp.

The doctors acted as watchdogs on each other by being available to help each other out of jams. Sometimes they were not successful, but you rarely heard about that. The hospital death committees do not make their findings public. You do not pick up your morning newspaper to find what your local surgeon's latest operating mortality rate for any given operation is. Nor do you know what percentage of your internist's diagnoses are correct. There is no way to know how well your psychiatrist's patients do. No one posts the box score on doctors' performances. The only way you know is if you are a doctor yourself, and even then you may not know how bad another doctor really is.

I had recently met Dr. Delwin, another psychiatrist, at a cocktail party. According to my host, who worshipped him, Dr. Delwin was "world famous" and frequently traveled around giving lectures at "famous universities." Dr. Delwin was a hyperactive, glassy-eyed man who had sweat right through his suit even though the evening was not particularly warm.

Delwin also had a reputation among some for knowing nothing and shocking everyone. After the usual niceties he started to tell me about one of his "remarkable" cases, meaning remarkable to him only, a teen-ager who was a behavior problem. From the sound of it the parents were in the midst of a divorce proceeding and contributed a great deal to the problem. They demanded that Delwin "fix" their kid. Dr. Delwin told me he had once read in *Life* magazine about using Dilantin, an anticonvulsive drug, for behavior problems, such as Jack Ruby, the guy who killed President Kennedy's assassin; and was treating the boy with massive doses, twice the normal customary dose. Delwin asked me what dose I "usually" use. I don't usually use the drug unless I am treating epilepsy, and I'm not usually.

Dr. Delwin did not know the dose and hadn't bothered to look it up. When I told him that 800 milligrams a day might be too much and might account for the boy almost being in a coma (Delwin called him "quiet"), Dr. Delwin said, raising his voice and putting on his speaking-from-my-clinical-experience tone, "Eight hundred milligrams doesn't seem like that much." I expected to hear him say next that he had patients on two thousand milligrams of Thorazine a day and that didn't seem to do any harm.

Delwin also told me about an article that he had once read which he said "revolutionized all our thinking about electroshock" and had bcome his rationale for such extensive shocking. It indicated that electroshock was beneficial in "many more diseases than anyone had ever thought before." It was written twenty years ago and was very possibly the last thing Delwin had read. Delwin didn't read it, actually, he only read the summary. "I could go through all those pages and read it," he said, "but it only repeats what is mentioned in the summary. Papers always do."

Why is Delwin allowed to practice?

First of all, Dr. Delwin generally is a respected man with years of clinical experience. That he has really lived the same year many times over and has learned nothing isn't considered important. If I marched down to the State Medical Society and said that Dr. Delwin is a quack and should lose his license, he would present a petition signed by all of the doctors he knows, the internists who do his hundreds of medical evaluations for EST, the psychiatrists whom he refers to, the radiologists who read his patients' X rays, and the staff members of the various hospitals he is affiliated with, all attesting to his worth and esteem. Some would sign because they think professionals have to stick together. Others would sign because they were no better than Delwin and feared that tomorow someone might come and attack *their* competency. It was usually hard to get one doctor to testify against another in a malpractice case and almost impossible to do when there is no injured party—that is, when a doctor is just plain incompetent.

This was especially true in psychiatry. Many psychiatrists were practicing something they incompletely understood and they would have a very difficult time defending themselves if they were questioned about it. Although most of them were better than Dr. Delwin, they would still feel very uncomfortable testifying against him, very unsure of themselves and afraid of having *their* mistakes exposed.

In addition to the many professional character witnesses Delwin could produce there would be an even greater number of grateful patients and their families, especially their families.

The family of an EST patient is often quite pleased with the treatment because it doesn't often bring the family's role in the patient's illness under close scrutiny. The patient is clearly identified as the "sick" member of the family and the family is reassured they don't need to feel guilty or in any way responsible. I actually heard a doctor tell the mother of a disturbed girl, "It's an electrical imbalance that's causing Elly's problem. It's as if her battery has run down and she needs some charging up." The mother was doubly grateful that she lived in an age when such a condition could be treated and was fortunate enough to have a doctor who understood such complicated procedures. The mother soon learned to tolerate her daughter more and more as the shocking every other day made Elly easier to get along with. After all, how can you get upset with a robot whose only fault is her forgetfulness?

Many patients who receive shock treatments also don't object to them; some, in fact, swear by them. They'd rather not look at their problems or confront themselves. They like the idea that they are going to have "treatments" which will make them forget painful ideas and feel better without working.

Such patients and their families would write letters telling how this sainted man had helped them when no one else could or would, when other doctors were unable to cope with all their demands and confusion.

In part, these people would be right. Delwin with his particular personality might be perfect for some patients in spite of himself. And, as I've said earlier, I suppose it can be argued that no one has the right to force anyone to face painful ideas and feelings against his will, but somehow, catering to families who want to evade their fair share of responsibility and to patients who don't want to understand themselves seems something less than the proper role of a psychiatrist.

I must point out that there were many excellent people who used electroshock and drugs, but it was unusual to find someone who relied very heavily on shock or drugs who was really able to use other forms of treatment. For such psychiatrists, the treatment they employed was chosen more often out of their limitations than appropriateness, their denial notwithstanding.

Certainly not quacks, but something short of the standards of openness and receptivity I'd been taught a psychiatrist should practice up to, were psychiatrists who were overly selective about their patients. For them the ideal patient was young (and therefore more likely to change), verbal (more likely to express feelings and conflicts), working (more goal-directed), bright (more interesting, able to appreciate the nuances of therapy, less likely to bore the therapist), highly motivated (less likely to drop out of therapy and produce a "hole" in the schedule which might be difficult to fill), had done well in the past (more reason to be hopeful) and was able to pay your fee (more likely to pay your fee). These were the kinds of patients these psychiatrists preferred to fill their practices with, especially if the patients weren't psychotic and weren't in the habit of calling at night—all of which was very nice if you happened to be one of these patients. If not, you might just be out of luck trying to get a doctor to accept you as a patient.

I remember several occasions (including one I'll mention later involving Stanley Lovett) when I tried to refer a patient to another psychiatrist who wanted to be *sure* the patient satisfied all his requirements. It sometimes got pretty ridiculous, such as when they told me, "I won't have an opening for a year." If a psychiatrist is especially interested in one kind of psychiatric problem, it's understandable that he selects patients; but to accept only one social class of patients tends to make therapy an exclusive club.

What happens to all the patients that very choosy psychiatrists reject, usually on the grounds that they aren't interesting enough? Some find their way to doctors who will accept them; others meet psychiatrists who are "too busy" with their "good" patients, with all those attractive verbal people who are so pleasant to work with. Accepting these patients does not make Delwin and his kind heroes if they mistreat them. Those who choose not to treat and those who mistreat are both villains, each in his own way.

There were also those who did qualify as quacks on the other side of the fence from Delwin—those therapists and analysts who always appeared to know everything and were still unable to help their patients. They gave long and involved explanations of everything happening in their patients' lives but they just sat silently by, passively, without trying to do anything except listen, while their patients raised hell, got pregnant, shoplifted, or ruined their careers or entire lives. Their favorite rationale was "the analyst's love is his silence." (Remember how Alvin Cushman's doctor loved him so much he fell asleep?) And they were the doctors who applied this arbitrarily to all of their patients even if being silent was not in a particular patient's best interest, just like Delwin giving drugs and EST to everyone. These analytic quacks seemed to take great pains in making fine diagnostic discriminations, but to what use if they did not alter their treatment plan? The truth was many were silent not because it was their way of loving the patient and in his best interest, but because they disliked interacting with their patients. It was not rare for such therapists to use their silence not only as a tool but also as a way of hiding their ignorance, or to avoid taking a stand because they themselves did not feel comfortable doing so, which was being dishonest and at least a bit of a quack.

The "mostly silent" therapist was an anachronism, hopelessly out of touch in an age where alienation and loneliness were the most common complaints of patients. It was very simple for a therapist to be quiet and just sit. Such silence would provoke anyone. Such therapists would quickly point out that their patients were projecting their feelings onto them and were developing a transference neurosis. The patients were merely acting just as predicted.

Patients in any therapeutic situation eventually learned to act the way their doctor expected them to because they wanted approval. The behavior that patients exhibited while in therapy had at least as much to do with the kind of therapy involved as it did with the basic nature of man. Most therapies claimed to have a special window on the true nature of man and to claim further that man was best seen from their therapeutic viewpoint. Each therapy ran the risk of becoming a self-fulfilling prophecy, because each type of therapist expected to see a certain type of behavior in the patient. Obviously when they saw the expected behavior which was the hallmark of their particular creed, they emphasized it, reacted to it, or showed pleasure that it had been demonstrated by their patient. Many other kinds of behavior were also shown by the patient. They were not noticed by the therapist, since he was not looking for them, and the patient was not rewarded by the therapist's attention and approval so he wasn't encouraged to repeat the behavior which was not characteristic of his therapist's discipline. The patient hungry for acceptance would repeat the acceptable behavior in time, whatever it was, simply because he wanted to be loved.

I suppose it can also be said that for every "bad" psychiatrist there is a "bad" patient—bad in the sense that he really doesn't want to work or eventually assume responsibility for his life and actions. Such people will usually look until they find *someone* willing to take over, including an inept psychiatrist.

The best therapists in one school of therapy are very much the same sort of people as the best therapists in another school of therapy. They are open and accepting and encourage independence in their patients. The worst are just the opposite. It makes you wonder about all these theories and who's really "right."

There is some rigidity, some dogma, in every therapeutic system, and it seems to me the extent to which rigidity and dogma are allowed to displace the humanity of the therapist is the extent to which all therapies run the risk of becoming quackery.

I met Marty DiAngelo and told him how upset I was with the situation at Kingswell and that I had doubts about staying there.

"I felt upset the same way that you do when I started," said Marty.

"But I don't want to get into something I don't believe in."

"No one is forcing you to. All you have to do is refuse, just say no. What's the big deal? You sound like you're overreacting a bit to the incompetence of these other doctors."

"Maybe I am."

"I know what's bothering you," said Marty, playing psychiatrist, "Mr. Brodner! I remember how upset you were when Jerry Gelb insisted that you try EST with him. You didn't want to. You went along with it even with that big smile of yours, pretending that you really believed in it. I knew you didn't. I think you felt incompetent then and didn't like the feeling."

"I know," I said. "I was very pissed off at myself for that. I kept on saying this man shouldn't be getting shock. Why are you going along with it? I wasn't sure of myself. I was trying to score points with Jerry. You're right, I did feel incompetent. I felt like a Dr. Lauria. I hated myself. I don't want to be in a situation like that again. I really made a big mistake doing that."

"Everybody makes mistakes," said Marty. "You've made a lot of them, too, David."

"Yes, I think I pushed some patients too hard. I've used patients to show how clever I was. I've made all the mistakes. I've missed diagnoses plenty of times," I said, all my weak points flooding over me.

"Have you ever killed a patient?" asked Marty. "I mean, where your actions specifically caused a patient's death?"

"Yes," I said, feeling even worse. "Once when I was an intern," I began, "I was the only one on call at a veterans' hospital."

"The one where you said they thought you were the chief resident and you were only an intern?" asked Marty. "I thought you did pretty well there."

"That doesn't mean I didn't make mistakes. I was called down to the operating room at three in the morning. An old man was on the operating table. After surgery they couldn't withdraw a tube from his larynx. Each time they tried he got a rapid heart rate and turned blue. The surgical resident asked me to help stop the tachycardia. I brought in an emergency cardiac monitor with all the attachments to stimulate the heart. The EKG was complicated. It looked like it could be used as an examination question for cardiology boards."

"Everything looks tough under pressure," said Marty, nodding. "What did you do?"

"I decided on the usual procedure. I pushed on the patient's carotid and he went into cardiac arrest. Bang, just like that. We couldn't get the heart going again. We tried everything. I felt like quitting my internship." I suddenly felt like a murderer, again.

"Look," said Marty, "Handleman is a jerk, but he's letting you use his office. So just practice the way you want to practice and let him practice the way he does. You have to be tolerant. OK, so you and I are better trained and more skilled than these guys, but that doesn't mean we have the right to tear them down. Someone's got to treat the patients in the Kingswells of this world. Would you want to practice out there in the sticks? I bet you wouldn't. So they make a few mistakes. You make them and I make them, too. That's why I asked about killing a patient. Get off your high horse, David, you'll fall on your ass someday and there won't be anyone around to pick you up."

"There's a difference. When we make a mistake we don't shut our eyes to the possibility we may be wrong. I'm willing to admit I'm wrong. I doubt myself all the time. I question what I think and believe. I question my methods. I question my right to make certain judgments. There are some days when I'm not sure of anything. But, goddammit, when I don't know, I try to find out. Some of these characters are insulted when you disagree with their opinions, diagnoses, or treatment plans. You know who I mean. The characters who are always referring to their *method of treatment* and are deaf to any other view. When they kill someone, they don't even know it! Do you know, I just did a consult where the doctor ripped my note out of the chart because he didn't want anyone contradicting him."

"That's the way it is. By the way, I almost forgot. There's an office that's being done over right across the hall from me in town. Why not consider it? Then you can taper off from Handleman's practice and do psychotherapy all day long like a nice little psychiatrist and leave these doctors to their patients and start worrying about patients of your own."

That was the best idea I'd heard all day.

CHAPTER TWENTY-SEVEN

SETTING UP, COVER-UP, AND THE COURT CLINIC

I TOOK one look at the office across the hall from Marty and decided on the spot I'd take it.

"You don't mind that it doesn't have a window?" asked the manager, picking lint from his jacket.

I hadn't noticed. It was a huge office, twenty-five by fifteen, with a large alcove where I could store records.

"I've installed air conditioning and ventilation to make up for it. There'll be a soft sound of rushing air coming in all year round. It's pleasant and drowns out any extraneous noise. It's the most soundproof office in the building."

I took it. Judy came down to look at the place, loved it, and said, "Where do I sign up for therapy?" We went shopping for furniture and bought a teak desk, a large leather chair for me with matching ottoman, two comfortable teak and leather chairs for my patients, some teak lamps and a swivel chair for the desk, which didn't squeak. Because I had no window in the office no plants could survive there and I had to settle for a huge plastic plant, which to my surprise only two patients ever noticed. Both said, "Plastic? Ugh!" I ordered a deep gold rug and left six Miro lithographs to be framed. We'd lucked into them for almost nothing some years before. A few desk and table accessories and we were done.

We tried to do as much shopping as possible in one day because Judy's legs had become so painful it was impossible for her to stand in one place very long. Judy had seen several doctors, including some of my old professors from medical school, but none of them felt she'd be helped by surgery. One even called them "mental varices." Judy decided to start figure skating again to build up her leg muscles. It helped, but she still had pain.

I used Marty's answering service because he said they were the best and would keep me from receiving unnecessary calls. I wasn't nearly so concerned about that as I was about not getting any calls at all. Who even knew that I was in practice? Who would send patients to me? Lauria, Delwin, Groper, Ciriello, Noyes, McKee, Sellers, Frogner, Scarpia, Albee? I filled out an application for a listing in the Yellow Pages. Physicians can't advertise, it's unethical. The medical society sometimes seemed more interested in controlling how you sold your services than the services themselves. All you could do was send out announcements, so I did that. It was pretty silly. I sent out about two hundred announcements. Some fifty were sent to personal friends, as a purely social gesture. Another fifty or so were sent to residents I had known in psychiatry and also in medicine. The rest were sent to other doctors in the psychiatry department and to other psychiatrists I had met along the way.

Some doctors send out announcements to almost everyone in their town or to every doctor in their specialty. Since I generally threw away announcements from doctors I didn't know, I expected that doctors who didn't know me would do the same, and so I didn't bother to send announcements to anyone I didn't know personally. The announcements prompted a dozen congratulatory phone calls, including one from my father who, of course, knew all about it and insisted on a "tour" of the office and waiting room. I could tell by his glistening eyes how much my dad had wanted to become a doctor himself. I received one paperweight, initialed, and one ash tray as gifts, but not one patient.

When they finally did come, they were mainly from Marty DiAngelo, who sent me three or four a week; all were college students from his busy clinic. Marty sent me so many patients, in fact, that I was almost embarrassed by it. "Relax," he said, "I need someone dependable to refer to." Marty was right about the others. Jerry Gelb sent me *one* patient. Eugene McKee, Gavin, Noyes, and all the other doctors I trained with did not send me one single patient, including Dr. Rutberg, who once told Marty he thought I was "extremely promising." I did get several referrals from a few local obstetricians, including "Back Passage" Maslow. I had forgotten to send him an announcement. Maslow was doing a lot of therapeutic abortions and he often sent me patients to determine if they had a psychological problem that justified interrupting their pregnancies. If a doctor sits long enough with any pregnant woman who doesn't want to have her baby, he will eventually hear several sound psychological reasons for terminating her pregnancy. After I evaluated a number of these young women I came to believe that no one had the right to force any woman to carry an unwanted baby to term and that the state was intruding in its citizens' private lives when it restricted their right to obtain abortions.

The law permitted therapeutic abortion if having a baby would be injurious to the mental health of the patient. If I refused to write a letter indicating that would happen, most of the women I saw would get an illegal abortion. They were desperate. Eugene McKee once decided in the OPD to allow a prostitute to have a therapeutic abortion although she had no psychological grounds for it, but she was planning to have it done illegally if he didn't write the letter. I objected at the time, not to the patient having an abortion but to the way the letter was, to my mind, contrived. I had a lot to learn. Dr. McKee felt this girl was appealing for help in the legitimate world for the first time and to refuse her would be saying no to her, telling her she could never get out of her life style.

As I saw more of these referrals, I understood how a doctor could uncover in his patients the indications he needed or wanted to see. It was possible to write two different reports based on the same interview with a patient, one saying the patient would have no bad psychological effects if she went on to have her baby, the other stating just the opposite; both reports would be well documented, of course.

A psychiatric diagnosis can depend more on the psychiatrist's attitudes than it does on the patient. Determining a patient's prognosis and treatment almost always did. I could see how the doctors who did EST tended to do more and more EST and drug therapy and eventually lost their willingness to use other methods. The answers a psychiatrist gets often depend on the questions he asks. It's easy to slant an interview the way you want, especially the first, when the patient is frightened and doesn't know what to expect.

In writing my letters I *tried* to be objective and to avoid being prejudiced. That was much harder to do than I imagined. The psychiatrists who were opposed to granting a therapeutic abortion on any grounds seemed more prejudiced than anyone else, because their professional judgment was influenced by their personal feelings considerably more than by the facts. They often had their minds made up before they saw the patient and looked for excuses not to write a report when they were examining the patient. According to some of the women who had seen them and been refused, and whom I saw later, they frequently also gave their patients a lecture on morality and promiscuity at the same time that they refused to write a report supporting a therapeutic abortion.

Handleman had now returned from his vacation in New Hampshire and was irritated to discover that none of his patients was currently receiving electroshock. Most of them had improved with medication and therapy alone. There was one exception, Mr. Grogan, who for weeks had practically begged me for shock.

"I need shock treatments again," Mr. Grogan said.

"Can you tell me what's wrong?"

"I just need shock. That's what Dr. Handleman always tells me," Mr. Grogan answered. For three weeks this was all that went on for the entire hour. Mr. Grogan refused to discuss his marriage, his job, his wife, his parents—anything. As soon as Handleman came back, he started giving Mr. Grogan shock as an outpatient, three times a week. In three weeks, Mr. Grogan was much better. Handleman saw him for less than fifteen minutes in that entire time. If an outsider had seen only that case, he would have been convinced that EST was the best treatment ever invented.

"How do you manage without shock?" asked Handleman. "Some of these patients are pretty rough. I just don't have the patience any more to sit down with a mute, depressed woman and fight it out."

"But you really only had one mute patient and she did well on Thorazine."

Handleman shrugged.

Watching Handleman I thought more about electroshock therapy and how it wasn't in and of itself evil. When it was used on patients with the proper indications it was an excellent form of treatment. The number of patients who could benefit from electroshock was small, probably much smaller than the number of patients who were actually receiving the treatment. The indications for any particular kind of therapy so often seem to be in the eye of the therapist. Doctors tend to look for symptoms and signs that point to a disease they have the tools and skills to cure. Surgeons find more surgical problems than internists and can give many more good reasons why surgery should be performed to cure patients than internists can and do. A plumber can usually find some work to do in any home, so can a mason or a carpenter; a reporter can find a story more easily than others. Discovering indications for your own particular expertise is only a human response. Same for doctors who use EST. They think about their patients mostly in terms of giving them electroshock and drugs. When they find enough indications in a patient for giving shock treatment, their minds are made up. They seem most interested in finding reasons for giving shock, not in trying to find out what really is wrong with the patient, even if something else is causing the same symptoms. It was not EST that was wrong but its indiscriminate use by, and the ever increasing narrowmindedness of, many of the people who used it.

I'd tried to take Marty's advice and be helpful to the doctors at Kingswell, but I guess in the process I'd made Handleman uneasy. Hell, no one likes to be shown up. Me included.

I also remembered doctors during my internship getting furious with their patients for not getting better because it made them look bad. Some doctors would almost disown patients when they were dying because they were frightened by their own helplessness or didn't want to be associated with a failure or a mistake; or maybe for both reasons. Sometimes a patient did die; after all, everyone does. A doctor doesn't have the control over life and death that he sometimes lets himself think he has. When a patient is dying he needs his doctor most, to ease his pain and to make him comfortable. A doctor lives with death and usually can tolerate getting closer to a dying man than most other people. If he gets angry, frightened, or suddenly very busy and avoids the patient and his family, he is guilty of desertion.

"There's nothing more we can do" is only partly true as long as the patient is alive. A doctor can spend ten minutes with a dying patient and talk about getting his affairs in order, his fears, how he feels, or his family. He can keep the patient's hopes up by suggesting a different medication he thinks will help, even if he doesn't say it will cure. A doctor can spend time with the family and tell them how to act with the patient. A great deal can be done.

A doctor who accepts his own humanness, who can admit failure and his own limitations and doesn't demand that his patients undergo a miraculous cure just to demonstrate his wonderfulness, can be very supportive to his dying patients. A doctor who believes in his omnipotence tends to avoid anything that undermines that belief. Nothing undermines it as much as a dying patient.

Every doctor makes honest mistakes. A doctor must believe that he can be wrong in order to pick up his mistakes. If you think you're perfect, why should you even bother to look? When a doctor takes a course of action that's wrong and the patient doesn't improve, and the doctor still persists just to prove that he was right, trouble inevitably results. Some doctors try to cover up their mistakes by lying to the patient or to his family. It's a conspiracy in which the other professionals remain silent, afraid they might be next. I'd seen too many examples during my training.

I remembered a hospitalized patient who went into cardiac arrest after his doctor gave him the wrong drug. The arrest team did a magnificent job reviving the patient. The doctor told the patient's wife, "You can be thankful that I could pull strings to get him into such a good hospital."

A mistake well-distorted could even become a laurel. One of the attending obstetricians at the obstetrics hospital I trained in while I was in medical school was losing his ability to concentrate. Usually one of the residents would deliver his babies for him. One evening they were all busy and the doctor was on his own. The delivery was a breech birth and he completely bungled it. The baby, who previously had shown no signs of fetal distress, was stillborn. The anesthesiologist was going to file a report to the death committee, but eventually calmed down. And what did this revered obstetrician say to the husband? He said, "Thank God, I was able to save your wife." The husband never stopped praising the doctor. . . .

I decided to terminate with my patients at Handleman's office as soon as possible and to bring the ones I could work with over to my own office in town.

I was never sure just how much my kids understood about psychiatry. One afternoon I brought Elizabeth, eight, and Penny, five, to my office while I tried to catch up on some paperwork. While I worked at the desk the girls turned on the air conditioner, flicked the lights on and off, and played with the telephone. Elizabeth climbed into the chair I sat in when I was with patients, and Penny sat down in one of the patient's chairs.

"Let's see," Elizabeth said, "what's your name?"

"Penny," said Penny.

"What's your biggest problem?" asked Elizabeth.

"I hate my little brother," Penny said. Ah, the candor of youth. Elizabeth wrote something. "How long have you hated him?"

"All my life," Penny said.

"Well, take some of these," said Elizabeth, handing Penny some candy. Medication on the first visit. She's going to be a Delwin!

The next morning I was interviewing a depressed secretary who seemed especially restless and kept moving in her chair. I asked what the matter was and she refused to answer. When she stood up at the end of the hour she had candy stuck to her dress. "What kind of a doctor are you?" she asked. I don't know why she was so angry. *I* didn't prescribe the stuff.

The seminars at the Forensic Medicine Institute covered the principles of criminal law and the treatment of the mentally-ill offender. The discussions tended to be very one-sided, and frequently very dull, and I took to playing devil's advocate to liven them up. Dr. Albee took it all straight. Once I said all children should be tried in court as adults because it was better than putting up with the juvenile division's terrible conditions and the limited access to adult legal protection that children suffered.

"Dr. Viscott's opinions do not reflect the opinions of his supervisors," Albee said, horrified.

"If you disagree, why not suggest something to correct the conditions and the violation of the children's civil rights?"

"Your methods are unreasonable," said Dr. Albee, not hearing my question.

"So are the conditions."

After the seminar Dr. Albee took me aside. "I'm shocked!"

I felt I had to spell it out to him, what I was trying to do by stirring things up a little.

"That can be upsetting to the others," Albee said, meaning he thought I was a troublemaker and was never really convinced I didn't completely believe in every recommendation I made.

Lawyers' personalities vary a great deal, but doctors involved in legal medicine often tend to be inflexible, protective of the system and very concerned with rules, laws, and controlling people. These forensic psychiatrists are often flat, dull people.

Dr. Grigsby was the psychiatrist in charge of the suburban court clinic I was assigned to for two mornings a week. He must have been the dullest of them all. It was part of the Forensic Institute's clinical program. Marty DiAngelo forewarned me that Grigsby was strange, maybe paranoid, and I should stay clear of him.

"If any two human beings will make sparks, you and Grigsby

are the ones. He'll try to clip your wings, force you to conform to his standards. Your hair is too long, for instance. He'll land on you for that right off the bat!"

When I first met him, Dr. Grigsby looked like he was wearing clothes two sizes too small for him. Apparently he'd gained weight recently, or maybe he liked the feeling of tight clothes, maybe it made him feel more under control. Grigsby was three years older than I, but had been only one year ahead of me in residency. He took a year off. Marty said he'd had his problems and let it go at that.

As soon as I sat down in his office Grigsby handed me a mimeographed piece of paper listing the clinic hours; the names and telephone numbers of the social workers, the clinical psychologist, Dr. Calligan, and Judge Singer's private number. "Here are the regulations. You are expected to see patients, write reports and send them to *me*. *I'll* present them to the judge and *we'll* decide what to do. You will get most of the adolescents, since you seem to have some background with them at the youth center."

Grigsby was talking to a colleague, not to a trainee. His own clinical experience was hardly greater than mine, but he felt he had to lord it over me. People unsure of themselves usually do that. Grigsby wasn't sure about himself at all. I didn't intend, though, to defer to him in every decision. I generally trusted my own judgment, and I would ask if I didn't know.

Judge Nemiah Singer, the presiding judge, was born a judge. I'm sure at age thirteen he had gray hair, carried a gavel, and was asked to be the umpire in baseball games. He was a very imposing figure of a man, as my mother would say. You just had to have respect for him; it was either that or to be frightened of him. He was also bright and concerned. I liked many of his innovations in his court: he held juvenile sessions in a small conference room. No spectators were allowed, only people who had a direct interest in the case. It was much more comfortable for the children we saw. He encouraged the kids to tell their story and sometimes, when he needed more information, he overruled a lawyer's objections even when the lawyer thought he might be infringing on the kid's rights. Often the information the kid then told him would make him decide leniently and the lawyer would appear surprised. (Unfortunately, the judge and I were later to have a confrontation that ended my association with the clinic. It was, ironically enough, over his mistreatment—as I saw it, admittedly—of an adult unjustly accused by a juvenile.)

Everything seemed to move along smoothly. I got along pretty well with the parole officers and the court personnel. I'd examine a patient and then discuss my findings with the parole officer and the social worker, or with Grigsby and Dale Calligan, the clinical psychologist. Calligan was really excellent, one of the very best clinical people I'd ever worked with, and had great insight into the thoughts and feelings of children and the workings of the legal process. Our talks were a relief for both of us from the routine issues of the court clinic. Calligan once spoke favorably about a report of mine in front of Singer and Grigsby. Grigsby predictably felt undermined. He looked sullen, angry, and I was expecting a flareup. I just didn't know when. . . .

Barry Glass was a fifteen-year-old high school student arrested for stealing a car; most of the charges were dropped since the car was the family's. But they still had him charged with driving without a license. He'd driven his dad's car into a local cemetery where he and three other boys sat around sharing a six-pack of beer one of them had taken from his family's refrigerator. They were pretending to be drunk and giving speeches standing on top of tombstones when the police arrived. The other three boys ran away, leaving Barry with his father's car. The police didn't press for a drunk-and-disorderly charge because only four beer cans had been opened and most were still more than half full. They were guilty of the very mildest form of delinquency. They did no harm, they planned no harm, they intended no harm.

Barry became very upset after he was arrested and began to cry in the car. The officer who took him home had planned to tell Mr. Glass to pick up the car and forget the whole thing, but Barry was shaking so badly the officer suggested the boy be brought in and evaluated.

Barry's school records hadn't arrived in time for me to read before my first interview with him. Barry told me his story, and I told him that I didn't find it so unusual.

"Why were you so upset, Barry?"

"I just felt that I'd catch real hell at home. I know I've let my father down. And now look at me. I'm here with a head shrinker. That means I'm crazy, doesn't it?"

Barry was shy and down on himself. He had a good vocabulary that he used correctly. He just seemed very unsure of himself, very convinced he was a disappointment to his family.

"Look," he said at one point, "I know I'm not as bright as the average person but that doesn't mean I don't have *any* rights."

"What do you mean, you're not as bright as the average person?"

"Everyone knows I'm not."

"You're brighter than average." I'd felt that earlier in the interview when he had said something that seemed especially insightful to me. "Really, you have a good head. You just seem terribly unsure of yourself, but there's no question that you're OK."

Barry lit up. We talked for another half hour. I told him that I couldn't find anything wrong with him except his putting himself down all the time, and asked him if he would like to talk about that again. I left it up to him. He thought he might. In my report I described him as an insecure young man who was easily supported by praise and esteem and needed reassurance. I said it might be useful to have the social worker see the parents. I also suggested that he was not to be considered delinquent.

Two days later Grigsby came storming into my office, demanding to see me. "Did you write this?" he gritted, holding up my evaluation of Barry. I hadn't even proofread it. Obviously Grigsby was following every move I made.

"Yes, what's wrong?"

"What's wrong? Your incompetence is what's wrong. You sat down with this kid for one lousy hour and decided that he was normal and sent him away."

"Yes, I thought he was upset about his image but could be easily reassured. I'll probably see him again to help in that. He didn't appear pathological to me."

"You didn't bother to review his school report?"

"It wasn't there when I saw him."

"And so you decided to go ahead solely on your clinical impression." Grigsby hated that.

"I felt the kid was normal in most respects and told him so."

"You told him that?" Grigsby sounded as if he'd just heard a key piece of convicting evidence. "Look at these," he said, handing me the school records. I read them quickly.

Barry Glass was in special classes in school although he was friendly with boys his own age, which is not the usual situation with retarded kids. His IQ was given at 76 and 73 on two tests taken in the first and second grade, but never again repeated. School IQ tests aren't terribly reliable. Barry did poorly throughout school and had been in special classes since the third grade. His work in special classes was no better than his work in regular classes.

"You still think he's normal?" Grigsby grabbed back the report. "What about these IQ tests?"

"They're wrong," I said. "This kid has at least a normal IQ and he belongs in regular class."

"You really believe you're above the rest of us here, don't you?" Grigsby said with a change of tone that startled me. He was yelling at me now. "You aren't really interested in this clinic, you're interested in you. You aren't in this because you want to be in forensic psychiatry. You're interested in a free ride. You goofed this case up inexcusably. I can't have a resident—"

"I'm not a resident, Grigsby. I'm a goddamn colleague, remember?"

"Don't interrupt me."

"Stop this temper tantrum, Grigsby. Tell me what I need to do to appease you."

"How dare you! How dare you speak to me like that! Who do you think you are? You mess up a case and then you want me to treat it as a light matter. I'll have to bring this up to Dr. Albee and to the judge."

"Bring what up? What the hell are you talking about?"

"You review this." Grigsby jabbed the report at me. "You tell me that this kid is normal, in the face of all these reports, and expect me to believe you. Read this, then rewrite your report. Start acting like a professional."

I took the report and started to leave.

"Wait, I'm not through with you," Grigsby shouted, following me into the corridor. "In the future you will report every case to me. You will discuss every session you have with your patients." He followed me right to my office.

I walked into my office, slammed the door in his face, and read the school report in detail. Apparently when Barry was in the first and second grades he had had severe allergies and couldn't work well in school. I guessed he was taking antihistamines. That would slow anyone down. The chart didn't mention that fact, but I was willing to bet on it. He was tested early in the fall and again in the latter part of May, the two worst times for allergy sufferers. Each time he did poorly. Somehow, although his work quality stayed poor, he seemed to maintain an achievement level that was higher than the other children in his special class. At the same time, he always seemed a year behind other kids his age in regular class. Retarded kids don't do that. Each year they fall more and more behind. Also, he was captain of the junior varsity football team and co-captain of the baseball team. Retarded kids aren't usually looked up to by the kids in other classes. Barry was, if they had elected him captain and co-captain.

I saw Barry again and asked his mother to come in with him. She told me that he *had* been taking antihistamines at the time of the IQ tests. OK, lucky guess! I told Barry that I believed it was all a big mistake and that he deserved a chance to straighten out the record.

"You don't know what a change has taken place in Barry since you saw him," Mrs. Glass said. "He's been so, well, confident lately. I've known all along that he was normal. You know, in the seventh and eighth grades he was at a special school."

"With all these weird kids," said Barry, making a face, "who drooled and touched you. It was awful." Barry obviously had a good memory.

Barry was tested. Overall, his IQ was 106, the bright side of normal. Barry was afraid of making mistakes. He probably could score higher. He saw each mistake as evidence he wouldn't do well. I could understand why.

I contacted Barry's school and saw his teacher and a member of the guidance department, who were surprised and cooperative.

Leo Albee asked to see me after the Thursday morning seminar. "I understand you are having difficulties at the court clinic."

"I'm having difficulties with Dr. Grigsby more than anything else. He's pretty uptight and vindictive and seems ready to pounce on mistakes or oversights—a very threatened man, it would seem."

"Never mind your diagnosis of Dr. Grigsby. I'm interested in your diagnosis, which he says was completely wrong, made without even bothering to look at a boy's school record. That's unacceptable. You should have examined the record."

"And changed my opinion? Even if I believe it's right?"

"A long school record is a more reliable guide to a child's development than one hour with a psychiatrist."

There was a knock on the door. Grigsby came in. Welcome to the Spanish Inquisition. Hi there, thirteenth-century fans.

"I was discussing the case with Dr. Viscott, Dr. Grigsby."

Grigsby nodded.

"What if the record were wrong?" I asked.

"See," said Grigsby, "what if everyone else were wrong and Viscott was right. Look at that point of view."

Albee shook his head, agreeing. "Sounds a bit like Brookfield. You have problems dealing with authorities, David. You should face it."

"I read the boy's record—I would have read it, anyway—but it didn't change my opinion. I thought Barry was a normal kid, a little unsure of himself, perhaps, and I said so. I decided to evaluate the situation further so I asked the family to come in and I saw the boy another time."

"You didn't tell me about that," Grigsby said, surprised. "I told you that you were to discuss your plans and everything you did in *my* clinic with me first. There's no need to bring the parents into this case until we've straightened out the matter together. They've had their heartbreak with this boy long enough." Albee nodded. It no doubt sounded like good sense to Albee, and showed Grigsby's decent concern.

"The mother felt that he was as normal as her other kids," I said. I was setting up Albee and Grigsby and I admit I kind of liked it.

"Mothers always deny such things, David. You know that," Albee said.

"I told Barry that I believed his tests were low because of his severe allergy and medication at the time he took the tests." Grigsby and Albee looked puzzled.

"What are you talking about?" asked Grigsby.

"The record indicated Barry had severe allergy and I noted that his IQ tests were in spring and fall, the worst times of year for most allergies. I guessed he was taking antihistamines and was sleepy."

"That's pure fantasy," Grigsby said. "That's what I mean, Leo. You've seen it now for yourself."

"His mother," I went on, relishing it, "said he was taking Chlortrimeton and one other antihistamine almost continuously for years." Albee looked at Grigsby. "That's not all. Barry was always depressed about being in the special class and never tried because he was afraid to fail and find out he was like the kids around him. So I had him tested."

"You were to consult with me!" Grigsby said.

"What difference does it make?"

"I'm chief," said Grigsby. He really said it.

"'Wonderful, hooray for you," I said, and just collapsed in my chair. Albee was angry at me He wasn't as rigid as Grigsby, but he still demanded that we keep up our facade of respect for the rules, even if the rules were idiotic. I looked at Grigsby glaring at me. "Oh, stop glaring, for Christsake," I said. "I had Barry tested."

"Don't tell me *your* clinical impression, just give me his IQ scores."

"One hundred and six," I said. Albee took his pipe out of his mouth. He looked worried. His horse was suddenly losing the race.

"You seem upset that this kid is *not* mentally defective."

"OK, Dr. Viscott, lay off," said Albee, deciding he'd heard enough.

"What is this 'OK-Dr.-Viscott-lay-off' routine? When you want to jump on me it's open season and any odds are fair. When I defend myself, I'm out of line. Would you tell me what this is all about? Or can't Grigsby talk for himself?"

"Dammit, shut up, Viscott," Albee said. "What are you planning to do with this boy?" he asked Grigsby.

"It's my patient," I reminded Albee. "Why not ask me?"

"I . . ." Grigsby started, trying to assert himself, "will examine this boy and if I think he is emotionally ready for it, I'll consider ways of correcting the situation. It's a slow process that took years to develop and will take some time to reverse."

"That's how I want you to go, Dr. Viscott. Slowly and following Dr. Grigsby's plans."

I looked at these two threatened men. Grigsby was acting like some sort of paranoid psychotic. Psychotic people, like pigeons, are everywhere. It occurred to me that Albee might have sponsored Grigsby for his court job. If Grigsby looked bad, so would Albee. "We'll need to take further steps to try to set things right—conferences with the school; start Barry back in regular classes, in the lowest curriculum, of course. He can catch up to the next curriculum in a year and he should be at his normal performance level by graduation."

"You have no right to go over my head," Grigsby protested, looking at Albee for support.

"I'm sorry, but practically everything I do seems to go over your head. That's not my fault, and I don't go around looking for faults in you. Get off my ass and leave me alone."

"It's my clinic."

"Then run it like a clinical director, not like a vindictive child looking to take out his hatred on the first person who comes along."

"Look," said Dr. Albee, gathering his forces, "you simply must follow routine—"

"I do follow routine," I shouted, "but like anybody worth anything I need *some* room for personal style."

"You didn't follow routine at the state hospital, or in Brookfield."

"Not strictly. The routine there was busywork. It was a place to hide from the patients. You followed routine there very nicely, Leo. Look what your methods did for Albert Carrol, or have you forgotten?" (Maybe a low blow, I don't know, I was mad.) I kept it up. "Look, this boy apparently believed in me. I was the first one in years who thought Barry was normal. Should I have let that belief die and held him off?" I remembered Peter Atkins, the boy who was admitted to Bamberg 5 in a family crisis, and how I had been stopped by Dr. Noyes when I wanted to discharge him. "This whole thing has been blown up way out of perspective by Dr. Grigsby. Personally, Dr. Grigsby, I think it's more a problem of your own that has nothing to do with me. Well, I've had enough." I left.

Grigsby and I avoided each other. It was the only way to travel. I refused to go over my cases with him. He went over all my records but apparently couldn't find much of anything to object to.

Definition of doing good work: when a paranoid boss can't find fault with you.

A few weeks later I was asked to review a case for Judge Singer. I interviewed Mr. Kane, who had a history of alcoholism a decade ago, with several arrests for drunkenness. Kane seemed able to take a few beers without much trouble. He and a friend had tickets for a hockey game in town and were waiting for a train in a local tavern. They missed the first train and went out to wait on the platform across the street. Mr. Kane had to urinate and didn't want to miss the train and the start of the game, so he walked around to the side of a building and, when he thought he was out of view, urinated. He heard some giggling and looked up to see three girls crossing a footbridge. One of the girls became hysterical at the sight of Mr. Kane peeing. She called her mother, and even before the next train came, a squad car arrived to pick up Mr. Kane.

Talking with Mr. Kane it was pretty clear he was telling the truth. His friend corroborated the story. Neither had a criminal record. I couldn't find any underlying problems that would have driven Mr. Kane to expose himself. I wrote a report indicating as much. Grigsby took the note to Singer. Singer was furious. Singer wanted to let Mr. Kane off but needed a psychiatric reason for doing so. I just couldn't find a psychiatric reason for peeing. If a young girl became upset like that girl had she was obviously upset about a lot more. The other girls just thought it was funny. Singer disregarded my report and sentenced Mr. Kane to three months. When I found out, I asked to see him.

"Why did you do that?" I asked. "Mr. Kane was innocent."

"Don't question me about my decisions. I don't need to discuss cases with anyone."

"Oh, come off it," I said. "I've had great respect for you and the way you handle most of the juvenile cases, but, hell, judges like doctors are just people. Mr. Kane didn't do anything. He didn't expose himself."

"He exposed himself in public. That's an offense and now he'll have to serve his time for it." Singer was very angry.

"That's not fair to Kane! Arrested falsely, convicted on a distortion and upheld by—"

"By what, Dr. Viscott? Finish your sentence."

"I'll do more than that," I said. "I'll finish my affiliation with this court. You and Dr. Grigsby—"

"Go ahead," said Judge Singer, showing me to the door.

"—deserve each other."

Actually, he was, of course, miles better than Grigsby, and my crack was unfair. But even so, I didn't feel I wanted to go on in a setting like that. I still continued, though, to go to the seminars to finish the year, and I still kept my job at the youth center. The Youth Division in the Department of Correction had been getting a lot of unfavorable reports in the press at that time. So had Brookfield. Dr. Cortina was attacked, and quit. Alcoholic Dr. Lear was fired. The youth center personnel felt unprotected and were very frightened. I stayed out of trouble. I just wrote my reports and tried to get the kids out as soon as possible.

I saw Greg Andrews at the youth center. He was a thirteen-year-old boy whose mother pressed criminal charges against him after she walked into his bedroom and found him and his twelve-year-old brother engaged in homosexual activities. According to Greg, he and his brother had done that several times before and took turns. The young brother didn't complain, in fact the brother admitted that he instigated most of the encounters. Some homosexual experimentation between boys of that age is almost universal. Certainly the younger brother seemed more involved in homosexual activities than Greg, who was dating girls and only using his brother as a substitute when they fooled around. The problem was that the brothers had different fathers, and the mother hated Greg's father. Pressing charges against the son was her way of letting some of her anger out against the father. The social worker spoke with her: she even admitted it. I suggested in my letter to the court that the matter would be best handled by sending Greg home and allowing each boy to talk individually to a psychiatrist for a few weeks just to reassure them and get them shaped up, or to begin treatment if it were found necessary.

Usually "Happy," the psychologist, gave me follow-up reports on the children I saw. I heard nothing for a week. When I asked, Happy reluctantly said, "I didn't want to tell you this because I was afraid you'd stir up trouble. Judge Meehan committed Greg Andrews for a year."

I immediately wrote another letter to the judge asking that he reconsider his decision, saying that such a disposition didn't seem to me to be in the boy's best interest and would only make him believe he was really a homosexual. It would also direct attention from whether the younger brother needed treatment (certainly more likely than Greg needing it).

The judge sent me a letter, telling me in effect that he had used his best judgment in the matter and that was that. He was the judge! I called him on the phone.

"Judge Meehan, I think we would be doing Greg Andrews real harm by committing him. He hasn't done anything so very much different from what most normal boys do at his stage of development."

"You call homosexuality normal? I've sent men away for committing homosexual acts for years. It's a crime in this state. It's a perversion. And with his *younger* brother, it's incestuous as well. What kind of psychiatry are they teaching you in medical school these days? I can tell you're young and haven't been around much. You'll learn."

"I've been around long enough to know that when a decision is unusually harsh it's going to unnecessarily hurt a youngster."

"That boy is committed. That is that."

I had my limits. Greg was about to be sent to a reform school. I could imagine him at some point in the future, genuinely afraid he might be homosexual because he remembered being committed for a homosexual act.

I remembered treating Duke, and I remembered that in therapy with children the therapist, in effect, became a part of the kid's experience that he could rely on and take strength from. I could help Greg best by getting him out of this situation, which could only undermine him if it were allowed to become a memory. OK. It would rock the boat, but dammit, if it were my kid—if it were me—I'd want someone to rock the boat for me.

"Your Honor," I began, hoping I was getting across a slightly threatening tone, "with all due respect, I believe you are acting inappropriately by committing Greg and may seriously harm him. If you persist in enforcing your decision, I will look for relief with every method I know, including going to the press." Judges are terrified of the press. They like their anonymity—their power needs secrecy.

"And just what are you planning to do?" he said, trying to sound casual.

"That depends on what you do. I think the press, made aware of one of your inappropriate decisions, might want to review all your past decisions dealing with juveniles to see just how appropriate they were. You know, it's interesting," I said, dropping my bomb, "judges are pretty much like everyone else. They tend to reveal their own prejudices and fears in the way they handle certain cases. You never know what a review like that might show."

There was silence on the other end of the phone.

"I'll get back to you, doctor." Judge Meehan was suddenly very quiet.

Greg's commitment had already been ordered, but the Youth Service Board recommended he be sent to a forestry camp, which wasn't for delinquents. Greg could commute home on weekends if he wanted or stay away from the family at the camp. It was the best the Board could do. Greg got to see a psychiatrist. His brother got to see a psychiatrist.

And I got to see Dr. Albee.

Albee had just been appointed chief of the division. He demanded that I see him at his convenience. I told him when I would be available. He was furious. If someone wants to clobber me, I decided, he can at least do it at *my* convenience.

Albee had a big new office with brand new furniture in a big building and a big new secretary. Inside the new office was the old Dr. Albee. Sitting with Dr. Albee was an elderly man. "You know Dr. Halperin, don't you?" asked Albee, introducing us.

"I've heard of you," I said, smiling and shaking hands, "but we've never met." Halperin had a fine tremor of the hands and looked chronically ill. His voice was hoarse, his breathing was labored. I guessed he might have emphysema.

"You don't know Dr. Halperin?" asked Dr. Albee, incredulously, as if Halperin were president of the United States.

"No," I said, "am I supposed to?" I knew Halperin had something to do with forensic medicine but I didn't know exactly what. Maybe Halperin used to write reports for one of the courts but I wasn't sure so I kept my mouth shut. No kidding.

"Dr. Halperin is your immediate *supervisor*."

"He is? I didn't know I had a supervisor." I really didn't.

"Well, he is. Dr. Halperin is the psychiatrist in charge of Region 3, and officially you serve in Region 3 as a senior psychiatric consultant."

"I really don't know what division I'm in. I just send in a voucher each month. I never look at it."

"You should look at it," said Albee, "it's important."

"It's just a technicality. It's how I get paid. Why should I care which department I'm paid under? I do the same work. I get the same pay." I could see Albee waiting for an opening.

"Dr. Halperin is responsible for the people under him, and you are one of them." Albee was building his point about the chain of command. Next he'd probably ask why I didn't go through proper channels and speak to Halperin or to him before going to the judge. Why should I let him build a logical argument?

"Look, Leo," I interrupted, "let's get to the point. You want to chew me out for calling up that judge and telling him I thought he was wrong."

"You listen to me," Albee said. "You are disturbing the fine relationship that took me years to build up with these judges, and I'm not going to let you ruin it."

"What good is a fine relationship with a judge if he still acts arbitrarily and won't listen to your advice? All you have then is a fine relationship with an incompetent."

Dr. Halperin started coughing.

"What good does your action do? You alienate the people you have to work with." Albee was pointing his finger at me.

"I suppose," I said, "it would've been better to say nothing and let this boy be committed just so your relationship with this judge wouldn't be damaged."

"You had no right to do what you did."

Halperin was shaking. I worried that he was going to become ill.

"I have a right to make a professional psychiatric decision and to try to have it carried out. If I see a correctable wrong being committed, why shouldn't I try to make it right? I'm sorry if I upset that judge for a few minutes, but that boy would be hurt his whole life. Maybe the judge needs to learn that his office doesn't make him infallible and that his decisions can be influenced by his own personal problems. Why should I stand by to watch a young man be ruined by an old man's own fears when I can help it?"

"It's not up to you to correct him. You listen to me. I've watched you working with patients and with staff people. I don't care what others think of your ability or skill, all I know is that my experience with you makes it clear that you are a distinct liability to me and to the entire department of mental health. You are precisely the kind of person we can't afford to have on our staff. You make trouble and disrupt people."

"Maybe that's what this department needs," I said. "I didn't get involved in these controversies because I wanted to. I think most fights like this are just useless and a waste of time. But to avoid a controversy just to spare someone in authority a painful moment of reflection isn't my style, especially when other people suffer because of it. That's simply wrong, Leo. You know it and I know it. I thought the law was written so that a guilty man occasionally goes free, just to prevent an innocent man from hanging. You can't let a judge commit people just because their behavior threatens him or reminds him of some of his own feelings that he can't accept."

"I won't listen to this kind of talk."

"I know," I said. "I expected you wouldn't. It complicates your untroubled life."

"What do you think we should do, Dr. Halperin?" Leo said, turning away from me.

Halperin coughed and looked at me very seriously. "This is a radical and irrational young man who is trying to change the entire system overnight." It sounded like the beginning of a psychiatric evaluation. "I don't think we can have him in our department. He seems to want a revolution."

Who was trying to do anything like that? I make one unconventional move and these people see it as an attempt to overthrow their goddamn system. Who would even want to bother? When you get rid of one bureaucracy, another always grows in its place. You couldn't get me involved in a situation like that. If there's going to be a revolution, I'll watch it on television, thank you. I figured I had better ways to spend my time.

"Well," began Leo, "I can't see the point of your staying on. I think you should resign." Halperin nodded. They had finished what they had come for.

"I disagree," I said. Halperin looked at Albee, confused. "I think I should stay at the youth center evaluating the kids just as I have been doing. I enjoy my work. I plan to stay there until I decide to leave and can find someone capable to take my place."

Leo looked stunned. "I said, I think you should resign," he repeated.

I was a free agent. I wasn't attached to the Institute anymore or to any academic program. I was my own man. "Leo, I plan to stay and do just what I have been doing."

"If you don't resign, you'll be fired."

"I wouldn't do that, Leo. Everyone has skeletons in his closet. Dr. Halperin, it's nice *meeting* you. Leo, I'll be seeing you."

I walked out, leaving the two of them to compare expressions in the wall mirror.

CHAPTER TWENTY-EIGHT

PRIVATE PRACTICE,
POLITICS FOR A FRIEND,
IN LOVE WITH A SPECIAL PATIENT

‖ WAS also working part-time at the University Psychiatry Clinic under the amiable stewardship of Marty DiAngelo. Marty had recruited three other psychiatrists and a clinical psychologist. All were excellent.

Marty had done a fantastic job organizing the clinic. He had begun four years before by working as a consultant to the university infirmary. He had come to know all the deans of the various schools and even the dormitory supervisors. He had made inroads into the psychology service, which was wary about letting any psychiatrist into their territory. More than anything else, Marty offered excellent care and a service, without any red tape, that helped students resolve their problems as quickly and with as little embarrassment as possible. Marty was everywhere, doing everything. He gave lectures in the dormitories on drugs, on alcohol, on sex, on VD, on finding a career, and on choosing a mate. His workweek was at least eighty hours. And his work paid off. He was accepted by the students, and in his footsteps so were the rest of us in the clinic. We all enjoyed working there.

There were so many students who needed to be referred elsewhere that we spent hours finding psychiatrists who had time available. I sent patients to D.J., who was in private practice, and to Bert, who was in child psychiatry. One day I decided to send a girl I had just evaluated to Stanley Lovett. She needed help in overcoming long-standing feelings of depression. I felt that Lovett, who was doing a little teaching and still in the Psychoanalytic Institute, would be happy to have a private patient. I called him on the phone.

"Stanley, have you any time open?"

"Time, you mean for a patient? I might have time." Nothing like a little enthusiasm.

"I'd like to send you Sally MacBride. She's an eighteen-year-old art student with a chronic depression that interferes with her functioning. She's very bright, very verbal. The family has money and is willing to pay a private therapist. So I thought of you."

"That's very kind of you," said Stanley. "Has she ever made any suicidal gestures?"

"No, just had the usual thoughts about wishing she weren't alive when she's depressed."

"How often does she get those?"

"When she gets depressed, once or twice a year over a period of a few months."

"Is the depression cyclic?" I would have bet he was taking notes at the other end of the line.

"It may be."

"Does she show any signs that would indicate she might regress and need hospitalization?"

"No, Stanley."

"Has she ever been treated before?"

"No."

"Is she well-motivated?"

"Yes, very, Stanley, she's a good candidate for treatment. Trust me. I hope you're not thinking of her as a candidate for analysis because I don't think she's interested in that and she doesn't need it. Stanley, I can't hang on the phone all day. Why don't you evaluate her? I can't promise she won't go crazy on you or that she won't need hospitalization. You sound like you're looking for a letter certifying that she is healthy and won't get into trouble and embarrass you. Stanley, she's a routine referral. Come on, you want her or not?"

"I uh . . . Let me look at my schedule."

"Stanley, I'll have her call you."

"Uh . . . I suppose."

A person just can't be too careful who he lets into his office. God only knows, the patient may be seriously ill and disgrace you.

I referred students from the clinic to psychiatrists all over town. Occasionally Marty or one of the other doctors I worked with sent me a student. I liked working with people in the arts. I seemed to have a natural feeling for them. More accurately, we seemed emotionally to be in the same place. I seemed to sense when a complaint was related to an artist's success with his work or to other problems in his life. The ability to make that distinction became very important.

Analyzing the unconscious meanings in an artist's work is not especially helpful. Analyzing an artist's creative process only transforms a non-verbal process into a verbal one. Because defenses often involve words and the creative process often does not, the creative process is much freer than the normal process of thinking. To give an artist a verbal understanding of the unconscious forces involved in his creativity may only ruin it. As the artist becomes more aware of these feelings that formerly found expression in his work without his conscious knowledge of them, he also becomes limited by the verbal inhibitions attached to those feelings. Inhibitions, like defenses, are also made up of words. The artist has a method of expressing feelings symbolically, without words. He has a method that already works. Why spoil it with words? The force that drives artists to create should not be analyzed, only those problems that get in its way. What good is it to know what your creations mean if you can't create anymore?

I got involved with an experimental theater group in town and worked with the director, who'd had formal training in psychodrama with Moreno, the inventor of psychodrama and one of the leaders of the group psychotherapy movement. The director was applying those techniques to her experimental theater group. I loved working with the group and was eventually accepted as an equal by them. I learned a great deal about artists and even more about myself. I rediscovered an old desire to write, to create, that I had almost forgotten. I began writing again and wrote a children's play the group performed.

The first full year of the student health clinic was almost over. It was a huge success. Marty had just received a large grant for next year. He asked me to stay on, but I wanted to devote more time to private practice, especially with people in the arts. I was getting a following of artists. I felt I'd let Marty down but I wanted more time to write and think.

One morning I found Marty sitting in his office with his head in his hands. He was staring at a letter.

"What's wrong, Marty?" He handed me the letter.

Dear Dr. DiAngelo:

It is with great pleasure that I offer you the position of Assistant Professor in the School of Medicine. Your duties next year will be to continue your work in the student health clinic in the position of Assistant Director. Dr. Robert Clarkson will be the new director of the unit. I trust you will give him your fullest co-operation.

Again, congratulations on being awarded tenure.

Sincerely,

Dr. M. Austin Noyes

"I don't believe it," I said. "Noyes plans to give your service to Bud Clarkson. Bud isn't used to working with young people. Besides, it's *your* service. You built it from nothing. It needs your strength and determination to survive. I can't believe Noyes would do a thing like this."

"Believe it," said Marty. "Bud Clarkson is getting the job because he's a psychoanalyst and I'm not. Also because he was analyzed by Noyes. And all these years I thought being analyzed by Noyes was a disadvantage."

"Talk about nepotism," I said.

"What can I do?" Marty said. "You know how chicken people are in that medical school. All these analysts and associate and assistant professors are too into the system to stick their neck out. I'm going to get the heave-ho and no one will do anything but say it's a shame."

"Psychiatrists have the least backbone of any group of people I know," I said, and sat down in a heap.

I got an idea. "Make an issue out of it instead of acting hurt. I got Noyes to back down once before in a hassle with Dr. McKee."

"What can I do?"

"You don't do anything. People have to rally to a cause." I sat down at the typewriter in my office and wrote a letter. I brought it out and read it to Marty. It was another Viscott special beauty, stating how Noyes had betrayed his staff, broken his word by giving a less competent man a break because he was an analyst and how taking away Marty's position demoralized the staff. It also said some embarrassing things about Bud Clarkson.

"But you can't circulate a thing like that. You certainly can't get people to sign it."

"I can try!"

I did. I spoke to everyone who'd listen. Nothing happened for some weeks. And then Marty came rushing into my office one day without knocking, right in the middle of a session. My patient jumped right up off her seat. So did I.

"Excuse me," said Marty, suddenly formal. "Can I see you please, Dr. Viscott."

I walked out and Marty closed the door. Marty gave me a big hug. "You did it, you sonofabitch. Clarkson turned it down."

"Marty," I said, "can I ask you a favor?"

"Anything, anything you want."

"Please put me down before I go into homosexual panic."

I'd now been in private practice full-time for nearly a year. I had developed an interesting practice that included several people in the creative and performing arts. I had completed my year at the Forensic Medicine Institute. I finally decided to leave the youth center and was replaced by Alvin Cushman. I was getting referrals from all over the place. It never seemed to slow down.

My office telephone rang twenty times a day. Actually I had a switch that cut out the bell on the phone, a yellow light flashed on the ceiling instead. Between patients I called my answering service and usually made one or two calls. I was overloaded with forty to fifty hours of patients a week, and I referred away a great deal of work.

My telephone at home rang on the average of ten times a night. I believed in answering or calling back right away. An uninterrupted dinner was a rarity. I usually had one or two severely ill patients and tried to keep them out of the hospital if possible. I believed that hospitals were places where patients frequently got worse. I would do anything I could do to keep a patient "on the street." Letting patients know that you are available to talk is helpful, but you also get called a lot.

What was I going to do about all these calls? I suppose it could've been worse. I suppose I could have been starving. I dreamed about phone calls and was awakened by ringing phones. One night, after ten calls from a psychotic woman, I just couldn't fall back to sleep. I imagined I had died and was buried in a coffin specially equipped with a telephone so that my patients could still get in touch with me. I could even hear one patient saying, "I knew you would have more free time to talk with me now so I called." I could hear my father calling, "Why are you lying like that in a coffin with such a good practice going for you? Is this what you worked so hard for in medical school, to lie around like that?" You can't win!

Something peculiar was also happening. Strange patients began to refer themselves. A dozen or so patients called in one month who totally refused to talk openly about their feelings. They often had one specific question that they wanted answered: usually it was unanswerable. They were rigid and demanding. Often they wanted me to tell them what to do every step of the way to solve a particular problem. These patients talked superficially for a minute and then expected me to speak profoundly for the rest of the hour. I couldn't understand it.

The telephone calls increased and also changed.

"Is this Dr. Viscott?"

"Yes."

"I need some help from you. I want you to make my daughter want to go to college. She wants to get married."

"Well, I'd be pleased to see her, if *she* thinks it's a problem."

"No, you've got to make her come to you."

"I don't understand."

"She refuses to come to you."

"Well, then there's nothing I can do."

"Aren't you a practical psychiatrist?"

"I think of myself as being as practical as the next fellow, but I'm not a miracle worker."

"Well, then *you'll* have to get her to come to you."

I received calls asking me to "make my husband stay home nights," "stop my daughter from screwing," and "make my boss give me a promotion." I couldn't understand it. I'd never had calls like this before. It was like one of those telephone gags we used to pull as kids, getting a dozen kids to call up someone to harass him. What *was* all this? One day the mystery was finally uncovered by another telephone call.

"Are you the practical psychiatrist?" Practical, common-sense psychiatry was the request of most of the new calls, but no one had ever called me "the practical psychiatrist" before.

"I don't understand what you mean, sir," I said.

"You the one who advertises as a practical psychiatrist?"

"Advertises?" I was puzzled. "Where?"

"In the Yellow Pages."

"The Yellow Pages! No."

I hung up and opened the Yellow Pages, which had just recently been delivered. I'd forgotten to look up my new listing. I thumbed through the book. I had just missed by one week getting listed in the Yellow Pages last year. Under "Physicians and Surgeons" was the following:

David Viscott, MD 1419 Grove 323-5656
Practical Psychiatrist

I started to laugh. It was supposed to read: "Practice limited to Psychiatry." I showed it to Jerry Gelb, expecting him to think it was terribly funny.

"Are you sure you didn't put it down that way, David?" he asked, looking for hidden meanings again.

"Jerry, why can't the Freudian slip be the telephone company's for a change?"

To this day Jerry Gelb doesn't believe me.

The telephone company did, and settled meagerly out of court.

Being a psychiatrist in private practice was very different from anything I'd experienced. You made your own hours, worked when you wanted. You saw a lot of very interesting pathology. Most important, you wasted very little time doing paperwork, administering people, or doing busywork.

Therapy wasn't always the same as it was in residency. I treated one woman who was terrified of meeting her new in-laws by taking her to a local caterer and helping her plan a dinner for eight. She saw me three times a week for two weeks while we discussed her feelings as we made the gastronomic preparations.

You never heard the same story twice in psychiatry. Every patient was different from every other patient, even if they experienced the same events. Each patient's defenses filtered the reality he encountered, and what was allowed to come through was *his* unique experience. I felt that each patient added something to my own understanding of what it means to be alive and feeling, and I tried to give what I could.

The year passed quickly. Judy was examined by a vascular surgeon (in the suburbs, by the way) who decided she had very severe varicosities and needed surgery. He couldn't understand why she hadn't been operated on long before. I told him the story. He suggested that perhaps the other doctors had missed something. Two weeks after her operation, she was back on her feet. In one month she had no pain. Her "mental varices" were cured.

Being a psychiatrist was sometimes a burden socially. Perfect strangers at cocktail parties told you their life story if you appeared to be even half-listening. Several times I was attacked by some shrink's ex-patient with the favorite opening blast, "You psychiatrists are all crazy yourselves." I tried to be polite, but I just didn't like being attacked for something I didn't do. And when I wasn't in my office I didn't think like a psychiatrist. I didn't want to relate to people as a psychiatrist when I was out socially. It would ruin my evening. Even so, people I met casually told me they were unfaithful, drug addicts, homosexuals, masochists, alcoholics, gamblers, or a dozen other intimate confessions. It seemed there was an epidemic of people hell-bent to reveal their pathology outside the treatment room—which, of course, is much easier than doing something about it in treatment or on their own. I began to wonder what "Back Passage" Maslow ran into socially.

Marty never told strangers he was a shrink. He took a cruise to the Caribbean and told the people at his table he was an internist. At their last meal together on board he told the others that for the sake of not rocking the boat (his joke) he didn't tell them he was really a psychiatrist. "One man threw up," said Marty, laughing.

Maybe you wonder if I ever fell in love with a patient? There were many I felt a great deal for, even loved, but there was none I ever become involved with in the usual sense—there was one . . . one girl I developed incredibly strong feelings about. All right, I guess you could say I did fall *in* love with her.

Jennifer Franklyn was twenty-one, and glowed. She was referred to be evaluated for a therapeutic abortion. The minute Jennifer walked into my office I felt she was special. It was a very distracting feeling. I couldn't understand what was going on. I felt very strongly toward her and didn't know why. It wasn't her looks that made her special. I've seen prettier girls. Not that Jennifer *wasn't* lovely. Jennifer was lovely, so lovely. She was also very pleasant and charming, but there was nothing uniquely new about that either. Jennifer had about her an almost overpowering sense of engagement, of involvement, of *being* that pervaded the room as soon as she came in. I'd never experienced that with anyone else before—even after knowing them for years.

Jennifer told me she was surprised to find herself pregnant.

"Why were you surprised?"

"When I was in the hospital they told me I wouldn't be able to get pregnant because of the radiation."

"The radiation?" I asked, my heart dropping to my feet. "What radiation?"

"I had radiation treatments for Hodgkin's Disease," said Jennifer, and noticing my pain, she smiled at me.

I felt dizzy and frightened. "What type did you have?" There were three types of Hodgkin's. *One* of them had a good prognosis.

"I don't know," she said. "They never told me. They didn't tell me anything. I started to lose all my hair during the radiation treatments." She handled her beautiful blonde hair. "It came out by the fistful. They said I would also have some fibrosis of my vagina and uterus. But they didn't tell me anything else."

"Why not?" I asked. I really didn't want her to talk. Every time she said something, it sliced through me like a knife. But I had a job to do, or so I told myself.

"I don't know. They just avoided me—all those doctors."

"Why didn't your obstetrician write a note? It appears to me that you have a medical reason for having an abortion."

"I don't know."

"I'll call him right now."

Dr. Shelby was in. "Why didn't you give Miss Franklyn a medical letter for an AB?" I asked.

"Oh, I don't know, I think it better that she get a psychiatrist's letter."

"Why?" I was afraid I knew.

"Well, that means putting down all the prognostic possibilities and . . . you know what I mean."

"Oh," I said, feeling sick inside. Shelby, like myself, couldn't face the idea of Jennifer having a fatal disease. It was too much for him to bear. Because Jennifer had never been told anything, I guessed that her other doctors had felt the same way. Jennifer simply had too much life, charm, and intensity. To think that she might be dying soon was just unbearable.

The other doctors had done their job, and they had done it superlatively, according to what Jennifer told me. They gave her every attention possible, left no possibility uncovered. Except for one problem. None of Jennifer's doctors could bring themselves to talk about her chances with her. Jennifer had talked with her radiologist, with her hematologist, Dr. Eastland, with her internist, and with Dr. Shelby; none of them could discuss what she was afraid to bring up.

Jennifer only wanted to know if she was going to die.

"Jennifer, what about you, why didn't you ask any of these people what was going on?"

Jennifer was silent, sad. Even so, she seemed to glow.

"You were afraid your doctors would tell you that you were going to die?" I said, forcing myself to say the words.

Jennifer nodded. Another patient would have looked down or away. Not her. Jennifer looked at me. *Please look away.*

"And you're just sitting there wondering whether it's today or tomorrow?"

"I just go in for tests. The doctors say the tests look good and tell me to come back in six months, or something like that. But I don't know what my future will be like. At the end of each appointment I can tell that Dr. Eastland or Dr. Shelby is about to bring up the subject. They start and then they seem to get upset and I end up, well, you know . . ."

"Yes, I do know. You end up comforting *them.*" I stood up and put my arms around her and hugged her. She was crying. I felt like it. After a while I said, "I'm going to find out exactly what is going on with all of these doctors and put all the information together. Then you and I will try to understand what it means." I sat down again. "There *is* something unusual about you that makes it difficult to deal with you. I happen to see in you a lot of the qualities that I love in people and just the thought of you not being alive is devastating. I imagine it's terrifying to you."

"You're the first doctor who's treated me like a human being, who's not been afraid of it."

"Who said I'm not afraid of it?"

Jennifer also needed a letter from a second psychiatrist. That's the law in my state. Stupid law.

Stanley Lovett ("The Selectivist") was the only psychiatrist I could find with an open hour later on that day. I sent Jennifer to see Stanley and gave her an appointment to see me again after she got out of the hospital.

Lovett called me at home that evening. He sounded very different. "David, that girl you sent me, Jennifer Franklyn, I don't know what it was but she is very unusual. I don't know how to describe her. She's such a beautiful person. . . ." I'd heard Stanley talk with this much feeling only once before. "In the year and a half I've been practicing I never did this before," he said, "but I asked her if she needed a ride home. I drove her ten miles out of my way and sat in the car and talked with her. Do you think I did the wrong thing?"

"She's incredible, isn't she?" I said.

"I don't know what it was," said Stanley.

"I hope to hell she had Hodgkin's paragranuloma," I said, trying to handle my feelings about Jennifer intellectually.

"Let me know," said Stanley, genuinely concerned.

I contacted everyone who had treated Jennifer. Dr. Eastland, her hematologist, was the chairman of the department at another medical school across town. He was internationally known. Some of his patients came from halfway around the world to see him. He was one of the best, and extraordinarily busy and stuffy. I didn't even expect I'd be able to get him to come to the phone. His secretary told me, "Dr. Eastland is very busy and I'll have to have his associate call you back. What is the patient's name, please, doctor?" Eastland was protected from intruders!

"Jennifer Franklyn," I said.

"She's all right, isn't she?" asked the secretary, suddenly very concerned.

"Yes," I said, "but there are some problems I would like to discuss with Dr. Eastland."

"Would you hold on, please?" asked the secretary. Eastland was on the phone in a second! Incredible!

"This is Dr. Eastland speaking, Dr. Viscott. You're calling about Jenny?" Jenny! In a sea of nameless faces there was one Jenny!

"Yes." When I told Eastland my problem, he sounded relieved.

"Well, I don't think an abortion is going to give Jenny any trouble," he said. "Why didn't Dr. Shelby write a note about her problem? I don't see why she needed a psychiatrist for an abortion, do you, doctor?"

"She really doesn't need a psychiatrist," I said, "but she needs a little help in understanding her disease, her chances. . . . I think everyone gets a bit overwhelmed with Jennifer. She's just too much alive, almost too feeling and real. The idea of Jennifer dying, I guess, is more than anyone can stand, doctors included."

"I couldn't agree more. What can I do for her?"

"Jennifer doesn't know anything about her disease or her *prognosis*. She doesn't know how long she has to live, she can't make plans, she—"

"I did spend a good deal of time talking with her, as I recall," Eastland said reflectively. "Perhaps I didn't mention her prognosis to her. . . . Come to think of it, I'm sure I didn't. You know she's planning to study in Paris, don't you? I spent a year studying in Paris . . . I suppose I was diverted by thinking about her living in Paris and her plans and the unfairness of illness. . . . That's unusual for me. I couldn't go on practicing if I did that too often."

I could well imagine. This busy, world-famous authority spending twenty minutes on the phone with a psychiatrist, of all people, telling me his fantasy life about a patient.

"What about her prognosis?" I asked again. That *was* a very painful question. So simple to ask, how long do you think Jennifer will live? It's only simple when you don't care that much.

"First of all," said Eastland, trying to be clinical, "Jennifer has Hodgkin's paragranuloma. A couple of nodes in the neck. Her mediastimum was clear. The radiologist is excellent. He called in two other radiologists before he gave her treatments. He apparently was very concerned too." Eastland became gentle again. "I tell you she's had the best care possible," he said, almost apologizing that he had no magic to offer.

"And . . ."

"I think her disease is arrested." Eastland had to become clinical again to answer the question. "I think she falls in the group with the highest survival rate. There's no guarantee, of course, but I expect her to live at least several decades." Then gentle again: "Put it this way, if Jennifer dies sooner than that it will *probably* be from something other than Hodgkin's."

"Thank you," I said. I really meant it, because somehow I felt spared.

"Anytime! Say hello for me," Eastland said. I said I would.

I told Jennifer the news and we went out to celebrate. We took a long, long walk across the river, had coffee in a sidewalk cafe, and talked. I saw Jennifer two or three more times because she wanted to talk about her plans for the coming year and because the idea of surviving was still very new to her. And I saw her once more because I wanted to see her.

As far as I know, Jennifer is married and living in Paris and is still doing well.

God, I hope so.

CHAPTER TWENTY-NINE

HEALING MYSELF,
FUTURE IMPERFECT

THE idea of becoming a psycho-
analyst had an aura of the mysterious about it. When I started my
psychiatric training I believed that analysts had more knowledge and
more power than ordinary psychiatrists, and for some time, as I've
mentioned, I considered the possibility of becoming one. I considered the time and the money involved and I also weighed the
prospects of being in training for perhaps five years beyond my residency. I finally abandoned the idea for good.

That's only half of it. I had both my hopes and my doubts about
the process. I was also a little anxious about being psychoanalyzed,
even though I felt I was pretty much aware of my own problems and
my own inner workings. In fact, I felt much better put together than
many of the analytic types I had met. Some of the analysts I admired
as teachers I found I had very little respect for as human beings.
Becoming an analyst might have made some people more powerful as
psychiatrists, but not better as people.

I felt some psychoanalysts stuck too rigidly to their system of
logic and accepted it as if it were dogma rather than theory. They
seemed concerned more with an artificial world of their own creation,
where the pieces could always be made to fit, than with the real
world that raged in their waiting rooms. Much of what analysts did
really didn't make much sense. Analysts, it seemed to me, rationalized
wasting a great deal of time and thousands of dollars of their patients'
money. Jerry Gelb once told me, "Sometimes I sit for weeks in silence
not understanding a single word of what the patient tells me." When

it finally made sense, Gelb would feel that the time spent was justified. Even if the patient's ramblings were really unimportant to begin with, the interest shown sometimes made them appear important. Why Gelb didn't ask his patients directly what they meant was beyond me.

Although most analysts would gladly admit that they don't know the answer to everything, they don't believe that anyone else can know anything they don't. They just assume that everything will eventually fit into their theory. How else can they justify to themselves their long hard years of work? Because analysts often believe that they know more than anyone else, they feel tolerant of other people's ignorance. Analysts are always tolerant of your ignorance. Tolerant of it! They're grateful for it because it makes them feel secure that their theories explain everything, if perhaps sometimes a bit too late.

Anyhow, I felt the people who were attracted to this way of life tended to the stuffy side, to be a bit passive, and rather egomaniacal. When one of the number was a regular sort of person, his peers called him "unusual." Analysts often seemed pleased with themselves, and why not? If you thought you knew everything and all the people you associated with felt the same way, you would feel very pleased with yourself too.

Analysts tend to stick together. The towns of Truro and Wellfleet on Cape Cod, Massachusetts, have a large summer colony of psychoanalysts, perhaps a hundred vacation there. They talk shop in the sun and drink themselves blind. I guess they feel the only people they can let their hair down with are other analysts. God forbid that a patient ever sees his analyst give his kid a belt across the chops, ever sees his analyst as a human being. Some analysts, of course, are less rigid, more open, more human with their patients. Many people today will just not put up with orthodox analysts' noninvolvement—perhaps it's a trend.

Nevertheless, having said and thought all this, I decided to go out and have my head shrunk. I asked Jerry Gelb if he knew of a good analyst he thought I would get along with who also had time available. After about two weeks Jerry called me at home. "I found someone I think would be just right for you—Dr. Frost. He's a very good person and a very competent analyst. He even lives around the corner from you."

I called up Dr. Frost and made an appointment to see him. Frost was a tall, balding man about fifty who looked, I thought, like an elongated version of my grandfather. "You look like an elongated version of my grandfather," I said when I met him for the first time.

He asked me why I was there.

I told him I had been thinking about a personal psychoanalysis for three years or so and had played the usual games postponing my decision.

What did I want? I wasn't really sure. I hoped to get a better understanding of myself, and I hoped in the process to become a better therapist. I saw Dr. Frost one other time and I decided to go ahead with it.

Dr. Frost just sat there and listened while I came four days a week, lay on my back, and spouted my guts out. I tried to say everything that came into my mind. I tried giving him a complete story of my life, including all the rough spots, the trials, the hurts.

He was remarkably silent.

I rattled on about everything, going into deeper and greater detail. Very little about myself actually came up that I did not know before. That was very surprising. I had already thought through most of the stuff I told him.

He was remarkably silent.

I noticed that I really didn't want him to say a hell of a lot and preferred to put everything together pretty much by myself with a few comments from him. So I rationalized a little. I was only human.

One day I picked Dr. Frost up on a point he had made, saying I thought he'd missed the real issue. He then picked me up on how sensitive I was about being misunderstood. It was a good point. Although I was well aware of those feelings, we talked about how little understood I felt, it *seemed* for a long time. I felt I understood myself and was interested in finding other people who understood me. I wasn't sure whether Dr. Frost really understood me or if he was just aware that I wanted to be understood. I went on talking about my feelings, my plans to write, and all my activities. . . .

He was remarkably silent.

In the spring I decided to buy a cabin cruiser. What the hell, I had always wanted one and I was making a lot of money and it sounded like a good idea at the time, and besides, I already owned a blazer and a pair of white pants. As part of the routine recitation of the what's-new-I-haven't-seen-you-in-three-days routine, I mentioned the boat.

The remarkable silence of Dr. Frost ended.

"What kind of boat?" he asked. An odd question for an analyst to ask, I thought.

"I got a Trojan, a cabin cruiser," I said.

"How long is the boat?" asked Dr. Frost.

I thought this *was* funny. Here I was spilling out my deepest feelings, hopes, dreams, and hurts to this guy for five months and he didn't say boo. I tell him about my boat and suddenly he's all hot to trot.

"Thirty-one feet."

"Big boat!" he said, sounding impressed. Was he sounding impressed or *trying* to sound impressed? I wasn't sure.

"Single-screw or twin," he asked. He *was* impressed!

"Twin, two hundred twenty-five horsepower gasoline engines," I said, smiling. This was very funny.

"What did it cost you?"

"That's a funny question," I said. "You're really into boats, I suppose. Well, with everything, and I mean *everything*, it was about seventeen thousand dollars."

"Hmm," Frost said.

I noticed after this that Dr. Frost had a pattern to the comments he made which I felt wasn't really related to my analysis. Dr. Frost commented about money. He said little things, like "How much," or, "Oh," or, "Really?" I had a shrink who reacted to comments about money. What did you do in a case like that? You told him. At least that's what I did.

"Dr. Frost, do you know you just did it again?" I said.

"Did what?" Frost answered after a moment—the moment it always took him to decide whether or not to answer a question.

"You made another comment about money. Are you aware that on at least four separate occasions this month you have focused on how much something has cost rather than what it meant to me or what I felt about it? Do you suppose you have a personal concern in this area? I'd like to know because I can't figure it out."

"Not intended," was all the man said.

"Intended or not, I lie here on my back trying to figure my own head out. Anything I say is considered fair game for discussion. I expect if you make a slip of the tongue or let your personality into your comments and I question it, you will give me a straight answer and admit it. Dr. Frost, I have to verify my own sense of reality here in analysis. I believe that what you just said has little to do with me.

If it is a slip, just admit it and let me move on to another issue. If it's my problem, let's discuss it."

He was remarkably silent.

"This is irritating as hell," I said. "I *know* you have a hangup in this area, Frost. If you'd just admit it, it would clear the air. I would admit something like that to my patients."

Frost played silent. I told him I thought it was stupid. "If my perceptions are right," I said, "I deserve to have them corroborated. If they aren't, I have the right to be told that."

Frost did not answer either way.

This might sound like a small point, but it was very important to me. If I had imagined this, we should have discussed it. If I was perceiving correctly, he should have told me, to avoid wasting time thinking and worry about it. Frost said nothing. I assumed I was right, but he refused to acknowledge it. Three weeks later I caught Dr. Frost in another slip about money. I was sure it was his problem and not mine.

I was also very disturbed. If my analyst wasn't honest about his own feelings and wasn't willing to admit when he was wrong, how could I trust him to understand my feelings and to be right when he told me I was distorting something? How could I be sure it wasn't his distortion? If I distorted something I wanted to know it. I hated wasting time on meaningless issues.

After a year of analysis we broke for the summer. I loved the boat and was out on it practically every day, rain or shine. Judy had a new disease, instant seasickness in all but dead calm conditions. I had a long time in a hot mariner's summer to think about what I was doing in analysis. I certainly was not getting enough out of analysis to justify spending a hundred dollars a week. Frost had precious little to add to my comments. He seemed to have all the time in the world to sit there and listen. I had been getting a big dose of silence, and wasn't convinced that it represented this analyst's love.

During that year I had more free time and had spent it working with the theater group and writing my first novel. I also became interested in television and developed some close friendships with several writers and directors at the local educational TV channel. I even worked with some of the artists to help them understand from a psychological viewpoint what was going on in their particular art form. I continued to find great pleasure in working with them and was delighted that they were beginning to respect some of my artistic notions as well as my psychiatric insights. Actually, they rarely contested my artistic judgments; they frequently rejected my psychiatric ideas. What else?

When I went back to analysis in the fall, I found myself very bored with the prospect of another year of talking while Dr. Frost sat silent, adding little to my own insights. My friends in analysis seemed to be uncovering more about themselves than I was about myself. But I still felt I was already very much more in touch with myself and more open to begin with.

I talked to Dr. Frost about my interest in the arts and in getting involved in them again. I had showed promise as a clarinetist as a child and started composing music when I was in my early teens. Before I decided to go to Dartmouth I seriously considered applying to the Conservatory of Music. I had always written poetry and stories, and that interest was still with me and still wanted to be expressed. I had mentioned all this to Frost before.

Frost said, "I think you are using your creativity as a way of avoiding getting close in the analysis."

"You think my creativity is a defense against the analysis?"

"Yes."

"That means if there were no analysis, there would be no need to be creative."

"That's exactly right." He was sure!

"Dr. Frost, I've been creative since I was a child and suspect and at least hope I'll continue to be somewhat creative until I die. What disturbs me is that you can make a comment like that about me. It means that after all this time, and during those hours you just listened, you really didn't understand. If you think my creativity is a defense then there's nothing left for us to talk about. Not even my feelings of not being understood. I think you have the right to be wrong. You're human. But I don't think you have the right not to understand, not at least to try to understand, what I am all about, or ask in order to find out. Being creative is my life. Everyone who knows me knows this. You, who supposedly know me best, don't know this at all. You don't really know *me* at all and you're unable or unwilling to ask." I couldn't believe this man. I was silent for two or three minutes, thinking this through. There was no question about it, I decided. This had been a big mistake.

"The analysis is over on Thursday," I said. This was Monday.

"But we are just beginning," said Frost, genuinely quite surprised.

"You may be just beginning. I'm ending. I can't pay the price for your not understanding."

I spent the next few days bringing up points I wanted to discuss to tie up things. Dr. Frost apparently had not taken me seriously. He asked only that, if I would like to have a fifth hour, he now had an opening on Fridays. Other than that, he said practically nothing.

At the end of the Thursday hour, I left. Frost did not even say good-bye. He played his role to the very end.

I met Dr. Frost once, a year later, outside a hospital where I had just admitted a patient. He asked me what I was up to. I mentioned that I had published a novel, *Labyrinth of Silence,* about life in a state hospital; a scientific paper, explaining an idea of mine about the creative process; and told him about another novel I was currently working on, as well as several other projects. His only comment was, "You always did have your finger in a lot of different pies."

But then, again, I guess I probably would have found fault with anything he said.

The year after I ended my analysis I joined a leaderless encounter group, not an encounter group in the usual sense of the word. It consisted of a clinical psychologist, a psychiatrist who had spent several years in training to become an analyst, a clinical psychologist who had worked with Reik, two theater directors trained in psychodrama, a clinical psychologist also trained in psychodrama. We stayed together as a group for almost two years, meeting once a week for four hours or more. In that time we got to know each other and we devised new techniques for reaching and helping each other understand.

In the group, I got a clearer picture of my effect on others, and I developed a greater sense of honesty about myself and about my feelings. I also felt understood, and very much at peace with myself. In the group we were bound only by the rules we wanted to make. Our relationships with each other were not restricted to the group and were not defined by a contract. We were real to each other and, in being real, became part of each other's lives in very real ways. Not all members of the group could take part in every other member's life. Some just didn't fit into another's life and it would have been insincere or contrived to try to make them. We did what we felt. In spite of the fact that there were no rules and although there was a great deal of closeness, we all managed to stay intact and maintain close relationships without sexualizing them. The group worked because we gave each other what we felt we needed—because we wanted to give, not because it was part of an agreement to do so.

In becoming a psychiatrist I discovered that we all spend our lives existing between two worlds that we can never really grasp, and so we live in an illusion of our own creation. Our unconscious frightens us because it holds the truth about our feelings and so we distort our memory of it. The dream is the creation of the dreamer, who fits the fragments of truth he has just seen in his sleep into a pattern acceptable to him. The world outside threatens us and is also unknown. We try to make the outside world seem familiar, altering what we perceive with our feelings.

Each of us perceives the world he must perceive. We invent our illusions to separate the world outside from the world within, thereby to avoid hurt and to feel comfortable. Even though the outside world is the same and feelings are universal, no two people share the same illusion.

Even if he may not express in words what he knows, the artist seems more in touch with the real world and the world of his own feelings than do others. The artist brings the world of reality and the world of feelings very close together. The artist also lives in an illusion, but he takes his illusion and gives it form and makes it real enough so that others can share it. In so doing the artist tries to make sense of his own life. By sharing what he has created with others he allows them to expand and enrich their illusion and perhaps gives sense to life itself.

In the end I found that nothing hurts more than a wound that cuts through the illusion and makes you see through yourself.

My wish to be understood became my drive to understand myself. I found that I was most myself when I was writing or working on something creative, when I tried to take a part of me, known only to me, and use it to create something for others embodying that part. It was like making the best of me more real, more available for other people to see. What I wrote became real to me and had an existence of its own separate from me. I felt more at home creating a world on paper than anything else. I had found a microcosm which I could always control and a world I could create in my own image. This little world was entirely my own. My life was greatly rewarding. I continued to learn about creative people by listening to them in therapy and by being creative myself up to the limit of my capacities.

I discovered that I enjoyed creating a work until it was almost completed, then I would be oppressed with doubt about its worth, even the worth of art itself. I would be afraid of losing something very private that I'd invested in the work. Even though at the beginning I might have wanted to share this with others, I was reluctant to let it go when I'd finished. Once a part of myself became public, I felt it would never be mine alone again.

I feel that way now as I write this sentence, knowing that soon this book will be printed and other people will be reading it and, in some way, the book will also be theirs. I will no longer own entirely what was once entirely mine.

And I suppose that's the way it must be. Should be. If this book is to have life, it must take some of my life from me. This may sadden me, and yet at the same time I somehow feel more complete in my being depleted. What was inside is now out. Whether this book lives or not is not so important to me now as my search for something new to say and share in the next one.

CHAPTER THIRTY

POSTSCRIPT:
SOME *FREE* ADVICE TO
PATIENTS IN PSYCHOTHERAPY

To GET the most out of your psychiatrist don't assume that he can read your mind. He can't. Remember that much of the time he may not know what is going on and will be trying to figure it out. He's only human and although he has a great deal of skill and training behind him, he needs your help and cooperation. Tell him everything that you think is wrong, even if you don't want to admit it to yourself. He's heard it all before and there is nothing you can tell him that is going to get him upset or make him think badly of you. Don't play games with him. Neither of you has the time for that, even if you do have the money to pay for it. Ask him what you could be doing in therapy to help the process along. If you find yourself telling him lies, admit that you are, right then on the spot! That's important because you can find out why and if you do you'll be put back on the right track. If you are trying to impress him or fool him, and catch yourself doing so, tell him. If you only feel you would like to impress or fool him, tell him that, too. It will give you a chance to look at the way you are with other people. A psychiatrist is there to hold up the mirror, but he can't function unless you give him something to reflect upon.

You can't tell if you are making progress unless you know what it is you want out of therapy. You should have some specific goals when you go into therapy. If you have trouble setting goals, ask your psychiatrist to help you determine your goals and help you decide which goals you value most. You can't solve all your problems in therapy, but making a list of goals will help you resolve what you need most.

Remember, being in therapy is no excuse for not trying. You deserve credit for struggling with the problems in your life and trying to solve them, but that is no reason to lord it over other people who don't have the courage or over members of your family you think are worse off. Remember, your problems are your problems and their problems are theirs. You can only solve your own problems and you can't change other people. Don't expect laurels for being in therapy, and don't use being in therapy as an excuse for behaving in a nutty or inconsiderate way toward others. If your psychiatrist is worth his salt he won't take that from you and you shouldn't expect anyone else to. In other words, don't expect special indulgences because you're in therapy. It doesn't become you. Also, you're going to discover a lot about yourself and your feelings about others. Your new opinions may sound reasonable to you but they won't always sound reasonable to others. You may discover that you are very angry at people; just be appropriate when you allow some of that anger to leak through. Otherwise it may be too much anger and you'll end up feeling guilty and screw up the entire process of allowing yourself to become more honest about expressing your feelings.

If you have questions about therapy, ask your therapist. You deserve an answer that makes sense in your terms. Psychiatry, you should know by now, is not mumbo jumbo. It's simply the hard and determined effort of two people to work together to help each understand the other and be more human. If you aren't given answers, ask why. Does your therapist know the answer or does he want to postpone telling you, or does he believe it's something you have to discover for yourself? Generally therapists will tell you on their own what they believe something means; but asking won't hurt.

If your therapist plays the role of the silent listener and you really need more than that, and you are getting worse, consider getting another opinion to check him out. If you are suffering and you hurt and you think that more should be done, ask for the name of another doctor. Remember, if your doctor won't give you the name of another doctor, ask why. If his answer doesn't sound reasonable, get another doctor's opinion anyway.

If you are feeling bad and your doctor keeps pouring pills into you, starting from the very first visit, and his answer to every future complaint is to increase the dosage or change the kind of medication, it's another reason to get a second opinion and as soon as possible.

Medicine doesn't cure anyone of psychological problems. It may help you cope, but you should expect more than that from your doctor. After all, that's what you're paying him for. And you should feel the same way about a doctor who refuses to give a medication under *any* conditions.

If your therapist is not helping you reach your goals, if you feel he is not your sort of person, a person who just doesn't have a feeling for you, maybe you should fire him. Remember, you hired him to help you, just like one hires a guide to find the way through an uncharted jungle. It's as if the therapist is blind but knows the way. You tell him what you see. He remembers the map. He tells you where to turn. He relies on your input to tell what is out there. He should help you decide what it is you're looking at. He should be a participant in the process, not an observer. How do you fire a therapist? You say that you are not reaching your goals, or that the two of you are such different people that you don't believe he has any genuine feeling for you and you would like to try elsewhere. And you say good-bye.

What should you look for in a therapist? Your therapist should be a person you have faith in, a person you feel you can trust and is the kind of person you would normally like to talk to, even if he weren't your therapist. He should be human, interested in what you have to say, and he should have feelings. He should be a person who does not hide behind the mask of a psychiatrist but is willing to share with you his feelings and opinions about what you tell him. He should be available when you need him and should be willing to let you try to make it on your own when you feel you want to try. He should be more interested in the healthy side of you than the sick side, even though he deals mostly with the sick side. He should remember his goal is to get you feeling better and in control of yourself and understanding yourself as soon as possible.

You don't want therapy to go on for years. You don't want to become dependent on your therapist. It's bad for both of you. You really don't want to have sexual intercourse with your therapist. It will only ruin everything and mainly you'll waste a lot of precious time fantasizing about it and talking about it.

Your doctor should not take telephone calls when you are in his office unless it is a bona fide emergency and a very rare occurrence. You don't want him ranting about all of his problems, although it may be necessary for him to tell you about a crisis in his life if it affects his attitude in therapy. You don't want a doctor who can't admit that he was wrong or that he made a mistake. He doesn't expect you to be perfect, why should he have to be perfect?

You want someone who will help you and who will be honest about his limitations, accepting them as part of his own humanness. Remember that because your doctor is human, it is possible to hurt him and to uncover his weak spots.

No therapist can be right for every patient, just as some people don't get along with others. Even though a psychiatrist is trained to get along with all sorts of people, why should you waste time trying to adjust to someone you just don't like if you could hit it off with someone else right away? If you don't get along with, say, three or four therapists in a row, maybe it *is* your fault and you *are* avoiding the problem. Either stop playing games and start trying, or see if you can manage on your own. You're not doing any good by faking being a patient.

Being in therapy is a good deal of work, which doesn't mean that you can't enjoy it. You can. Not all insights are painful, not all memories are sad. Therapy at its best should be very real, very much like life. It should be a place where you learn to feel more and see more, and where you learn to build an alliance with the healthy side of yourself and learn more of the truth so that you can act in your own best interests.